# Instinct Based Medicine™

by Dr. Leonard Coldwell

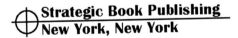
Strategic Book Publishing
New York, New York

Strategic Book Publishing
An imprint of Writers Literary & Publishing Services, Inc.
845 Third Avenue, 6th Floor – 6016
New York, NY 10022
http://www.strategicbookpublishing.com

ISBN: 978-1-934925-56-0, 1-934925-56-X

Printed in the United States of America

Cover Design: Kurt Bredt

Book Design: Roger Hayes

# Instinct Based Medicine™

## "Let's Heal Together"

## How to survive your illness and your doctor!

A step-by-step guide to optimum health for the beginner and the professional therapist from Europe's leading researcher and self-help authority for cancer, stress-related illnesses, depression and chronic disease.

**by Dr. Leonard Coldwell**

Leading researcher and education self- help expert for cancer and stress related illness

Major Degrees:
NMD, ND, Ph.D. CNHP – Retired not practicing in the USA

# Disclaimer

The techniques presented in this book are powerful, natural stress reducing and immune system enhancing, self-healing methods and self- help educational information, but they are not a substitute for medical care from a physician. Results will vary for each person, but these methods are so powerful that there use is occasionally capable of relieving pain from serious underlying disease processes. The information offered in this book is for your personal use in stress reduction and for self- help education, to create the health and wellness you deserve. Do not neglect taking care of what is causing the stress. The author believes that the root cause of all illness is mental and emotional stress. This book is written to provide you with the education, knowledge, training and coaching to take charge of your own life, health and happiness and to enable you to define and eliminate the root cause of your health and life challenges. Remember, stress is a signal from your body telling you when something is wrong.

This book is based on the authors experience working with tens of thousands of patients and millions of seminar attendees. It is the final conclusion of the knowledge Dr. Coldwell accumulated as the leading expert for stress- related illness and terminal chronic diseases in Europe. The author put the main and updated information from his nine best- selling books into this book so that you have the most comprehensive information and tools available today.

Here is the legal disclaimer the law requires:

Consult a doctor if you are injured or if you suffer form medical conditions. This publication presents only the author's opinions which are based on his knowledge, experience and beliefs. The techniques and theories offered here do not represent a scientific consensus in stress alleviation or prevention or self help. Results will be based on an individual's specific situation and will vary for each individual. Dr. Coldwell's stress reduction and self help will not work for everyone. You use all information and techniques published in this book at your own risk and based on your power of free will.

**Legal Notices**

This book is designed to provide information about the subject matter covered. While all attempts have been made to verify information provided in this publication, neither the author not the publisher assumes any responsibility for errors, omissions or contrary interpretation of the subject matter.

. This publication is sold with the understanding that the publisher and author are not engaged in rendering medical professional services. If you have a medical condition, you should seek the services of a competent medical professional. The purchaser or reader of this publication assumes responsibility for the use of these materials and information. Adherence to all applicable laws and regulations, federal and state and local, governing professional licensing, business practices, advertising and all other aspects of doing business in the United States or any other jurisdiction is the sole responsibility of the purchaser or reader. The author and publisher assume no responsibility or liability whatsoever on behalf of any purchaser or reader of these materials.

The purpose of this workbook is to educate. Any perceived slights to a specific individual or organization is unintentional.

The information in this book is not a substitute for a doctor's visit. It is not intended to treat, diagnose or prevent any illness. If you are in therapeutic care, ask your doctor or therapist first before you do any changes or use any of the techniques described in this book. This book and "**Instinct Based Medicine**™" is the way to make better-educated decisions, to find the root cause of life's challenges and shows ways to eliminate these causes. It also is intended to help you to establish your personal level of optimum health in the shortest amount of time.

# Table of Contents

# Foreword

I am excited that Dr. Leonard Coldwell has the guts to share with us his knowledge about the dangers of the medical profession, and shows us how we can use the self-help system that he created to cure tens of thousands of patients and helped millions of others through his books, CD, programs and seminars so that we are aware of the dangers of modern medicine and able to uncover and eliminate the root cause of all illness.

Dr. Coldwell is my personal physician in Europe and his input over the years was extremely valuable for me and the creation of my mega best selling book, Natural Cures They Don't Want You to Know About. Dr. Leonard Coldwell is the original natural cures doctor. We are in constant contact, consulting with each other all the time. I am glad that Dr. Leonard Coldwell is now willing to share with the world his secrets for health and healing. In Instinct Based Medicine, Dr. Coldwell uncovers the horrifying truth about the medical profession and shows us how to find and eliminate the life circumstances, behaviors, decisions and actions we live with on a daily basis that endanger our health.

Dr. Coldwell uncovers the shocking fact that the medical doctor is the number one cause of death in America. He boldly tells you what you need to know to avoid becoming permanently damaged or killed by modern medicine. The information in this book can save your life and the life of your loved ones. It will extend your lifespan, quality of health, happiness and success in tremendous ways while teaching you to avoid the fatal consequences of modern medicine.

I congratulate my dear friend, Dr. Leonard Coldwell, on the making of this book, Instinct Based Medicine: How to Survive Your Illness and Your Doctor. This book is destined to change the lives of millions of people world-wide and will finally spread the truth about vaccination, medical incompetence, weaknesses and the fact that education for the medical doctor is purposefully manipulated to keep patients sick and dependent on drugs that make the pharmaceutical companies trillions of dollars.

Dr. Coldwell understands that this is not the medical doctors' fault. It is the fault of a greedy system based on the foundation that John D. Rockefeller gave the medical educational system with his only intent to turn the medical doctor into the advocate and salesperson for the chemical drugs he produced. The FTC and FDA are the bodyguards for this fraudulent medical system and if you don't learn about the dangers of this corrupt and dangerous system you will never be able to protect yourself or the ones you love.

Finally, in the second part of his book, Instinct Based Medicine, Dr. Coldwell uncovers the secrets of his healing success that until today were only known by a very select few students that Dr. Coldwell trusted and trained in his IBMS™. My research shows and it is my professional opinion that Dr. Leonard Coldwell has the highest cancer curing rate in Europe. The same is true for many other illnesses including: MS, rheumatoid arthritis, muscular dystrophy and countless others. He has worked with over 35,000 patients and more than 2.2 million seminar attendees, and is the author of 8 best-selling books. He has published thousands of articles and taught millions of people how to help themselves gain their lives, health and happiness back. Dr. Coldwell is, in my opinion, the leading expert for stress related illness. In Instinct Based Medicine he gives you, for the very first time, the tools and knowledge on how to take charge of your own life, health and quality of life.

I applaud Dr. Coldwell for his boldness to take on the most powerful and protected profession in the world, the profession of modern medicine. He knowingly goes into this war with the dangerous group to help and protect you from death and harm by modern medicine, and to give you the tools to understand and control your personal health.

Dr. Leonard Coldwell is absolutely right when he states that mental and emotional stress is the only cause of all illness because permanent stress leads us to all the behaviors and lack of energy that makes us sick. Dr. Coldwell has the effective solutions for you!

This groundbreaking book will reach and help millions of people! I ask you to support Dr. Coldwell in his approach to educating and protecting the public from the dangers of modern medicine to give everyone the tools to control their own life and health. Please support this book and help spread the message. I wish my dear friend, Dr. Leonard Coldwell, the biggest success with his book Instinct Based Medicine!

Kevin Trudeau
NY Times Best Selling Author and Consumer advocate
May 2008

# Instinct Based Medicine™

Even though you will read a lot about the weaknesses of traditional medicine and alternative or natural medicine, I do not condemn either. I will share with you what I personally learned from my more than 35 years of dealing with cancer and other terminal illnesses in my family members and from the work with over 35, 000 patients. I also learned a lot about life and human behavior from my 2.2 million seminar attendees and I also had a lot of valuable input from my over 7 million readers of my columns, articles, my nine best- selling books and publications and appearances on TV, radio and the print news media. First, I was a rebel, then an arrogant doctor then I learned what life and health really are and I became a student of health and life. I learned that everybody has to take control and responsibility over his or her life, health and happiness. I finally learned that the only way to cure somebody is to educate, train, coach and support them. Nobody cures anybody else. Only our own body has the possibility to heal and repair itself. We have to take the responsibility to make sure our body has the right ingredients to be able to do its work as best as possible. The same way you have your oil in your car changed regularly and you choose the best oil or gas for your car, you should learn to give your body all it needs. The oil change equals the regular cleansing process and the gasoline the diet we choose. However, I don't want to mislead you because all of this together makes up only 14% of our health — although a

13

very important 14%. The other 86% of our health is based on mental and emotional stress and the lack of energy, quality of life and happiness.

The only cause of illness is lack of energy and the main cause for long- term, damaging lack of energy is mental and emotional stress. Stress is caused by living in constant doubt, fear, worries, hopelessness, lack of self confidence, self love or self esteem and making compromises. The most healing energy is produced when you are happy, fulfilled and successful. Remember, the body can only heal in a state of sleep or total relaxation and if you give your body the cleansing, nutrients and rest it needs.

# Introduction

## Full of Pride

Whenever I think of my endless years of suffering I see the little boy who sat beside me, holding his hands on my stomach and praying aloud, begging God to heal me, hoping that my pain would disappear. I think of that little boy, now a few years older, who tried to understand books on natural healing and attempted to apply them as metaphysical or medical works. Then I remember the endless suffering I endured for many years. How often did I feel the need to end my own life? This boy gave me the courage and incentive to keep on fighting. How often did I reach the end of the rope, while a physician tried once more to relieve my colic cramps with medication so that I could stop screaming from pain? I think of our horror, when a doctor gave us the unbelievable, cruel news that I suffered from chronic inflammation of the liver and liver cancer, saying I only had two years to live, and that if I were a horse he would put me out of my misery.

Out of our fear and helplessness, and out of his love for me and his strong belief in God, this boy's strength and devotion emerged and he tried to do everything possible – absolutely everything - to cure me and to keep me alive.

Today, I remember the first successes we shared; how he lessened my pain and how happy we were that I had lived one day without hurting. I remember the intensity with which we repeatedly begged the doctors for causes and remedies. I think of the many books this boy read, often late into the night, and how he researched all the possibilities available at the time to try and improve my condition.

I think of how this boy sat with our old family doctor and had the relationships and functions of the body explained to him how he wrote to authors who had published books on healing and talked on the telephone to people who had conquered so-called incurable illnesses.

This boy became the "in house" doctor of our whole family. He treated my sister Christel, who had developed a severe heart ailment resulting from an attack of polio in her youth. He treated my sister Martha, who had developed a kidney condition. I think of the helplessness this boy experienced and the intensity with which he fought to save the life of my mother, who had cancer in her lymph nodes. It became commonplace for all family members, friends and relatives to ask this boy to relieve them of their aches and illnesses.

The day we realized that three years had passed since the doctor had given me two years to live, I remember how I felt at the time when I was told there was no hope of healing, and now I had already lived a year longer than I was suppose to and found myself on the path toward improvement and healing. It still moves me now.

Even today I experience an immense feeling of gratitude, love and happiness when I think about the miracle which this boy worked in my life. I have no greater wish then as many ill people as possible come to know this feeling and recognize that there is always hope as long as you are willing to search for a way and fight for success.

By the time he was eighteen-years-old healing people with so-called miracle cures for asthma, rheumatism, gout, shingles, psoriasis, and more were normal every day occurrences in his life.

I became his secretary, scheduled his appointments for him and took care of his patients. I followed his path of development, which he pursued in the same unusual way as when he was a child. He lived with healers and miracle healers, with medicine specialists and other people who helped him to develop this unbelievable ability which he carried within himself. In those years as his secretary and adviser, I saw so many miracles that I lost count. He healed people with cancer, multiple sclerosis, asthma, rheumatism gout and even those with severe depression, anxiety and unbearable fears generally regarded as incurable. He cured them all and did not even think much about it.

Then one day, this now mature young man mentioned to me that there must be a way to help more people, faster and more effectively. He no longer believed that he cured those people; rather the infinite power of the human mind that exists in every one of us does the healing. With this recognition he went into the world, studied, learned, researched and developed, in my opinion, the most effective system in the world. He put together a manual to guide every individual on his own path to total health. This system called **Instinct Based Medicine System™, (IBMS™)** is a guide for self-healing and self-training, so that every person can find his own personal path and gain and maintain perfect health and vitality.

He dedicated his life to the desire that there should only be independent, successful and happy people in every walk of life. He wanted to help all people in taking charge of their lives. He wanted to share his information and knowledge on help and self-help through his teachings. This man, whom I introduce to you now with such love and trust, is my son, Dr. Leonard Coldwell.

Please read this book with an open heart and open mind, for the revelations, the knowledge and my son's success were born of his concern for my life. His strength resulted from the fight for my health and from the pure spiritual freedom of a person who strove from his earliest childhood toward solutions. He refused to believe in the so-called incurable illnesses or unsolvable problems. He worked sixteen hours a day in order to perfect the system he developed. He worked to improve its effectiveness in hopes that every man and woman could understand and utilize it as quickly as possible. He had to fight not only for the cure but most of all against the medical establishment that constantly tries to destroy him with lies and defamation. I wish you God speed for the innate power which we all possess.

Mama Coldwell

# I dedicate this book to

## Tina

## A personal word

I am writing this book because the medical profession murdered my grandmother. They killed my unborn sister and countless family members and friends. They gave my mother liver cancer due to medical malpractice and slaughtered my father. They gave my father's second wife a vaccination shot and she has been in a wheelchair ever since. Personally, I have had a lot of negative experience with the medical profession and learned it is nearly always about the money and power. I learned that medical doctors don't have the right answers about healing and perfect health. They don't know where illness comes from and how to heal it but they have a lot of unfounded opinions. For example, for decades they said cancer has nothing to do with diet yet they don't know where cancer comes from. If they don't know how cancer develops how can they dismiss diet?

Medicine is a religion not a science because it is just based on beliefs and not on scientific facts. If I ask ten different doctors for their diagnosis and treatment plan, I get 10 different answers. If I ask a specialist he always comes up with an answer that is within his personal field of expertise. How can that be science? If you want to get and stay healthy you have to help yourself and stop trusting others with your health and life. Make your own educated decisions about your own life and health; don't let them kill you with their diagnostic tools like radiation machines or contrast solutions.

Remember you are the only one that has to live with the consequences of your decisions, I learned they don't care if you undergo surgery as long as it makes them money. They act like they care but in my experience they don't. You, and not them, suffer and pay the price and their bill. Statistically, a medical doctor has the shortest lifespan of all professions — 56 years of age in average. Doctors have one of the highest suicide rates and many of them are alcoholics or drug addicts. Many M.D.s are incompetent and helpless. Their main subject to talk about in private is often how to make more money on the same patient. I have rarely heard them discuss a more effective cure. It is even common for male doctors to make derogatory comments about their female patients. I leaned that if you have 10 different plumbers or masons you can be lucky if there is one good one among them. The same is true for the medical profession. It is just another trade.

Since no one has proven a higher cure rate for cancer and all other terminal or chronic disease then I have, I believe all my success and experience will provide you with a very good overview of the world of therapy.

Of course there are exceptions! Of course your doctor is different (until you are in real trouble — and you find out the truth about your M.D.).

On the other hand, I have never heard a doctor just starting out say lets hurt or kill some patients today. Very often the M.D. starts out with a lot of ideals and good intentions but when the reality of life (the bills and the need for a new Porsche) kicks in, there usually is a gradual change in the approach and the thought process of how to run a medical office. The kickbacks from the pharmaceutical reps for the use of their chemical drugs and all the other perks they can get in selling specific treatments and tools are overwhelming. Many fall for the "free vacation" camouflaged as an educational conference in Las Vegas or Hawaii. I have even heard that the eight- year- old child of a doctor was hired as an advisor to a specific company and paid a full salary because the doctor (the father) promoted a specific treatment from that company.

I know there are some good doctors out there, but I want you to stop believing that everybody that has a medical degree or works as a therapist is trustworthy or even has the competence or knowledge to heal. I tell my patients: Don't believe anybody. Question everything until you have answers that make you feel confident and safe with the diagnosis and treatment. Never, ever have surgery (except emergency or life saving surgery) before getting opinions from at least three other experts. It could be that the M.D.'s wife or husband needs a new Mercedes or nice spa vacation and your surgery is providing the finances for it. Let me tell you that I have many close friends that are medical doctors and good people but not necessarily good physicians and they all need money!

As a last word of hope: There may be a few therapists out there that are really different and filled with ideals, love and competence but I could not find them. If you know one please let me know and I will put his or her name on my website. www.instinctbasedmedicine.com and www.drleonardcoldwell. com

Because I believe there are still enough doctors out there that would love to heal and help their patients while still making enough money on them, I offer the only logical and in my opinion right solution for the good of us all: Let's heal together!

I offer in this book not only the tools and information for the patients but also for the therapist that has a real interest in healing and optimum health. I will show some of the major challenges in the medical world and also in the alternative field. But my final goal is to find a way for all of us, working for the greater good of human kind, to work together with our knowledge and education to find the right way for every individual that seeks our advice or help.

I retired from the field of therapy in 1999 in order to invest my time in research, teaching and my work for the Dr. Leonard Coldwell Foundation. I also wanted the freedom to say whatever I believe is right. As long as you have a license as a therapist, you are bound to use the systems that are set in place. The systems that make the money for the pharmaceutical and medical industry and, in my opinion, have nothing to do with healing, prevention or health.

If all patients are cured (and they could be) the entire illness profession would be bankrupt. Please be aware of the fact that minerals and vitamins can cure many illnesses that are based on nutritional deficiencies, toxemia and acidosis, which means that your body pH is below 7.36 and therefore acidic. Your body needs to be slightly alkaline to be healthy and illnesses like cancer cannot develop in an alkaline and oxygen rich environment. However, the pharmaceutical and medical industries and their almighty powers have made sure that laws were passed that all nutritional supplements provide a disclaimer that states:

"This product does not heal, prevent, treat or diagnose any disease." Even if the nutritional supplement, vitamin, herb or mineral could heal an illness or symptom, by law, only the pharmaceutical drugs can cure the above mentioned diseases and their symptoms. To make sure that the pharmaceutical industry does not loose any money because of natural products it has its bodyguards the Federal Trade Commission  and Federal Drug Administration creating laws and regulations that forbid herb and supplement companies to mention any connection between health benefits and their products. If they state what kind of illness their products cure and which symptoms are eliminated they would go to jail and their products would be destroyed. Besides stress relief, I only used natural products to cure my patients, mainly natural cleanses (cleanses that are based on certified organic whole foods). For information go to www.instinctbasedmedicine.com

# Instinct based Medicine™

## The guide for healthy action

Nearly every health and self healing book I have ever read is written in a manner that is too complicated, too specific, too hard to understand, too manipulative, too out of this world, too new age or too much like traditional medicine. After writing nine best- selling books and seeing why they are so successful, I decided to write an educational book about health and self help for all those people who don't have as much knowledge about medicine or natural healing as a fully educated practitioner. This book is written for the person with common sense and the will to achieve optimum health without getting killed by the medical profession, pharmaceutical industry or the hocus pocus new age "wannabe healers" and the new crowd of naturopathic practitioners with no formal education, experience or real life knowledge about health.

In my experience, the fact is only .8% of all therapists are willing, competent and able to help a person with any health challenge. The medical profession just wants your money. They get rich by all the unnecessary and mostly dangerous tests and the senseless and usually harmful therapies. No medical doctor I know has even the slightest idea about healing any illness. They treat symptoms instead the cause of all illness. Many try to make sure you never get really well so that they have you as a "customer" for life. A doctor's office has about 300 patients. If they all become healthy, the doctor is broke. So how much interest does the doctor have in your everlasting health and well-being? The pharmaceutical companies have little interest in creating a drug that would really cure the cause of an illness and, therefore, make their drugs unnecessary.

Please be aware that there are many strange people in the field of alternative healing but, at least in this field, we find open-minded people that are interested in natural health and healing and that means we can have hope.

Let's be aware of the psychologists, who usually studied psychology to find out what is wrong with themselves. Psychology is not even a science. It is nothing more than the accumulation of often unfounded ideas. Sigmund Freud, the founder of what later became psychiatry had more problems than all his patients combined. Freud's psychotherapy and psycho-analysis is the most absurd technique taught in medical schools. Most of his theories have already been proven wrong and more people committed suicide as a result of this psycho junk than in any other therapy form. To whine and complain about your past does not make it better. It makes it worse and gives you more mental illnesses. It is teaching you to learn to live in denial and schizophrenia. Psychiatry never cured anybody. All they do is numb the poor patient with dangerous psycho drugs or brain surgeries and turn them into zombies so that they are just unable to function or feel anything at all. Of course, the pharmaceutical industry really loves these patients because they get addicted to their drugs and they make money on their victims forever). These companies don't even care that they turn children on prescription drugs like Ritalin into drug addicts. Not even to mention all the horrible side effects all these drugs have on patients. They give people dangerous, addictive drugs with horrible side effects instead of teaching them how to control their behavior and their emotional states with natural techniques.

So now, you ask, what is left if they're all not worth the money and time? Listen to your instincts. Learn to develop and use your common sense and try, if possible, to stay away from any doctor. Why do you think most 100-year-old people questioned in a study reported they never went to a doctor except in the case of an accident?

Many studies around the world have found: The more often you visit a doctor the higher the possibility of developing serious illnesses. In addition, you will most likely die from the side effects of treatments and medications than from the illness. Studies show that at least one in four people develop a dangerous or even deadly bacteria infection in a hospital. It is a known fact that the overuse of antibiotics has caused a deadly, super-resistant bacteria.

The only way to survive the influence of greed of the illness society is to get as educated as possible about your own health. Would you give a stranger the power to do what they like with your money and everything you own without questioning them about the risks and dangers and if there are any guarantees? Why do you do this with your health and your doctor?

We are so brainwashed and manipulated by the media to trust and believe in our doctors and their advice and treatments. That is where the root of all dangers and most suffering lies: the childlike acceptance that the doctor knows best because he or she is an expert.

So what makes him or her an expert? The fact that he read a couple of medical books that usually are already outdated before he leaves medical school? He is taught about hypothetical theories that have no conclusive or scientific evidence and no proof that they work.

The so-called medical field is nothing more than a religion because it is based on the momentary belief system instead of scientific facts. For example, there has never been any proof that artificial vaccination is safe or effective. There is countless evidence that it is harmful for people and causes many illnesses and even death. They say polio, small pox and other deadly illnesses were eradicated through vaccination. However, in countries where people were not vaccinated the illnesses disappeared even faster. These illnesses disappeared through better nutrition and cleanliness and not because of vaccinations. Why did the public have to pay billions for vaccination damage when 36,000 people died shortly after being given the swine flu vaccination if vaccination is safe?

For me, the connection between vaccination and autism is just a fact. But, as you know, there are many people making a lot of money on vaccination and they —or the scientists they pay— contend that vaccinations are safe and effective. I just question those findings (see www.nvic.org).

Nearly all men who got vaccinated in the 1960s with a vaccine that was derived from ape kidneys later got prostate cancer! I believe that Sudden Infant Death Syndrome can be connected to vaccination. Most absurd is the flu vaccine. That cannot work! The virus is in constant change and to get vaccinated with the virus from last year is just not worth the effort, risk and money. Many scientists agree: it cannot work.

All they teach in medical school has usually nothing to do with facts and science. It is based on the momentary belief system of the medical profession which is usually manipulated and controlled by the pharmaceutical industry and the medical society for power and profits.

I just read a publication *Death by Doctors*, from Gary Null ND and others, which stated: The main cause of illness today is from the side effects of prescription and over-the-counter drugs. In addition, the main cause of death today is the medical doctor.

Think about your neighbor or colleague at work. Think about everybody you know. Think about the plumbers, or handyman you know. How many of them would you trust? How many are competent, trustworthy and honest?

Do you think doctors are different? They are people like you and I and all the other people we know. So how many good ones do you think you will run into by coincidence?

Now here is the main question: Why should you believe and trust me and what I have to say? The answer is very simple. I had countless illnesses myself that I conquered without the medical crooks. My mom, as well as seven of her siblings, had cancer. My Mom was told she was terminal with liver cancer more than 30 years ago. My grandmother, as well as my father, died of cancer. By the age of 14, I had already had more contact with illness and horrible death than most people will ever experience in their lifetime.

I learned though my own experience and from patients that cured themselves, from extraordinary people that had stunning healing results. I accumulated and put together the essence of what I learned to become one person with the highest cure rate ever.

Why should you trust me? Because I made a pact with God. I promised him, that if he helped me cure my mother from terminal liver cancer, I would spend the rest of my life helping other people with their health. I am not a religious freak or radical – I believe in God but not in any specific form of organized religion. I am a Christian the way I understand it. I respect each person's religious beliefs as well the right for people not to believe in religion or God at all.

My mom was cured and today, over 30 years later at the age of 72 is one of the healthiest most energized and enthusiastic people you will ever meet. She was my very first patient. By the age of 18, I had more success than anybody out there. Of course, they authorities wanted to take me to court for practicing medicine without a license, despite my near 100% success rate. So, I went to the schools of brainwashing, false ideas, pseudo science and lies (the official schools for physicians) just to legally help dying and sick people to get and stay healthy.

The people that make money on our illness and suffering don't care about results. They care about the power to brainwash, control and manipulate you in their universities. They want control over everything you think and do. They tell you how you have to treat a cancer patient (killing radiation and chemotherapy and disabling slaughter called surgery). If you don't harm your patients the way their therapy and treatment plans tell you to, you lose your license. I just learned that in California a doctor's license was revoked and he was imprisoned because he cured multiple patients with vitamin

B-17 instead of harming or killing them with the mandatory "treatment."

They make sure that natural healers and their individual successes and cure rates are unknown. If a natural healer dares to cure an illness or patient that is supposedly incurable, they are all of a sudden a quack or it was a false diagnosis to begin with, or it was just luck that cured the person. Modern medicine will not even look into my unconventional ideas or treatments. The traditional medical establishment is afraid of being proven wrong. If that were to occur, then what? They would have to throw away all the lies and get rid of all the brainwashing from medical education. Never! So it is better for them to ignore you. If this doesn't work, they try to defame you, and destroy your reputation. Today, the internet provides a new way to distribute lies to destroy your reputation. People look at these lies instead of facts. Websites that supposedly expose people are set up to control the opinions of the masses. Have you ever asked yourself why someone would go through all the effort and financial costs to set up a free website to defame people and their ideas? It is all about control and power and the pharmaceutical industry and other power groups paying people to set up these defamation sites. There are scientists and doctors that are specifically paid to fraudulently debunk credible alternative doctors or natural treatments to preserve the income for the pharmaceutical industry.

If all of this fails they try to take you, or mainly your system, over. Now they say it is too powerful to be used by untrained people and they come up with a curriculum for "your system". They haven't the slightest idea of what you are doing but they want to control it and make money from it.

Sometimes, they simply want to pay you off. Representatives of the pharmaceutical companies offered me a lot of money if I would stop performing my work and writing my publications and change my opinions in their favor.

The most dangerous M.D.s of all are the so-called integrated practitioners! They act like they give the patient the best of both worlds in combining traditional medicine with natural healing methods. There is no way to combine traditional medicine and natural medicine. Because traditional medicine harms or even kills and natural medicine helps the body to heal itself. If one therapist would really use both therapy forms they would cancel each other out and destroy the patient's health even more then if just one form of therapy would be used. I learned with thousand of cancer patients that if you do both you will die guarantied. They pretend to give you the best of both worlds, but if it comes down to it they tell you to get antibiotics and vaccinations and other harmful treatments. The real danger of these people is that they imply they have knowledge about how to create natural healing (which they usually do not) and that you are safer with them because they use harmful chemicals only if necessary and otherwise use helpful and harmless natural medicines.

Riding the wave to make money is one thing. Fraudulently pretending they are natural healers but, in fact, promoting all the dangers of prescription drugs and therapies is misleading and dangerous for the patients. In addition, as a pretend expert they undermine the value of supplements and natural medicine and further promote the use of chemical toxins. It seems to me that their only goal is to sell their own products. They also mislead people to believe you can safely mix chemical drug based medicines with natural healing methods.

Then there is sunny boy Sanji Gupta (the always charming smiling TV doctor that every mother wants to have as there son-in-law) who spreads the propaganda of the pharmaceutical mafia. With his youthful appearance and nice smile he sells the messages of the pharmaceutical industry.

In October 2005 in a live interview with Bill Maher, Gupta was asked isn't it known that if your body is healthy, you cannot get sick. Gupta, stunned for a moment, blatantly lied and said that even if you live a healthy lifestyle you can get sick, especially get the flu. This is absolutely not true at all! You cannot get sick from any microbe if you live a healthy lifestyle and your body is detoxified, alkaline and oxygen rich, de-stressed and full of energy. Gupta is the most effective sales person out there for the pharmaceutical industry, chemical drugs, medical tests and procedures.

Who are they? They are the individuals and groups of people that make money on your suffering, pain, illness, helplessness, hopelessness, lack of knowledge and education and, most of all, capitalize on your fear— the fear of illness, suffering or death.

## Take charge or your health!

I am about to share with you the most suppressed and overlooked secrets to optimum health. My educational, self-help and self-healing system, the **Instinct Based Medical System (IBMS™)** can help you to identify and remove the root cause of every disease! That is the only way to optimum health! My system does not just treat the symptoms because they disappear anyway after the root cause of the health break down is defined and eliminated. In this book, you will learn exactly what it takes to experience optimum health and how you can reverse the progress of virtually any disease.

In my opinion, disease is only caused by lack of energy that is originally caused by stress. Usually mental and emotional stress, that is caused by living in fear, with doubts, worries, feelings of hopelessness, helplessness, and lack of self esteem, lack of self love and  self acceptance. Over 86% of illness is caused by stress alone. Only 14%, if even that much, is caused or supported by acidosis caused by bad diets and nutritional deficiencies and the accumulation of toxins in the body, dehydration, lack of oxygen, and lack of movement or exercise. Some people say you get cancer from radiation and that it is not from stress. In my opinion, that is an accident caused by an outside force. I believe the cause of every illness is mental and emotional stress.

Don't wait a second longer to educate yourself about your body's natural healing power, and start using it immediately! Making educated decisions is the best defense against illness and the best way to reverse back to optimum health.

Do you suffer from a so-called incurable disease? Have your doctors told you that you have only a short time to live? Or that you have to learn to live with these limitations or pain? Are you suffering from anything labeled chronic or terminal? Then this book is for you! Even if you just want to maintain optimum health you'll find how to achieve that here in this book.

Do you suffer from depression, lack of energy or are you on any kind of medical drugs or treatment? Have you been told you have to live with some kind of medication for the rest of your life? Then this book is definitely for you!

You have to take charge of your life and health, your energy and happiness right away! Regardless of your age or physical condition, you can recover from virtually any disease and achieve optimum health if you are willing to do whatever it takes to achieve your goal and as long as you are willing to do it yourself instead of expecting me or someone else to do it for you.

I have treated directly or indirectly over 35,000 patients in my clinics, workshops and my **Modern Therapy Centers™ MTC™**. Over 2.2 million people have attended my seminars. More than seven million people have read my books, columns, and newsletters. My speeches have been broadcasted worldwide to millions of people with huge success and a phenomenal response. The Life Coach Company found in a study that I am the most recommended alternative doctor in the world. As you may know, my system is endorsed by Kevin Trudeau's mega bestseller "Natural Cures They Don't Want You to Know About" countless times and my system **(Dr. Coldwell System™)** is recommended for nearly every illness. The main authority on Fibromyalgia, Dr. Bowersox, also recommends my system for his patients in his book. I have been called on as an expert for TV, radio and newspaper interviews countless times.

My personal experience and belief is that every illness is curable. It doesn't matter if the doctors have given you a short time to live, or if they insist that your disease is terminal or incurable. You can recover from disease!

The only exception to the success of my system is, if a person is so damaged by medical treatments – surgery, radiation, chemotherapy, etc. – that there is not enough substance left to work with. The only prerequisite is that you must be committed to do whatever it takes to get better. I will show you how to do it!

This book will teach you how to take care of yourself mentally, emotionally and physically. From start to finish, I will show you how you can rid yourself of disease using nothing else then the natural function of the body. Your body is genetically conditioned to survive and to heal itself. In the pages to come, I will show you how to activate your body's natural healing powers. You will learn about stress, and how to use my system to reduce or even eliminate negative stress factors in your life. Your eyes will be opened to the dangers of doctors and medicine. I will also reveal my secret technology that will enable you to think clearer, stay focused, and get healthier faster than you ever thought possible. The natural state of the body is to be healthy,   not somewhat healthy, or tortured by pain or symptoms of illness.

You should be excited about the journey ahead of us. Dear reader, you may not be feeling well right now, but by the time you finish this book, you can be a new person. Your eyes can be bright and shiny. Your skin can be clear, radiant and glowing. You will have pep in your step. Your energy level can skyrocket. You will be optimistic about the future. Your feelings of anxiety, fear and depression can be replaced with a zest for living. You won't even struggle with willpower anymore, because you'll be so self motivated to achieve and maintain optimum health.

I have seen thousands of people recover from so-called incurable disease, and I am absolutely convinced that you can do the same. I even have seen spontaneous healing where patients recovered in minutes from some terrible disease or symptom.

Is this too good to be true? It almost sounds too easy, doesn't it? You'd think that everyone would want to be healthy. Doesn't everyone want to be their best? Doesn't everyone want to function at a peak, optimum level?

When it comes right down to it, few people are willing to make the lifestyle changes that are necessary for optimum health. Many people are not willing to take charge over their own life and don't want to take responsibility for their own recovery and healing process. Many are too afraid or just too lazy to make the necessary changes in their life and some just don't want to take the responsibility for their own life and health. Most of our society is conditioned to pop a pill for whatever ails them, or to have someone else fix their problems for them. Surgery is often a convenient alternative. Unfortunately, surgeries always cause long-term damage, lower the immune function and the long term effects are often detrimental. Pharmaceutical drugs all have side effects that are often worse than the illness itself. In my opinion, they nearly always do more harm than good. Medicine treats only the symptoms and does nothing to identify and eliminate the root of illness. (Of course, all my statements exclude emergency and restorative medicine.)

Some people don't strive to be healthy because they don't care enough about themselves. They lack self love and self-esteem and don't even make the effort to be the best they can be. Very often they are overweight, sick or immobile and don't do anything about it. Sometimes they even get to this state on purpose out of self pity, self punishment or even self hatred.

**Common justifications not to act include:**
- "This is the way I am."
- "This is part of growing older."
- "I'll learn to live with this pain or discomfort."
- "It's not that bad, let's forget about it."
- "Maybe if I ignore it, the pain will go away."
- "I don't feel any pain; it's just my imagination."

- "Eating right and taking care of myself is too much work!"
- "I'd like to know more about getting healthy, but I don't know where to start."
- "I am confused by the variety of information available. Who can I trust?"
- "It will get better on its own."
- "It's just bad luck."
- "The doctors will cure me or the medication will help."

## For a better understanding

This book is written for the person searching for health and happiness who is willing to do his own part to accelerate health and happiness and who is willing to take responsibility for his own well-being. This is for the person who wants the information to make a quality decision about their own health. The information in this book is the result of more than 36 years of suffering, studying, research, trial and error, devastation, countless tears, pain, hopelessness, helplessness, fear, endless struggle, determination, doubt, worries, three decades of therapy and unmatched results of thousands of cured patients mostly in a terminal state (some even with a life expectancy of three to nine months). People, who were given up on by the medical profession after they tried everything unsuccessfully.

Parts of this book were originally written for my patients and their families so that they could learn to understand why and how their loved ones became sick and how they could help them to get healthy again and stay that way.

This book is necessary to make everyone aware of the fact that we are the only people who can make ourselves sick, and we are the only people who can make and keep ourselves healthy.

After working for about 15 years as a general health practitioner, I found out, that it is not the doctor, the medication or the surgery that cures patients. It is the patient himself, his own immune and self- healing system. This system is genetically prepared to survive. Only in emergency situations, in accidents or rare unusual situations, does it need outside help. Nature builds every living being self-sufficient. I don't believe that diseases are genetic. If you are born healthy, you can stay that way. People can have genetic predispositions for health malfunctions but they don't have to get the problem.

After I recognized that the therapist can only be a teacher, trainer or coach for the patient, my entire way of thinking, as well as my belief system, changed dramatically forever.

My colleagues hated me for that statement. They wanted to play God. They love the admiration and blind obedience and the endless income from their patients. I found they are more interested in their own egos and financial welfare, then in the welfare of their patients. There are some exceptions of course, but a sparingly small amount.

I had to learn to fight the media that is brainwashed by the medical profession and controlled by the pharmaceutical industry that pays for advertisements. It is very scary that it seems to be all about money. The patient is only seen as a paying customer.

Threats and all kind of attacks against me and my message were a daily part of my life, even attempts on my life happened. I needed to hire my own lawyer just to go through a normal day. I had to spend a lot of money to fight all the legal attacks. One company even offered to pay me a huge amount of money if I would cancel the publication of one of my self-healing books.

No one cared that I had cured more patients from cancer, asthma, diabetes, muscular dystrophy, depression, rheumatoid arthritis and all kind of nutritional deficiency and stress- related illnesses than all of my enemies together. No one cared about the thousands of cured patients that are a living testimony of my message, meaning that every illness is curable cheap, fast and easy. The patient just needs to do his part

It is not only the therapists I have to fight. I have to fight the patients. When they heard that their own behavior, their own way of thinking and acting, their decisions, their own compromises made them sick, often I thought, they wanted to physically attack me. They felt offended. They felt guilty or just denied even the possibility that they had anything to do with their own illness and suffering. But it is just a fact and also it opens up the opportunity to cure yourself because if you believe you are responsible for your own illness or symptoms you also have the power to create your own health.

Of course, nobody wants to be sick, and no one wants to have the responsibility to have made himself or herself sick. It is so much easier to believe that it is destiny, genetics, or bad luck to get sick, or God's way of testing you, than it is to accept the fact that we are the only person that is responsible for our health.

Every patient I've ever treated, who did not have chemotherapies, radiation or surgery, became healthy again as long as they were willing to take responsibility for their own life and make the necessary changes.

Of course we need our doctors. But I am not one of them anymore. I put all the essence of what I learned from life, my patients, and my mentors into one single, easy- to- understand self-help system: the **Instinct Based Medicine System (IBMS™)**.

To my knowledge, this system is the only scientific educational holistic self-help system worldwide that works on the cause of the problem and helps to eliminate the root cause of the illness.

This unique system is an educational health coaching system. It gives the student all the information, the capabilities, the tools, the training and coaching, to reach his optimum state of health. It does not manipulate or interfere in any way. The IBMS™ gives everyone the opportunity to find the root causes of their own life challenges and gives them the education, training and help to achieve all their goals through themselves.

My system helps the student use what he has naturally since birth. It only uses the normal body functions and the natural way things are suppose to work in our body. We didn't need surgery or chemotherapy in the previous hundreds of years, but now we have them and the illness rate and death rate due to these illnesses are higher then ever.

I learned by curing my mother from terminal liver cancer with a life expectancy of two years that we only need the power of our own body and mind to get and stay healthy. Why was the rate of cancer 7% in 1900 and today it is 56%? They say people live longer. That is absurd because these patients usually do not get cancer at an older age. I believe if my father would not have had a colonoscopy done he would still be alive today because he had not had problems before. The doctors found a tumor and tricked him into surgery, chemotherapy and radiation and his horrible dying process began instantly. My grandmother was perfectly fine with a tumor in her breast for 28 years until they talked her into surgery, chemo and radiation treatment and her painful and inhuman dying processes begun instantly after surgery. She died after suffering for two years with the worse pain I have ever witnessed.

Therefore, I created an educational self-help training system that enables everybody to achieve their optimum level of health. The results prove it works.

If you want someone else to cure you or someone else to take responsibility for your life and health, this book is not for you. If you want to learn how to take charge of your own life and health and view your doctor more as a source of information, diagnoses and help, as your partner (if you even need one) then my system is made for you. Remember, the natural state of your body is healthy not sick.

Today after being trainer, coach, consultant and speaker for the largest companies in Europe, as well as for countless medical associations, groups and health insurance companies and after more then 30 years of experience as a therapist and teacher, I am proudly known as the Health-Educator. Professor Dr. Peter Lange, president of the Charitee in Berlin, Germany (the German equivalent of the National Institute of Health) said, "My colleague, Dr. Leonard Coldwell, is the David Copperfield in his field." The most effective way to help somebody is to encourage that person's self-confidence, strengthen their believe in themselves and their own abilities and to provide education, training, support, motivation, hope and understanding and sometimes even a good kick in the rear end.

The context of this book is only based on my own personal research, conclusions, experience and is my personal opinion. This concept is created by trial and error and the essence of all existing techniques and therapy methods known today. This concept is only result oriented.

My intention is to help as many people as possible to become completely healthy, self sufficient, as well as so strong and educated that no one on earth will be able to manipulate them ever again. I want my readers to be able to make the best educated decisions for their health possible.

I hope to help create confident happy, healthy people who know their own potential and are willing and able to use it. That is my goal.

I stand for health education in schools and for healthcare instead of illness care and symptom treatment. That is the reason I founded the Dr. Leonard Coldwell Foundation for Drug and Crime Free Schools and Health for Children more than 15 years ago.

When I was fighting the fight to save my mom's life from liver cancer more than 30 years ago, I prayed constantly to God, to help me and my mom. I promised God if he helped me to save my mother, I would dedicate my life, to make sure, that other mothers and their children wouldn't have to go through the suffering, pain and horror that we went through. This book, as well as the **Instinct Based Medicine System™**, is one of the ways I am keeping my promise.

To avoid misunderstanding: I believe in God because he is a daily reality for me. I don't believe in organized religion because this power has been abused since its inception. It is not the idea or concept that I have a problem with, it is the person that takes control over organized religion that due to his own interpretation and needs creates the problem. I believe in the creation of evolution in science and religion because without God there is no nature and therefore no future or development. The use of my system is based on the Christian belief of free will. The use of my techniques is scientifically proven and still based on my Christian beliefs. I am not a radical or extremist. I believe that everybody has the right to his or her own beliefs and conclusions. Most of all, I don't believe that any person or religion has the right to tell people what to do or not to do. I believe in free will and that nobody has the right to judge another person.

## Medicine is the fastest growing failing profession

When I was a child I had constant abdominal pain on my right side. Doctors tried a couple of times to convince me and my mother to have my appendix removed because in their eyes I was much too young to have gallbladder problems. This misdiagnosis caused me 28 years of pain and I have lost the ability to eat anything besides rice, potatoes and similar type foods.

First of all, it caused me to almost die and I have had an inflammation of almost all my organs. They finally figured out that my gallbladder was full of stones and that it was about to burst.

They wanted to perform surgery on my shoulder but my persistence against surgery and my chiropractic knowledge stopped me. I discovered that the cause of my shoulder problems was a disc between the fifth and sixth cervical vertebra and after a chiropractor fixed this problem, my shoulder pain disappeared completely.

They also wanted to do surgery on my ring finger because I have had chronic pain in the joints. A chiropractor fixed this completely in three weeks. They wanted to take my tonsils out when I was a child because they were working perfectly and they were inflamed because they were trying to get rid of all the toxins in my system.

The history with my tonsils led me to develop the **Instinct Based Medicine System™**. When I was a child, doctors told me about having to cut my tonsils out and I knew that this was not something that I wanted. I also heard that when the tonsils were inflamed you couldn't get them removed. I learned very quickly that I needed my tonsils to be inflamed when I went to the doctor so that they wouldn't cut them out. I learned pretty fast that it is very easy to control your body in every possible way. I could produce tonsillitis in 5 minutes if I needed to. Today, I still have my tonsils and my appendix and I am really happy about it. If you let the doctors do whatever they want to do they are basically experimenting on you.

The medical profession is always looking for ways to make more money. They try to perform surgery all the time. Lots of people don't have their appendix or their tonsils. They also try to put tubes in small children's ears to prevent ear infections. In most cases, those ear infections are caused by vaccines and the surgery is worthless anyway.

# Chapter 1

*There are no incurable diseases — Only incurable people*

## My mother's terminal cancer

When I was seven years old, I remember my mother crying constantly from intense pain. I watched helplessly as doctors gave her painkillers and shots so that she would be more comfortable. Due to complications from gallbladder surgery performed by a medical doctor, my mother developed liver cirrhosis of the worst kind. Her liver was inflamed and she was constantly in horrible pain. When I turned 12, my mother's liver cirrhosis progressed into terminal liver cancer. The doctors gave her a maximum of two years to live. They stated that there was no hope; no one had ever recovered from this kind of advanced cancer.

The doctors suggested that she had to learn to live with the pain and make the best out of the time she had left. Imagine what this meant to a little boy like me. All I could think about was if my mother would still be alive when I got home from school that day. In fact, the first thing I did when I got home from school was open my mother's bedroom door to see if she was still alive. I did this every morning as well.

While she was in the hospital, I was constantly worried. I was afraid that my mother would die. I cried more during this time of my life than any other time.

My mother and I only had each other. My biological father had left us because he did not want a sick wife. It was probably best that he left because he abused my mother and made our lives miserable. We were better off without him but we were financially really poor.

With no means of financial support, I became the sole breadwinner for our family. I cleaned restaurants before school and worked in a sandwich shop after school. It was the only way that I could put food on the table and a roof over our heads.

I also paid for medical treatment and alternative therapies that the health insurance did not cover. We had nothing to lose. The medical profession had completely given up on my mother and refused to treat her anymore. The only things they gave her were painkillers.

Of course, my experience with the pharmaceutical and medical profession occurred in Germany. Things may have turned out differently if we were living elsewhere but there is no way to tell now. I tried desperately to find a cure for my mother's cancer. We tried everything from alternative medicine to homeopathy to healers from all over the world... nothing seemed to work.

I read every book about healing that I could get my hands on. I went to countless seminars, studied herbs, hypnotherapy, and tried all kinds of medical and alternative therapies, even new age stuff. I was desperate to help my mother and was willing to try anything. I did try it all, believe me.

I was constantly experimenting on my mother. It was trial and error, and we had nothing to lose. Finally, our retired family doctor sat down with me to explain the functions and connections regarding medicine. She studied with me, explained medical procedures and helped me to understand the way of medical thinking and theories. While studying naturopathic medicine, I discovered that new age stuff does not work. Unfortunately, neither does modern medicine. But, if we combine our forces of natural healing and the result-producing knowledge of modern medicine we can create the perfect way to health.

## My teenage years

By the age of 14, I had been to every health seminar I could afford. I got a lot of help from the professors and speakers after I told them my story and why I was attending the seminars. When they discovered that I was a hardship case, many even gave me the money back that I originally paid for the seminar. Some even took me under their wing and taught me privately everything they knew. People can be so generous when they know that someone is in real trouble. Today, I carry the knowledge and experience of hundreds of years of my mentors combined experience, knowledge and success with me.

When I was 16- years- old, I had already earned degrees in naturopathy and relaxation therapy, isolated muscle stretching (similar to chiropractic methods) and hypnotherapy. I gave workshops and seminars and treated patients. I was the youngest self- help coach and educational therapist in Europe. My success was astonishing. I could afford to travel around the world to meet the most successful therapists and healers in the world. I traveled to the Philippines, Brazil, Australia, Africa and many Asian countries to study with the best of the best. I spent all of my time and money educating myself.

I did not study illness, symptom treatment, death or drugs like most traditional medical doctors. I studied health: how and why it happens. I studied people who produced results unknown in traditional medicine. I studied patients who successfully recovered from a serious or terminal illness. I wanted to know what–made them healthy again. I also studied senior citizens who were remarkably healthy and vital, in spite of their age. I was looking for answers and not excuses.

I experimented with all of these new findings on my mom. When I turned 16, my mother was still alive. If I had believed the doctors, she should have been dead two years earlier. By this time, my mother had completely changed her diet. She was eating lots of fresh vegetables and fruit. My mother realized that her stressful relationship with my father was the cause of her health problems. He was verbally and physically abusive, which caused her anguish. Now that he was gone, we could start over. Mom was on the road to recovery, but not completely well at this point.

At 16, I operated a "natural healing center" out of my home. All of the people in my neighborhood (including the kids from school) witnessed my mother's remarkable transformation. Now, they sent their sick loved ones to me.

At 17- years of age, I had my first book published. Today, that book is in its 49th printing.

When I reached the age of 18, I had already helped over a hundred people recover from all kinds of "terminal" or "incurable" diseases. My success grew rapidly and I was so well-known that many jealous medical doctors, lawyers and journalists tried to defame me and stop me from helping others. They accused me of false advertising. They created websites to defame my character, question my professional credentials and completely discredit my work. They hired and paid people to work against me on every level, to try to break me. The problem was that I was working for free and had a nearly 100% success rate and nothing is stronger than the proof of success. It is hard to ignore a cancer patient who, in the opinion of the medical profession, had only years left to live but is now, decades later, perfectly healthy.

At 18 years old, I knew more about health than most people in the health profession. I was known as a "miracle healer" although nothing I did had to do with miracles. It's a tremendous compliment, but I can't take credit for anyone's miracle, healing or recovery. I simply use the tools that I learned from my world travels, research and own success. I never take credit for anyone's miraculous recovery. The credit belongs to the patients, clients and students themselves. Perhaps, I should say, these people created a healthy internal environment in which their bodies could heal themselves. Neither the medical or pharmaceutical profession likes what I have to say. They hate my results so much that even today they try to do everything to destroy me.

## Finally the ultimate Victory

When I was about 22 years old, my mother completely recovered from cancer. My spirit soared high enough to fly. Her healing was everything I ever wanted out of life. Now, it was time for me to set a new goal. I wanted to help heal as many people as I possibly could with natural health remedies. Most of all, I wanted to keep my promise to God!

My mother is still alive and healthy today. She is 72 years old and continues to run my business and foundation in Germany. My mother married a wonderful man named Lothar (for me my real father who was also later murdered by the medical profession), and had another child. My mother's recovery was the beginning of helping thousands of people recover from terminal and incurable diseases.

## Becoming a Naturopathic Practitioner

I finished my studies as a Natural Healing Physician (ND). We have two types of physicians in Europe. One is a strictly medical physician and the other is a Natural Medical Doctor, which deals with alternative medicine with herbs, vitamins, and nutrition. Later, I added degrees as a Doctor of Naturopathic Medicine (NMD) and a Ph.D. in psychology as well as earning more master's degrees in many fields of alternative or complementary medicine as well as in clinical hypnotherapy. My education goes on as well as my degrees. The last degree I added to my list of accomplishments is that of Certified Natural Health Practitioner (CNHP).

My education taught me that healing is based on the basic laws of nature. Recovery involves activating or re- activating the natural healing powers that we all have within ourselves. Given the right internal environment and programming the body heals itself. Everyone has the healing power of nature within themselves.

## Putting self-help into practice

My professional practice continued to grow. I had so many people asking for help that I worked 14 to 16 hour days, seven days a week. I worked around the clock, but that wasn't enough time for me to help everyone. People were sleeping on the sidewalk in front of my house, just to get a chance to talk to me. Many of them were on their deathbed, with no hope for survival. I tried to help every one of these people, but I nearly collapsed from exhaustion.

That's when I realized that I needed more self help therapists to absorb the workload. I hired and trained many alternative health practitioners, so that more people could be treated effectively.

As we treated hundreds of people, I started to wonder why some people would recover quickly, whereas others didn't heal at all. I realized that there is no such thing as incurable disease. There are only incurable people. Many of my patients were deemed hopeless, incurable or terminal by the medical profession. To my delight, most of these patients recovered using natural remedies. Most importantly, I found that if we tried to cure the patient it was a slow and often unsuccessful experience. However, the second we started to educate, train and coach the patient to cure him or herself, we got instant results. The greatest development at this time was the proof that my system is reproducible and can be used or taught by anyone appropriately trained by me personally.

A lot of desperate people turned up on my doorstep. Some were victims of the medical slaughterhouse. They were more harmed and adversely affected by medical treatment than the illness itself. The comment that I heard most often was, "I was fine until the doctors started to treat me!"

In some cases, these people were still able to recover. The point of no return is when treatments, surgery, chemo or radiation therapy or drugs has completely destroyed someone's mental and physical ability to recover. That is when it is too late to turn things around.

Other people are incurable because they're not willing to discipline themselves, eat the right foods, and follow my regimen of cleansing and nutrition. Everyone must be willing to take responsibility for their life, and do what it takes to recover from illness. All healing comes from the inside out. There is no healing force from outside the human body. Every terminally ill person needs to make the decision that they want to live and be committed to following a healthy regimen. Most of all, people have to understand that it is the accumulation of many things that we do wrong that makes us sick and rarely, if ever, only one major mistake. Therefore, we have to take care of our body in a holistic way to achieve long- term optimum health. The first and fundamental step to help your body be strong and healthy is the correct supplements. Most supplements can do more harm than good which is why I've provided a list of companies, supplements and cleanses I believe are safe and most effective. See:

www.instinctbasedmedicine.com →
www.drleonardcoldwell.com.

The most important and most effective cleanse I do myself twice a year and suggest to all my family members and friends is the Tri-Decathlon Delux.

Most people are simply putting toxins into and onto their bodies faster than the body's cleansing system can remove them. When the toxins build up over time, this becomes dangerous. The Tri-Decathlon Delux is a 13-day full body and colon cleanses that works by supporting your body's own built-in cleansing system. This 13-day supply of pure food keeps new toxins from getting into your body. During the first few days, your body's cleansing system will have a chance to start catching up – from there, you body's own built-in cleansing system will continue to cleanse deeper and deeper throughout your entire body right down to the cellular level. It's an entire whole body cleanse that reaches every organ and tissue in your body – supporting nature is what works best – this is the most effective, healthiest and safest cleanse available on the market today. For more cleansing information go to www. instinctbasedmedicine.com

## Learning from world travels

In my life I've studied abroad with gypsies and healers in Brazil, Philippines, Nigeria and Asia. Professor Treder the leading hypnotherapist in Europe also took me under his wings. He taught me everything he knew from his 50 years of experience in hypnotherapy. From Professor Teppewin, I learned about the science of therapeutic mind conditioning.

Note: It is very important to me that you know that, today I am the main opponent against hypnotism. It makes creates addiction, multiple personality disorder, schizophrenia, and is a crime against humanity. Even worse is Neuro Linguistic Programming (NLP) invented by Richard Bandler and John Grinder that, potentially, can cause cancer and many personal tragedies.

Later, I collaborated and improved my newfound knowledge with research and practical application. I wrote a book entitled, "The Unlimited Power of the Subconscious." The book teaches you to awaken and utilize the unlimited power of your mind. The book also led to the development of my **Instinct Based Medicine System™**, which I used in counseling and coaching to help clients identify and eliminate the root cause of their problems. Interestingly enough my motivational book: "You are born to win" helped a tremendous amount of people take charge of their life and to get healthy again. It is a motivational book that gives people a better sense of how great, unique and wonderful they really are and provides tools to develop self esteem, self confidence and a sense of self worthiness everybody deserves.

## The day my life changed forever

My grandmother was very close to me. She was a good church-going woman who raised seven children and worked with mentally handicapped children most of her life. She brought all of them through the horrors of the Second World War, being a refugee alone without my grandfather. He was in a Nazi concentration camp because he refused to hang Jewish people on Hitler's order. My grandmother spent her entire life, even after retirement, caring as a nurse for mentally retarded children. For over 28 years, she had an enlarged cancerous lymph note in her breast. It did not grow. It did not hurt. However, during an unnecessary and dangerous, so-called routine check, the doctors scared her into surgery. That's what they always do. They work with the fear of death —their most powerful marketing trick.

My beloved grandmother had no problems for 28 years. Nothing had ever bothered her and there was no acceptable reason for surgery, chemotherapy or radiation. But they did it all. My grandmother said later that she did not understand what the doctors were telling her. She was just scared. In the hands of experts, who spoke to her in a way she could not understand she agreed to surgery. They assured her that everything would be fine.

The most horrible slaughter that I have ever seen began. Two weeks after the surgery, chemo and radiation my grandmother did not look like herself anymore. I even passed her by once when I went to visit her in the hospital, without recognizing her.

She was full of unbearable pain. Her hair and fingernails had fallen out - the long beautiful hair that she was so proud of. Her arm was swollen four times its original size. It later did not even fit into the casket. Her entire skin was ripped open. Blood and mucus was coming out all over her skin.

This woman who was so admired for her strength, energy and power, all of a sudden looked 100 years older in just weeks. Whoever saw her could not hold back the tears.

My grandmother finally died a horrible death after a long history of new surgeries and new unproven drugs if the medical profession is at the end of its usual poisoning and cutting, they come up with the story of the new drugs that are still in research and pump people full of new chemicals. They always say that it is too late for that patient, but the research could help others in the future. So my grandmother gave them the okay to put untested new poison into her body.

In her casket, my grandmother looked like a 6,000 year old mummy.

When my mother asked the doctor what was going on with my grandmother he answered, "We didn't know it would happen that fast." My mom and I yelled nearly simultaneously: "You didn't know what would happen?"

Then why did you do it to her, was our next question. The stumbling answer was the typical excuse; that they had tried to save her life. Then the doctor said we had to accept it. I told him he had to take responsibility for my grandmother's death. At which point, they threw me out of the hospital. I am absolutely convinced that if my grandmother had never had a mammogram in the first place, she would still be alive today or at least lived another 20 years.

Remember, my grandmother was completely fine before she went and gave herself into the hands of the medical profession; She even still had her period. Then, within days, she started to die over a period of two years.

That was the day I lost all trust, confidence and belief in the medical profession. Beginning that day, I started to collect from other people all kinds of life stories about what the medical profession had done to them. A story like my grandmother's seemed to be repeated over and over again.

When you think about that they told my mother over 30 years ago that she had a maximum of two years to live, they stopped treating her except for the painkillers, you will understand why I went a different route.

My grandmother could not understand the doctors with their secret language. Then, they abused the trust my grandmother had in them. Plus, the doctors constantly told her not to worry, that everything would be fine. The possible side effects only happen to one in 50,000 patients. What a blatant lie.

## Through slaughter, poisoning and medical malpractice they murdered my dad.

My father passed away recently after a long battle with colon cancer. His death is a sobering reminder that conventional medicine is a miserable failure when it comes to treating chronic illness. Drugs and surgery are not the answer. It is too late for my father, but I share my experience with you so that you won't make the same mistake (My biological father, who lost his leg due to malpractice, died of stomach cancer in the same way that my "real" father died of his colon cancer treatment.)

Over the past four years, the medical establishment poisoned, burned and slaughtered my father. Doctors gave him bad advice and frightened him into surgery, which ultimately cost him his life. It grieves me deeply, because his death could have been prevented.

I've spent the past 30 years showing people how to activate their body's natural healing power. I have seen thousands of people recover from disease, but I could not save my father because he was fraudulently and purposefully misled by doctors, who preyed on his simplicity and fear.

My system could have awakened the extraordinary healing power of his body, and its natural ability to heal itself. Instead, my father trusted his doctor, and it cost him his life.

When my father was diagnosed with colon cancer, I urged him to leave Germany and come to America so that I could treat him. Colon cancer is something that I usually cure within three weeks with an almost 100% success rate. I assured my Dad that recovery would be fast and easy. I was completely convinced that I could cure him!

My Dad was a simple, hard working, honest man who wanted to be straightforward with his doctor. My Dad told his doctor that he was going to America to get cured by his son.

In response, the doctor said his tumor was so large that it would burst in the airplane. The doctor persuaded my Dad to have surgery immediately. "The surgery is simple and easy," he insisted. "The hospital does this type of surgery every day. Get the surgery first, and then fly to America."

My trusting father believed his doctor. He was convinced that the doctor was the ultimate authority, having his best interest at heart. The doctor said that he was doing me a favor. It would be easier for me to treat him if the tumor was gone. So my Dad decided to surprise me and followed his doctor's orders.

Nobody told my Dad that the tumor had grown into his spine and was impossible to remove. The doctors were fully aware of this and they still proceeded with surgery. Later, I found out that the doctors wanted to keep my Dad away from me. They were aware of my track record as a natural health practitioner. I was a threat to their way of doing business.

Death is a hard pill to swallow. Conventional medicine took the life of my unborn sister (with a use of a "new drug" while my mom was pregnant without telling my mom that they used the drug,) my grandmother, father and countless family members. Why do they trick and deceive us into destroying our mind, body and spirit? They're motivated by profit and greed. At the very least, they are incompetent and ignorant. Conventional medicine is a mega trillion-dollar industry. It employs millions of people and produces astronomical profits for hospitals and the pharmaceutical industry. Any alternative that is safe, natural and effective is a threat to the entire system. It cuts into their bottom line.

Doctors are also usually completely ignorant about nutrition, vitamins and energy. They parrot the same old stuff that they've read in medical textbooks or learned in college. For this reason, they have a limited frame of reference. Their teachings are outdated and obsolete. Most M.D.s do not have any formal education in diet and nutrition.

My Dad's tumor was at least 20 years old but now he needed surgery immediately. He had no pain or discomfort and this tumor could have remained for years without injury.

On the operating table, the doctors cut my Dad open and disfigured him in the worst possible way. They removed the tumor, but left a large portion of it in there. After the surgery, Dad suffered from chronic pain. He developed a problem with his lungs. The doctors overlooked my Dad's methothelioma, which he developed at age 18 from working with asbestos. His condition was previously in remission (with the help of nutrition and vitamin supplements) but now it was back in the form of a respiratory infection. He nearly died and then he got pneumonia. His life was on thin ice again.

To "help" my father, the criminals in white lab coats performed emergency cervical surgery. They persuaded him to try chemotherapy, which is a poisonous form of chemical warfare that is leftover from World War I and II. Later they burned my Dad with radiation, another ineffective treatment. None of this cured or treated anything. Radiation and chemotherapy treatment is based upon the absurd hope that if you kill bad things then your cancer will disappear and your health will return. The problem is that chemo zaps and kills vital organisms and the cause of cancer is never considered. With these treatments, my father was poisoned, burned and nearly died.

Most cancer victims die from the side effects of treatment, rather than the disease itself. Of course, a death certificate will probably list heart failure as the cause of death, but the side effects are to blame.

My Dad's tumor grew more aggressively after the surgery and eventually exploded. Typically, surgery suppresses your immune system, which causes the cancer to grow even faster.

That's when the doctors insist that your cancer is rapidly progressing and getting worse.

A doctor's manipulation tactics are so obvious. First, they give a devastating diagnosis, then life-or-death scare tactics to lure you into surgery. This is followed by chemo and radiation all of which will drain your wallet dry.

Doctors know that if you talk to other cancer victims and their friends and family, you'll hear plenty of horror stories: treatments gone awry with unimaginable pain and suffering. You will discover that many cancer victims have died. Ironically, what most doctors are afraid of is alternative, non-invasive healing methods that may actually cure people. That's scary, because it affects their bottom line.

Even scarier is that doctors can't identify the root cause of cancer and how to cure it. They lie to people when they insist that cancer treatments are effective. They do more harm than good. No cancer victims have been cured because of chemo and radiation. Cancer survivors have recovered in spite of their therapy. Even if you deny all treatment you have a 27% chance that your cancer will go into remission. With the help of alternative medicine, you have a 50% chance of recovery. As a natural health practitioner, I have a 92.3% cancer recovery rate with patients who had no prior medical treatment. The medical profession has a cancer recovery rate of 3%. That is significantly less than the 24% who recovered with no treatment at all.

Before his death, I was able to see my father one last time. He had countless surgeries, chemo, radiation treatments, and the doctors even created a separate exit for his bowel movements.

At that time, I realized that it was too late to help my Dad. There was not enough left of him to initiate health and healing. I tried everything I could to give him a couple of more years of pain-free living, but the side effects of the medical treatment were completely devastating.

Dad's last year was unbearable for him and the family. The medical treatment left nothing but an empty hollow of a man. Chronic pain made life unbearable and grim. After the medical establishment drained his life savings, they sent him home from the hospital, and my 70 year-old-mother was forced to take care of him around the clock. He was not even a shadow of the fierce, funny and lovable man that he once was. Now he cried constantly from pain, his body was stuffed with plastic tubes for artificial respiration and elimination. He was totally incapacitated of doing anything on his own. The doctors sent him home to die. This infuriates me! The worthless medical treatment cost him everything he had. They took his life savings as well as his livelihood. They even kept Dad from visiting me for alternative treatment and made notes of this in his medical file.

A doctor's potential to harm has been recognized since ancient times. The first written set of laws in human history, the Code of Hammurabi, was created nearly 4,000 years ago in Babylon. The Code established rewards and punishments for medical practice, and other professions. A surgeon who successfully saved a patient from a tumor received 10 shekels; one whose patient died under the knife had his hands cut off. "First, do no harm" became the main code of the medical profession. It shouldn't be, "first, make all the money you can and then move on to the next victim." These doctors should be punished, not financially rewarded for their losses.

When conventional medicine murdered my father, I declared war on the cruel and de-humanizing way that sick people are abused, tortured, disfigured, slaughtered, poisoned, radiated and killed in the name of modern medicine. The medical agenda and motive is clear. They don't know what cures people, but they are willing to risk lives in order to make money and stay in business. This hypocrisy and double-standard includes government agencies, politicians, medical profession and, most of all, the pharmaceutical industry. It should be brought to a grinding halt. This will only happen if people have the courage to take a stand, challenge the establishment, think for themselves and claim full responsibility for their health.

Sometimes it is so much harder to help your own family and friends (as the Bible states: the prophet in his own land....) because you are too familiar and close to them. They know you as a child and as simple human being and instead tend to trust a stranger.

Consider the number of people who die each year from:

- Unnecessary surgery: 12,000 deaths[1]
- Medication errors in hospitals: 7,000 deaths[2]
- Other hospital errors: 20,000 deaths[3]
- Infections due to hospitalization: 80,000 deaths[4]
- Non-error, negative effects of drugs: 106,000 deaths[5]

## The struggle at the beginning

Of course I have made many mistakes in the search for my life's purpose, my true personality and my personal development. However, that was a good thing because you can learn from personal experience and your mistakes. Someone who has never been ill or has never suffered pain cannot understand and help others in a similar situation.

I consider myself someone who constantly strives for perfection in his professional and personal development. I have never stopped working at perfecting my system of self-help and self-healing and developing myself and my personal skills.

With this motivation, I read every book I could find about healing, orthodox medicine, natural healing, metaphysics and related matters, in the hope that I would find a way to heal my

---

[1] Leape, L. "Unnecessary surgery." Annual Review of Public Health. 1992, 13:363-383.

[2] Phillips, D Christenfield, N, Glynn L. "Increase in US medication: Error deaths between 1983 and 1993." Lancet: 1998: 351-643-644.

[3] Lazarou, J; Porneranz, B. & Corey, P. "Incidence of adverse drug reactions in hospitalized patients." JAMA, 1998, 279: 1200 – 1205.

[4] Lazarou, J; Porneranz, B. & Corey, P. "Incidence of adverse drug reactions in hospitalized patients." JAMA, 1998, 279: 1200 – 1205.

[5] Kohn, L.; Corrigan, J. & Donaldson, M. "To err is human: Building a safer health system." Washington, DC. National Academy Press, 1999.

mother. By the age of sixteen I knew more about various healing methods than many therapists. I attended back-to-back seminars and explored every possible means to gather more information on the subject of healing. I studied natural healing, explored all available information, researched, learned and discovered!

I discovered something "new" that is actually as old as humanity itself: The only help is self-help and the only way to healing is self-healing.

It is of course difficult to say to a person, who is severely ill: "Get up and walk!" Sometimes it is almost impossible to tell a person plagued by pain: "Start to fight, find the causes that have led to your illness, take charge of your own fate, recognize your mistakes, weaknesses and errors and eliminate them. Activate the powers of your subconscious and heal yourself— now, here, today, immediately!"

I have known many people that I could not approach like that. Nonetheless, many of them gave me just enough information to allow me insight into their illnesses. For example, my grandfather returned from a prison camp in Russia, ill, maltreated, and exhausted. His liver had shrunk to a small round ball and doctors agreed that the end of his life was near. He also suffered from black lung from being a coal miner all his life. However, my grandfather began to fight back. He read books about natural nutrition and behavior regimens based on natural methods. He managed to change his attitude and took the responsibility for his life in his own hands! He reached such a high level of self-awareness that he was able to tell his subconscious: I shall not die; I shall become healthy, healthier than ever before! He used this program with admirable perseverance and discipline. My grandfather regained his health and became extremely vigorous; his mind remained active until he died at the age of 86, after the medical profession murdered him. He had to go into a hospital with some lung problems. They put him in a bathroom until a room was ready. He had a high fever and the bathroom was not heated in the middle of a very cold winter. He had no real sheet and just the hospital gown on. They forgot about him for almost 24 hours in this cold bathroom. When they finally found him, he had pneumonia and high fever and died shortly after that.

Looking at his outstanding healing process and observing similar experiences of other people, it became clear to me that there is always a way. You must just be willing to search your path, recognize it and follow it faithfully.

My Uncle Fritz also showed me that the impossible can become possible. At this time, my knowledge about the system of healing was already well developed. Uncle Fritz became my first real success. He had retired early because he could no longer lift his arms due to a chronic inflammation of his shoulder joints. I succeeded in helping him. Many of my relatives, friends and acquaintances have been cured of all kinds of health problems through my method of natural healing. These problems included migraine headaches, stomach ulcers, intestinal problems and more.

Around that time, life confronted me with a task that left me in fear and horror.

My then girlfriend was diagnosed with an advanced case of cervical cancer. I already thought of myself as a great "healer". However, I knew then that I had to improve and escalate all the information that I had learned up to that point. I was fighting illness, time and fear. After six months, however, my girlfriend was completely healed. Today, many years later, she is physically fit and full of vitality.

My mother's case showed me how difficult the task of healing is and what it entails.

Despite her cancer, she opened a coffee shop with my father even though money was in short supply. My biological father had problems of his own: he had lost a leg due to medical malpractice and could stand only with the help of a wooden prosthesis. Sometimes he bled; sometimes he cried from excruciating pain. Managing the coffee shop required that both of my parents spend a lot of time on their feet. They opened the coffee shop because they hoped to earn enough money for the pursuit of alternative methods of healing that their health insurance would not cover. Indeed, my mother went to see many doctors, chiropractors, miracle healers and quacks in Germany, Holland, Switzerland and Austria. Anyone who has been in a similar situation understands what I am talking about. What happened? Nothing! But I did notice that my mother's energy level increased slowly. I witnessed how her confidence and strength steadily increased. Together, we discovered that the botched gallbladder operation was the cause of the horrible suffering she endured for so many years. A second operation revealed that only half of the gallbladder had been removed and that a new stone was lodged in the remaining portion of the gallbladder, blocking the passageways and poisoning the liver. Consequently everything in that part of her body was poisoned and destroyed.

At this point I entered an entirely new phase in my work! My mother and I began to practice the method that led to my current **Instinct Based Medicine System™** with an iron will, self-discipline and faith. The miracle healing of my mother took place. Even my sister developed cancer over 28 years ago but is in perfect health today.

I hope that you too will experience such a miracle, if you are suffering in a similar manner. We all deserve to be healthy and live without pain. You too are probably a mother, father, brother, or sister to someone and your family is concerned about you and shares your pain.

I am telling you all this, because these events led to the next step in my research. I came to the conclusion that self-pity is a destructive force from within that can destroy people. Only the sick person can cure himself. If you want to help a patient you must motivate him, because he alone can facilitate the healing in his body, soul, and spirit. Indeed, only the individual's own will, spirit and motivation can set the necessary healing process in motion.

There are, of course, many outstanding therapists, whose accomplishments deserve unlimited recognition. When you are ill, consult a doctor immediately but don't trust only one opinion ask a lot of questions and most of all make your own educated decisions. It is your health and your life. Don't trust it in the hands of others! However, the doctor should not be viewed as a healer, but rather as partner in a joint effort to bring the afflicted individual's body and soul, which are out of sync, back into a state of natural balance. Even the best doctors can only prescribe a therapy or medication which might help to suppress the symptoms, but they cannot and will not heal you. The healing process lies within the individual's body, his immune system and his self-healing power. . Remember that the medical profession is like any other trade there are always more incompetent people than competent ones.

By now you should understand that idleness, crying and self-pity will not make you healthy. Education and self-help is the only way.

I know what I am talking about because I have been through hell. For many years I lived with continuous pain and illness. Doctors and physicians could not help me even with surgery. I had chronic bronchitis, severe eye problems, chronic spine problems, gallstones, colic, liver problems and a two year infection that affected almost all the organs in my body. I invested more than 1.6 million dollars into my teeth and had close to 4,000 hours in the dentist chair with no satisfying solution until today. The pain and suffering I experienced made me wish for my own death. I am telling you this so that you won't think: yes, it is easy to talk. I speak from personal experience. I have not only had serious medical problems, I have studied and practiced health. They wanted to take my appendix out because they did not correctly diagnosis my gallbladder problem. That was the start of the invention of the **Instinct Based Medicine System™**.

Another fundamental experience that led to the development of my **IBMS**™ was when I saw a psychology professor perform a hypnotic experiment. He suggested to the hypnotized person that the normal and cold half-dollar coin he put in the person's hand was a piece of hot coal. The person developed a blister without any physical reason. That was the day I understood if the body can create a burn blister without any real reason the body can get rid of a tumor in the same way just by mental stimulation. That was the breakthrough and I cured my mother and countless patients after that.

Today I am a very healthy, energetic and highly motivated individual. I have found the key to good health and am willing to share my findings with you.

My method is by no means the only valid one and each individual must develop a system that works for him. However, I want to give you the tools so that you can build your own path to health and happiness.

Millions of people have already benefited from my method — follow their example! The only thing you need is the will to be healthy. You must begin by taking responsibility of your own life. Start now!

Just as there is a cure for every sickness, there is a cure for every malady, like fear, failure and doubt. Whenever something does not work, change your attitude, your behavior and try again and again until you have reached the success you desire.

Never be satisfied with limitations and certainly never accept any limitations in the quality of your life. Never forget that a fight continues until you stop fighting. Everything becomes hopeless only when you give up the hope and the fight.

The insight I gained through my practical work, my studies and research, showed me that each and every cure has to be a "self-cure" in order to be effective and lasting. Real help can only be help if it is based on self-help. For that reason, I have created the self-healing-system which is described in this book.

Of course, the examples here only give a glimpse into the function and working of the self-healing mechanism and its consequences. However, this book provides enough information for you to recognize that there are ways and possibilities to heal "apparently" incurable diseases and to solve your problems so that you can lead a happy life.

## My challenge to you

I hope that my story has inspired you to take action. There is no healing force outside the body. No doctor, drugs or therapy can cure you. Doctors and drugs only suppress the symptoms; they do not cure a person. It is a person's mental, emotional and physical behavior that makes him or her sick or well.

Now is the time to activate your natural self-healing powers, so that your body can recover from disease. Regardless of your age or physical condition, you can recover from virtually any disease. You can cleanse your body and enjoy life again. The next chapter covers the building blocks of health: food, water and exercise.

Are you ready to begin your journey? Get into the driver's seat and buckle your seat beat. You're on the road to recovery and wellness.

I learned if you give your life or health into the hands of the medical profession you are doomed! If you want to get healthy and stay that way you have to rely only on yourself.

## You can only depend on yourself

You have to study health. Get the right teachers and coaches and heal yourself and keep yourself healthy. Use the medical profession to help diagnosis illnesses, for emergency care and maybe control over the progress of your healing process, but otherwise don't trust them blindly with your life. Let them give you advice and listen carefully. Ask a lot of questions. Educate yourself. Keep asking questions until you feel comfortable with the answers and your decision. A doctor is just a person and can make mistakes. He could be lazy or uninterested or even incompetent. Everything is possible. At least keep the possibility in your mind that your doctor is not God and does not have all the answers.

Do you want to depend on the profession that makes only money when you are sick?

Do you want to trust your life to the profession that needs you to stay sick and suffering to survive financially themselves? I endorse chiropractic, but I know a lot of chiropractors that make sure their patients never really get pain free so that their income is safe for the future.

If everybody is healthy, they all are broke. The pharmaceutical and medical professions live from your pain, suffering and illness. They have not the slightest interest in permanent cures or in a world of only healthy people. That is the reason why they brainwash you all the time to believe they have the answers! They brainwash you to think that if you are sick they are the only ones that can help you.

Do you know that some teachers and schools get $500 or more per year for getting a child on the chemical form of heroin called Ritalin? And that every child on the ADD or ADHD drug Ritalin is a drug addict for life after just a few days? Please read the book: *Talking back to Ritalin!*

Money is the reason why they mislead you all the time. They tell you if you treat the symptoms you will get healthy. No, you will not! The only way to get healthy is to get rid of the root cause of all illness (mental, emotional and physical stress) and not to put chemicals into your body or suppress symptoms by surgery, chemotherapy, radiation or other toxic techniques. Chemotherapy and radiation cause cancer. Surgery often leads to the spreading of cancer into the entire body or weakens the immune system that much that the patient dies.

Do you want to learn how to get healthy and stay that way, doing it yourself? Or, do you want to give your life and health over to the hands of others that live from your illness, pain and suffering? There are publications that state that the medical profession is the number one cause of death today.

This book is the result of personal experience, pain, suffering illness and death, the result of personal victories over so-called incurable and chronic disease and the result of failure and success in a way nobody else has ever produced or experienced.

You can use and trust the medical and pharmaceutical industries and make them even richer through your endless suffering or you can take charge of your own destiny and create the optimum health you deserve.

The pharmaceutical companies are publicly traded companies. Their fiduciary duty is to make more money for their stock holders. That is the law.

You think your diet makes you sick? No, what the food industry puts in its products does. Plus, we have to deal with genetic manipulation of food which will cause even more problems.

It is basically stressing that makes you sick! Stress can make you dehydrated and can kill you. Stress shuts off your digestion and that can make you nutritional deficient. Of course, you can poison yourself with the wrong food and have accidents that lead to long term health challenges but that is just a tiny percentage and not the main cause of illness and suffering. Eighty six percent of all illnesses are stress related. Only 14% stem from other reasons.

Do you think lack of oxygen makes you sick? Yes, but the lack of oxygen is mainly caused by stress in the first place. By shallow breathing you constrict your breathing capacity that can lead to stress related restriction of blood vessels, muscles and organs. In the end, every single disease or illness can be traced to stress as the root cause of malfunctions and deficiencies.

Where is this stress coming from? It comes from living in fear, hopeless, doubt, compromises against our self, living with lack of self extreme, self love or self respect, living in bad relationships or suffering daily in a bad job, having no future and so on.

So how do you fix this problem? Follow the easy step- by-step process in this book to educate yourself Learn how to make the right decisions and how to take charge of your life and achieve everything you deserve by creating it yourself!

You learn how to uncover the root cause of every problem in your life and how to fix it. You learn how to eliminate unnecessary stressors out of your life and learn how to minimize your stress level in your life. Learn the **Instinct Based Medicine System™!**

Remember diet, lifestyle and everything else is only responsible for about 14% of illnesses. Stress causes 86% of illnesses and is therefore the main, if not only, cause of illness.

# Chapter 2

## *Medical Doctors – Quackery with license*

### Medicine – The outdated profession

Between 700,000 to 900,000 people die each year due to medical doctor errors. Doctors are the highest single cause of death in the western world and the side affects of over- the-counter and prescription drugs are the main cause of illness.

Between 200,000 and 300,000 patients die each year in hospitals on unnecessary infections or complications. Thousands of surgeries on the wrong organs or the wrong limbs are done each year.

Statistically, medical doctors have an average lifespan of 56 years and the highest suicide rate worldwide. How come we ask these "professionals" for advice and help? A study of 100-year- old people showed that most of them never saw a medical doctor except for accidents.

Each year, week and sometimes every day we hear about new developments in medicine. We hear about new and better diagnostic, surgical or therapeutical techniques. We also hear about things within the medical profession that they thought were true at one time that they are proving untrue, dangerous and even deadly. The rate of cancer went up from 7% in 1900 to 56 % in 2005. The same is true for nearly every other illness.

67

We constantly hear about medication that was thought to be safe that is now dangerous to our health. We hear about the dramatic negative impact caused by vaccinations. Opinions have changed regarding diet, exercise and many other aspects of life and health. We are trained and programmed to believe that this is positive development. We completely miss the obvious. Through their new developments and discoveries they prove that they themselves are not scientific and are dangerous. Medicine is experimental and until people are hurt they don't know the truth. Most of the time, it is too late for the unlucky ones.

Who wants to be a patient who has surgery, say a heart transplant, and later finds out that it was not the most current or safe? The things they did to you will be updated, so what they did to you was probably wrong and dangerous.

All of this proves that medicine is not a science at all, it is a huge experiment. It is based on beliefs. This makes it basically equal to a religion. The doctors are fed by the money-hungry pharmaceutical companies and don't even know what they are doing.

They tell you that vaccination eradicated small pox, polio, and other diseases but fail to disclose that in countries where people were never vaccinated these illnesses disappeared at the same time or even faster. They just disappeared because of better nutrition, more cleanliness, less physical stress and better life situations and not because of vaccination.

The medical profession is trained and educated by a group of business people that want to sell their product. These people make over 1.5 trillion dollars a year on illness care and the treatment of symptoms. The growth and income is based on the need for people to remain unhealthy. They want life- long customers. If they had a cure it would be a huge loss for their businesses.

The terrifying horror in all of this is that the media is brainwashed by the pharmaceutical industry and they, in turn, brainwash us. If a treatment or medication really works it shouldn't need any advertisement. It should advertise itself through results and successes.

The only things that really help the body to heal itself are natural elements like a healthy diet with plenty of water and fresh juices, correct breathing and exercise and nutritional supplements with no side effects.

If you read the side effects on the side of the pill bottles you should be scared of them. The proven side effects of vaccinations alone should scare everyone away from them.

A national vaccination information center in Virginia put together a very useful website that I believe everyone should look up. Please go to www.nvic.org and get all the necessary information that you need.

Many doctors or therapists that I know who are producing results and actually cure patients are usually outsiders who don't follow the usual treatments of the pharmaceutical industry.

Everyone who produces results produces them based on their life experiences. Most of the time, these people have overcome life threatening illnesses that they themselves have cured through natural therapies like self help and preventative techniques. These are the key elements for healing.

No artificial element, chemical or drug can do what the bodies own immune system is capable of doing. If the body is aided with more natural devices it will remain healthy.

The pharmaceutical and medical industries use their money and power to make sure that the public does not receive the information about herbal and nutritional supplements that will prevent illness. They can't make money this way so they make sure that it is not allowed for the producers of these herbal products to tell you the real benefits. They would rather sell their products.

This is evident in marijuana experiments. The pharmaceutical industry does use this product but it is made to be highly addictive and dangerous to whoever uses it.

Because the pharmaceutical company cannot patent, control or overcharge for a plant that grows like a weed, and is cheap to produce, they try to keep the natural product out of our hands. They, in turn, produce an artificial product that they can sell for a large amount of money. The government shouldn't have the right to have any say on our health; however, they make things mandatory which guarantees them trillions of dollars a year.

John D. Rockefeller made sure that he created sales people to sell his product. These people were trained and manipulated, these people are medical doctors.

The scandal book, "Healing Forbidden, Killing Allowed", shows the entire development of the medical profession. It exposes their crooked ways. It shows their human experiments.

Now, look at the trick they use to scare us every year with the horrible flu of 1918 when millions died. The only reason why the politicians are playing this game is that they want to spend a lot of taxpayer money on worthless flu vaccines. And would they do it without personal gain? How much do they get from the trillion dollar industry of vaccination?

Fact: In 1918, when the worse flu outbreak hit, it was the end of the First World War. Dead and rotting bodies were all over. The water was poisoned. No food or only rotten food was available. It was cold and there were no warm clothes. Personal hygiene was impossible. People starved. That was the environment in which these people died. We don't have and will not have these conditions worldwide ever again.

If we go back in history, we see that every time the government has interfered with the medical profession about a decade later it comes out the government sabotaged us.

Putting mercury in sick people was one experiment. Today we know that this is one of the most dangerous, life threatening things you could do. These mandatory treatments led to more deaths than imaginable.

We know that George Washington died a horrible, drawn-out death because of the leeching process and use of mercury that was preformed on him.

The only way to achieve health is to keep it out of the hands of the government. The government is capable of destroying everything that it touches. We need to create a sort of health council that is staffed by scientists from all fields and only three different medical doctors for every group of 100 people. We should have every kind of alternative therapist who produces results in this group as well. Politicians should not be allowed in this group.

The pure fact of greed that was proven in the 2003 debate about the cost of drugs is evidence   they are crooked. That coupled with the fact that you can buy the same drugs in Canada for 60-70% cheaper than in the U.S.   I am not a communist and it is ok for every company to want to make money. However, it is not ok to kill and disable people just for the sake of profit. This is a horrifying thought.

## Hurry or you are going to die.

The medical profession always acts on fear and guilt. They scare you into treating things by threatening you with death. They always make it seem like there is such a rush to operate.

The fear of dying scares you into getting surgery. The problem has probably been there in your system for years, it's just that now someone has told you about it and you are scared of what will happen next. It is only in the rarest cases that surgery is needed immediately. Usually a tumor in the breast will grow for seven years before it is detectable by a mammography machine.

In my opinion, more women get breast cancer because of mammograms and the painful poking and prodding of the doctor.

With the invention of the mammography machine, the cases of breast cancer exploded. Not because more women had breast cancer, but because doctors wanted more money.  In 1980, it was proven that there were too many unnecessary breast surgeries. Leave it to your body to get rid of the toxins.

The medical profession and the pharmaceutical industries do not pay for studies that prove they are wrong. If you use common sense you will see that nature cannot create a problem

71

that nature cannot fix. You should think about what doctors are doing. Out of all the people treated for cancer, almost 80% died because of side effects.

The death certificate usually states that someone died of cardiac arrest; you never find out it was caused by side effects of surgery or medications.

You can only survive doctors and the pharmaceutical companies if you educate yourself. If you don't let them trick you into taking things you will live longer. Tell them you need to talk it over with your loved ones. If it is regarding your money or your health or your life, never trust an expert. An expert wants your money. You will always find out what people are really about by looking at their life.

If it is regarding your life, you are the only one who can make the decisions. If something was fine for years why is it so important to get operated on immediately?

It takes seven years for breast cancer to grow to a point where it is possible to diagnose it and believe me there is no reason to rush into surgery within days.

There is a completely artificial concept of high risk groups. It is very funny that medical professionals say that if someone in your family had cancer then you are at a higher risk. I find this odd because only about 33% of people who have cancer are in a high-`risk group.

How can it even be a high risk group if only 10 or 33% of the group gets cancer? This means that 70% of the group is not. It is absurd; they are really the low risk group in comparison.

All of these categories are only there to scare people into expensive treatments and tests or life- long medications. On the other hand, I see Susanne Summers and how people tried to push her into chemotherapy. They said she didn't do it because she didn't want her hair to fall out.

Then, there is the issue of genetic predisposition for certain illnesses which are completely misrepresented. No genes on earth can cause any kind of illness. This is because genes determine only the pre-disposition not the illness! A gene does not make you have an illness. Usually it is the learned behavior from your parents on how to deal with life, stress and diet that causes the same illness in you.

Of course, there are a certain amount of cancers that appear to come from an outside source. This is considered an accident. If you live near a nuclear plant and are harmed by the radiation then this is not an illness this is because of an accident. This is like someone shooting you in the head. No matter how healthy you are, you will die.

The Lung Cancer Specialty Hospital in Hanover, Germany determined that patients with tuberculosis who were treated by chemotherapy and radiation only lived a couple of days longer than the ones who were not treated. Those treated suffered much more from the side effects. The other group had a much better quality of life and patients were pain free until the day they died.

You can no longer allow the special interest groups to finance our politicians and hope that these people will protect us from the pharmaceutical sales people who are lying to us. It might be possible, but I do not believe it. If the medication works well and does its job then word of mouth advertisement should be sufficient to help the sales grow and it will help more people. Why do pharmaceutical people need advertisements? If it works it will sell itself. It should be illegal to advertise any kind of pharmaceutical drug or treatment. If your doctor doesn't know about it, it probably doesn't work. However, if it does work then your doctor should already know about it. So what is the reason for advertisement? The reason is that they want people to take medications for every little thing that goes wrong in their life. They want us to try to fix things with a pill instead of going to the root cause of the problem and changing the way that we live so that we can be healthier. Most of all, pharmaceutical companies would not need to hire good looking women to convince doctors to prescribe their medicine. If the results were positive, the doctor would use the product anyway and not because he has financial interest in the sale of the drugs.

This basically looks like a huge conspiracy with the common denominator being money and power. Everyone who makes money off of the pain and suffering and death of people should never be allowed to have any control over political influences. The government should always stay out of decision making when it comes to treatments and never make anything mandatory. The governor of any state who is on the board of directors of a pharmaceutical company should not have the right to make it mandatory (as planned in Texas) to give your children any vaccination that has many dangerous and unknown factors. For example, the HPV vaccine does not prevent cervical cancer and has major side effects.

In my opinion, from a legal standpoint the government is practicing medicine without a license. Whenever the government interferes with something it gets messed up. Everyone knows this.

A 2003 study published in Europe stated that the cost of medications was the second highest cost for health insurance companies. This means that we could cut costs drastically by using health supplements and protecting ourselves from drugs. We don't need expensive treatments and medications in about 90% of the cases.

## Under the control of organized medicine

This path has created a multi-billion dollar disease business in America. According to almost every study done, it hasn't helped make us healthier. Major, life-threatening diseases like cancer, heart disease and diabetes are striking more people than ever. Practices like chemotherapy and radiation therapy— labeled "barbaric" by many health practitioners – are, in many cases, killing the very people they're supposed to help.

We need to start to eliminate the dangerous side effects of the chemical compounds pushed by the pharmaceutical companies. We need to stop thinking in terms of treating illnesses, and start thinking in terms of creating wellness.

Most importantly we have to realize that health is our body's natural state and the goal of health care should be to allow the body to function as it was designed to function. Medical doctors and drug company executives are not smarter than nature. Real health is something we create from the inside, not something we can achieve from pills or surgical procedures. Healthy people don't ring up billions of dollars in drug store purchases and doctors visits, so the medical and pharmaceutical industries began promoting the idea that our number one health care goal was to treat diseases rather than increase our wellness.

Albert Schweitzer, M.D. – "Each patient carries his own doctor inside him."

In 1997, Lucian Leape, M.D. of the Harvard School of Public Health reported that three million people per year die or are seriously injured as a result of medical errors.

A natural approach to health is considered the number one "threat" to the medical monopoly.

This fear has sparked a billion-dollar cancer industry, with drugs, clinics, hospitals and research projects all making piles of money and empty promises. In a report published in the New England Journal of Medicine, researchers admitted that, "Despite decades of basic and clinical research and trials of promising new therapies, cancer remains a major cause in morbidity and mortality …The effect of new treatments for cancer on mortality have been largely disappointing."

The researchers examined statistics on cancer death rates in the United States form 1970 through 1994 and found that age-adjusted mortality due to cancer in 1994 was six percent higher than the rate in 1970  up a mere seven percent from the survival rate in the 1960's.

It is estimated that nearly 1.4 million new cancer cases will be diagnosed in 1997 and approximately 560,000 people will die from the disease. These figures make in clear that the American people are not benefiting from the billions of dollars already expended for "research."

Patients who were subjected to chemotherapy were 14 times more likely to develop leukemia. Chemotherapy was also associated with a six times greater risk of developing cancer of the bones, joints, and soft tissue.

Scientist Jim Devlin says, "No doctor cures anything. No hospital heals. No medicine truly makes one well. It is the force within one's own body, the life in the blood stream which affects all cures."

Men in a study who took aspirin had half the number of heart attacks as those in the group who didn't take it. The study also found that those taking the aspirin suffered more strokes.

The Arizona Cancer Center and the University of Arizona College of Medicine conducted a six-year study and found that participants taking selenium supplements had a 37% reduction in cancer incidence and a 50% reduction in cancer mortality. Of the nearly 200 cases of cancer diagnosed, the selenium group had 63% fewer prostate cancer, 58% fewer colorectal cancers and 46% fewer lung cancers than the placebo group. There was not a single case of selenium toxicity reported in any of the patients being studied. Yet, the medical community immediately issued dire "warnings," urging patients not to take the all-natural nutritional supplement!

Men and boys who are subjected to chemotherapy for Hodgkin's disease may end up with mutations in their sperm cells that could lead to birth defects in their children. It was confirmed that chemotherapy can cause a deviation from the normal number of chromosomes in sperm cells, called an aneuploidy. There is growing concern that genetic defects are introduced in the germ cells of these young patients.

Modern medicine has created the attitude that growing old is a disease which, in and of itself, needs to be treated.

The study, conducted by Dr. Steffi Woolhander, found that more than 1.2 million Americans were taking diazepam, or Valium. This is a long-acting sedative that can cause grogginess and forgetfulness.

According to the Alzheimer Association, four million Americans have been diagnosed with the disease, which translates into $90-$100 billion in yearly health care costs. Older people taking a certain type of drug for anxiety or insomnia are at increased risk for motor vehicle crashed.

There is no proof that the potential benefits of mammograms outweigh the risks. The fact that radiation from yearly mammograms during ages 40-49 has been estimated to cause one additional breast cancer death per 10,000 women.

There were abnormal findings for more than 48% of the study population. Yet, only 13% were later diagnosed as actually having breast cancer.

One of the greatest drawbacks of screening women of this age is the anxiety an abnormal mammogram can cause, according to Ron Schwartz, M.D. and Gerard Kerins, M.D.

The uncontrolled and inappropriate use of antibiotics is one of the primary reasons for the outbreak of drug-resistant strains of infectious diseases. Despite warnings from the World Health Organization, doctors still rely heavily on the drugs. Devastating diseases – including AIDS and Ebola – may be blamed in great part on the overuse of antibiotics throughout the world.

In essence, the medical profession – through its use of antibiotics – has bred numerous "super bacteria" which are resistant to many of the current antibiotics. These illnesses are most commonly caused by viruses – and antibiotic drugs are of "little or no benefit" in those cases! Antibiotic-resistance bacterial pneumonia is already becoming more prevalent.

Clinicians often prescribe antibiotics to treat acute bronchitis despite scant evidence that this approach is effective,

Bronchitis, which is an inflammation of the linings of the major lung airways, can cause persistent cough as well as difficulty breathing and other discomfort. Many medical doctors continue to use antibiotics as a treatment despite proof that acute bronchitis is usually triggered by viral infections – which do not respond to antibiotics.

The Lancet, a renowned medical journal, found that antibiotics did nothing more than the placebos used as the control. Symptoms had greatly improved or disappeared in

83% of the antibiotic group and in 77% of the placebo group, which was not considered a significant difference.

The World Health Organization may be a direct cause of the outbreak of worldwide epidemics such Ebola and even AIDS. The medical misuse and overuse of antibiotics has been implicated in the development of several "super bacteria," as well as the outbreak of new epidemics and diseases around the world.

The drugs can inflame and even rupture patient's tendons. In a randomized trial of three approaches to sore throat – a 10 - day prescription of antibiotics, no antibiotics and a delayed prescription if the sore throat had not begun to improve after three days – the authors found there was no difference between the three groups in the incidence of complications.

One medical study showed that 70% of all infants in the U.S. are subjected to their first course of antibiotics during the first 200 days of their lives. The study showed that children with recurrent middle ear infections — that is, three infections within six months or four in a year – fare about the same as children given a placebo, with 61-64% remaining free of new infections during the study period.

We've been brainwashed to believe that this means pumping drugs into them from the moment they're born. Most children are born into this world with perfectly healthy bodies, which innately "know" how to maintain the highest level of health possible. They have the right chemicals, in the right amounts, to function properly in this world. Yet, medical science is arrogant enough to think it can improve on the original design and immediately bombards the body with dangerous and sometimes potentially deadly chemicals. The result is not improved function, but impaired function. That tiny body not only has to adapt to its environment, it now has to assimilate foreign chemicals in its system.

Chronic ear infections, asthma, childhood diabetes, and "new" diseases like attention deficit disorder, are all at epidemic proportions and getting worse.

Lacy Keele, a five year old whose mother treated her cold with Tylenol, died of an overdose. Lacy's liver shut down and she died– making her another statistic on the list of many children who are inadvertently poisoned each year with common over-the-counter (OTC) remedies and prescription medicines. This is a new kind of drug abuse epidemic which is threatening the lives and health of hundreds of thousands of American children. Well-meaning parents believe the lies told to them by medical doctors and drug makers and are pumping their kids full of toxic substances – many of which are specifically marketed to children!

The three main areas of concern are common cold medication, including aspirin and non-aspirin pain relievers such as Tylenol, antibiotics, and behavior modification drugs like Ritalin and Prozac. Almost all surveys conducted in this country have revealed that at least half of all children routinely receive either OTC or prescription drugs, particularly for common childhood ailments, cold and flu. The sad fact is much of the billion-dollar cold medication industry may be based more on hype than on health care.

"Viewed from this perspective," they noted "the high use rate of these medications may be a tremendous waste of money and may unnecessarily expose children to toxicity." according to *The Lancet*.

Antibiotics, available by prescription, don't work at all on cold viruses.

"A child's ear infection offers a classic example of how over-treatment with antibiotics can lead to the development of drug-resistant strains of bacteria. For years, amoxicillin – a penicillin-like antibiotic – was the standard treatment for acute otitis media. However, these infections usually clear, without treatment, in two to three days," according to *The Lancet*.

Many health care professionals have expressed deep concern about both the short-term and long-term effects. In the past two years alone, prescriptions for children on antidepressants have risen almost 80%. Today, more than 1.3 million children are being drugged up on these medicines. The growth rate in prescribing for children is three times faster than for adults! Since 1990, the production rate for Ritalin has quadrupled. Some 1.5 million children are taking it on a regular basis – more than two-and-a-half times the number who received it just five years ago.

Compounding the crime, the pharmaceutical industry relentlessly pumps out drugs which are marketed directly at children, often using marketing techniques which exploit a parent's sense of guilt or helplessness.

More than half of all medications widely given to children have never been tested to assure they are safe. The presidential announcement brought to light what some see as a shameful indictment of the drug and medical industries, two multi-billion dollar conglomerates which are more interested in profit than in the lives of our world's children. Due to the lack of tests, doctors often guess at dosages, exposing children to toxic amounts of drugs. Doctors gave infants reduced doses of adult antibiotics. Later, it was discovered that the drug accumulates in children's livers – 23 of the babies died.

In 1977, it happened to nearly 2,300 children and nearly one third of them died. It wasn't some strange disease or microbe that killed them – it was aspirin. When children are given aspirin during a variety of viral infections they risk developing a condition known as Reye's syndrome. Tragically, the medical profession knew about the link between aspirin and RS years before those 2,300 children were stricken. Even though the Centers for Disease Control had RS "under surveillance" from 1973-1976, they did nothing to warn the public. While they stood by and watched, as many as 550 cases of RS were reported each year. Whenever there was a major outbreak of influenza, the number of cases rose. At its worst, fatality rates reached 40%. Despite mounting evidence, the makers and marketers of aspirin refused to admit their drug could be killing so many children.

High doses of Ritalin administered to mice caused up to four times the expected incidence of cancerous liver tumors. A listing for Ritalin in the 42$^{nd}$ edition of the "Physicians'

Reference," is filled with warnings. The "Physicians' Reference" lists for Ritalin are: nervousness and insomnia; skin rash; fever; anorexia; nausea; dizziness; palpitations; headache; drowsiness; blood pressure and pulse changes; tachycardia; angina; cardiac arrhythmia; abdominal pain; weight loss during prolonged therapy; Tourette's syndrome; toxic psychosis; leucopenia and /or anemia; and scalp hair loss.

According to a 1997 pediatrics journal report, there was a staggering 44% increase in recurrent ear infections in the United States. Insertion of tympanotomy tubes can be risky. Complications include prolonged discharge from the ear, as well as tearing and permanent scaring of the eardrum, which may be associated with low-grade, long-term hearing loss. After looking at research results, many parents are finally realizing that the medical approach to treating ear infections is not only ineffective but dangerous. A 1997 medical study showed that 70% of all infants in the U.S. are subjected to their first course of antibiotics before they are even six months old. Little evidence has been found to suggest that children given antibiotics had a shorter duration of symptoms, fewer recurrences or better long term outcomes than those who had received a placebo. However, since an estimated $3-$4 billion is spent every year for medication and surgery to treat the problem, it is unlikely that the medical and drug industries will support either preventative measures or alternative care possibilities.

John Hopkins researchers resolved a longstanding controversy by showing that allergy shots offer little or no benefit to children with year-round, moderate-to-severe asthma. "Despite widespread use of asthmatic drugs, the mortality and morbidity due to asthma is increasing worldwide, suggesting the lack of really effective drugs for therapy," said Dr. Kazuhiko Kondo.

Despite the severity of Churg-Strauss Syndrome, the Federal Drug Administration had no plans to prohibit use of zafirlukast/Accolate and told patients not to discontinue its use without consulting their doctors – who prescribed it in the first place. Thousands of children who do not suffer from a true growth hormone deficiency are nevertheless being subjected to potentially risky growth hormone therapy – just because they are shorter than average.

The "blue smile" syndrome is just the latest of numerous reports of serious side effects from a popular acne treatment. Links between minocycline and liver disease, hepatitis, lupus and incidents of auto-immune disease have been found.

We should, instead, heed the advice of most health care advocates: stay out of the hospital at all costs!

News of the increasing number of medical errors which injure or kill patients – particularly in hospitals – is shocking. In London not long ago, medical tragedy was given a very real face – that of a premature baby who died within an hour of being given a hundred times the intended dose of morphine.

Half of all adverse drug events (ADE) are preventable. Plus drug-related morbidity and mortality costs the U.S. more than $86 billion each year. That's more than the cost of cardiovascular care or diabetes care in America.

It is estimated that the annual additional cost associated with preventable ADEs occurring in a large tertiary care hospital is $2.8 million and that the cost associated with all ADEs is $5.6 million.

Interestingly, it is the high cost that may prove to be the real incentive for hospitals to decrease these unnecessary – and at times tragic – mistakes.

One study indicated that about 12% of the mistakes involved giving patients drugs to which they were allergic, 11% involved giving the wrong drug and another 11% involved prescribing the wrong dosage.

In Massachusetts, for example, there are only three investigators to oversee the state's 120,000 licensed nurses; ensuring their competency has become nearly impossible.

When patients are admitted into hospitals, one of the biggest health problems they face isn't necessarily the one they went in with. They must battle infections they are likely to acquire during their stay. Now there is an added danger.

Bacterial infections resistant to a potent antibiotic are increasing in hospitals and are associated with a high death rate, according to infectious disease researchers at Northwestern University Medical School.

In a study of 53 patients with enterococcal infections, Valentina Stosor, M.D., and colleagues found that all 21 cases of vancomycin-resistant infections were acquired in the hospital. All the patients had received treatment with vancomycin previously. Of this group, 75% of the patients died- most from complications of the infection. Twenty five of the other 32 cases – which were not resistant to vancomycin – also acquired the infection in the hospital. In this group, 40% died from their illness. All patients had received a variety of broad spectrum antibiotics before developing the bacteria in their blood, possibly weakening their immune systems and making them more vulnerable to the infection. Both studies said the hospitals did not adequately disinfect bronchoscopes according to guidelines established by the Association for Practitioners in Infection Control.

One patient named Larson died in January after doctors at two different hospital emergency rooms failed to correctly diagnose the aneurysm that killed him. Although he complained of severe chest pains, ER doctors at one hospital told him he was suffering from food poisoning. Doctors at the other said it was a virus.

It is certainly possible that better understanding of the side effects of medications and of the appropriate time to resume normal activities would reduce the risk of unplanned re-admission or improve other outcomes of care following hospital discharge.

In fact a computerized analysis of the nutritional value of the house diets offered in 57 universities' teaching hospitals showed that only four met all seven of the recommendations of the National Research Council. Measurement was made of content in four component areas: fat, saturated fat, cholesterol and sodium. Results revealed that 22 of the hospitals exceeded the acceptable target for fat content, 27 for saturated fat, 46 for

Dr. Leonard Coldwell

cholesterol, and 31 failed to keep within safe limits of sodium content in the food.

What conquered polio? If you're like most Americans, you probably believe it was a vaccine which rescued the human race from this tragic illness. But there is mounting evidence that the terrible polio epidemic of the 1930's and 40's was a normal, temporary episode of the disease which was already running its course when the polio vaccine was developed. The disease petered out around the world at about the same time – even in countries which did not employ the vaccine. Similar epidemics have come and gone throughout history.

In fact, however, those vaccines are now threatening the very immune systems they are supposed to support. Every year, medical studies are sounding warning alarms that we may be causing irreparable damage to the human system – especially in children – through unnecessary and potentially harmful vaccines.

Their efforts to hide the truth about the dangers of vaccines have been so successful that few parents in America are even aware that the government was forced to set up a special compensation fund to reimburse the families of children who were killed or injured as a result of mandatory vaccines. Instead, the public is told only that their children's health depends on these drugs. How long will we continue to believe the lies?

The group warns that the government's recommendation to inject all healthy children with the new live virus vaccine may cause more serious disease when they become adults.

A mild disease for most children, chicken pox is caused by the varicella zoster virus, a relative of the herpes virus. A vaccine was originally developed to protect high-risk individuals – particularly children with leukemia, kidney disease or immune suppression, etc. – from serious complications such as brain damage and death.

We know this vaccine only gives temporary immunity – perhaps five-to-ten years' worth. There is a real danger that if everyone gets vaccinated, chicken pox will become an adult disease where it can be much more deadly.

At the same time, no one knows if the live vaccine virus will lay dormant in many vaccinated individuals and reactivate later in life in the form of herpes zoster (shingles") or other immune system disorders.

The death rate for chicken pox is 1.4 per 100,000 cases in healthy children but rises to nearly 31 per 100,000 cases in adults. According to the U.S. government, chicken pox results in more than 9,000 hospitalizations annually and causes between 50 and 100 deaths – mostly in adults.

## What Is the Status Of U.S. Medicine?

American physicians are convinced that our medical services are the finest in the world. I know I was. We do not read the world literature so it comes as a surprise to learn that German physicians have been administering natural products for more than 100 years.

The truth is shocking! The United States is ranked seventeenth out of 32 developed nations for life expectancy at (75 years old). Japan is the highest with a life expectancy of 79.1 years old. One of the major factors contributing to slightly improved longevity figures in the U.S. is the survival of the 40% of U.S. citizens who are using supplements to keep themselves healthy and out of hospitals. If these 40 % of U.S. citizens who are using natural products to keep themselves well were factored out of the statistics the U.S. might rank near the bottom among all developed nations.

The United States spends twice as much per capita on health care costs as other developed nations. We have advanced technology to diagnose and perform very expensive coronary bypass surgery. Many years ago the eminent Harvard University cardiologist, Dr. Eugene Braunwald, expressed grave concern that coronary bypass surgery was becoming an established procedure *without any solid evidence that it was effective*. This very costly and somewhat dangerous procedure is no more effective than good medical care which attacks the causes of arteriosclerosis.

The "war" on cancer has been lost as chemotherapy and radiation are no more successful now than they were 25 years ago. Fortunately, a few people have heard about natural approaches to malignancies and are recovering without the terrible side effects of conventional cancer therapy. When the general public learns that most oncologists would refuse to undergo chemotherapy in the event they developed cancer more persons will look for far safer natural treatments of malignancy which provide better results.

Immense amounts of money are expended on pharmaceutical drugs that are heavily publicized but have no ability to cure a disease. A good example of this is the use of expensive toxic anti-retroviral drugs for HIV when the simple repletion of selenium, niacin, tryptophan and glutamine appears to be very successful in stopping this nutrient-consuming illness from progressing. Conventional medicine does not have good therapy for the common lung disease emphysema. The effective alternative therapies for emphysema of nebulized glutathione, intravenous hydrogen peroxide, and cetyl myristolate remain unknown to most practitioners.

Pharmaceutical firms are spending large sums of money to develop new drugs that will correct the blood sugar in type 2 diabetes when an electronic engineer, Thomas Smith, has pointed the way to eliminating this problem by dietary measures.

Multiple sclerosis is being stabilized or improved by hyperbaric oxygen in most English patients whereas the United States does not authorize this therapy.

The true status of U.S. medicine is *dismal*. Does this reflect arrogance? My suspicion is that it is all about money. We are spending large amounts of money and getting poor health. Patients that get treated with drugs and do not get cured are enormously profitable for pharmaceutical firms, physicians, hospitals, pharmacists and medical laboratories.

## Why Is The Medical Profession Resisting Natural Therapies?

In 1902, Sir William Osler stated, "The greater the ignorance the greater the dogmatism." Today, approximately 40% of U.S. citizens have taken the responsibility for their health care into their own hands and are taking vitamins and supplements that they feel will preserve their health and help them avoid illness. The significant fall in death rates from heart disease (585 to 268 per 100,000) and strokes (181 to 62) almost certainly reflects the benefits of these supplements. There are no pharmaceutical drugs that reverse the causes for this disease (arteriosclerosis) it is caused by free radical damage, atrocious diets, and exposure to a multitude of very toxic substances such as mercury, xenoestrogens, fluoride, chlorine, pesticides, herbicides, aluminum, etc.

There are many good reasons why physicians have not started to use natural therapies:

- Physicians do not receive education in medical school about the merits of natural treatments. Medical meetings and medical journals are heavily subsidized by the pharmaceutical industry so no information about the virtues of natural treatments will not be brought forth in these arenas. Review articles about diseases will either omit information about natural therapies or the material about natural treatments will be presented in such a biased or negative way that no physician would want to use it.
- Most physicians believe that the only valid therapies are pharmaceutical and everything else is a scam.
- Powerful governmental agencies exist to protect the earnings of the pharmaceutical industry and are not very interested in the health status of the general populace. Money wins out so dangerous therapies are released on the public without any attempt to

prove safety (genetically modified foods, irradiation of food, fluoridation of water, vaccines, etc.).

- Supposed tax free foundations concerned about public health set up research studies to disprove the value of natural therapies which is easy to do by using impotent products, stopping the study before sufficient time has elapsed and using statistics to skew the results. Unfortunately, some research scientists are just like accountants and lawyers and their services can be bought. When these unfavorable results come forth they are widely disseminated on television and through other media by skilled public relations experts to convince the public there is no value in the substances. The key to unraveling the truth about these sordid pieces of research lies in discovering whose funds set up the foundation (aluminum, tobacco, agribusiness, etc.).

- Physicians who decide to try natural substances are forced to learn new skills, which is not easy.

- Inertia can be a strong influence. When things are going well for physicians why would they want to rock the boat. Human nature tends to oppose change so medical advances often take 50 or more years until they are implemented.

- Several alternative medical practitioners have been badly harassed by governmental authorities (Dr.Stanislaw Burzynski, Dr. Max Gerson, Dr. Carl Reich, Dr. Royal Rife, etc.) forcing them to leave the country or defend themselves in expensive lawsuits to avoid losing their licenses. A leader in natural health, Dr. Jonathan Wright, had his office ransacked by Gestapo-like federal agents who seized all his patient records.

- There is a legal concept that is widely appreciated by physicians as a way to avoid lawsuits. This concept is you are at risk if you are using treatments that your colleagues are not using. Naturally this impedes change!

In the light of all the negative influences mentioned above it is not surprising that so few M.D.s and other practitioners have embraced natural therapies. However, truth always dispels darkness and lies. When the general public learns that most oncologists would refuse to take chemotherapy if they developed cancer fewer persons will consent to this dangerous therapy.

My guess is that less than one infectious disease specialist in a hundred has ever heard of sulfoxime and dioxychlor. These two remarkable antimicrobial substances are very effective in eliminating systemic fungal infections, mycoplasma, yeast and anaerobic infections without side effects and at minimal cost. Their developer, Dr. Robert W. Bradford, will probably never be invited to speak at an infectious disease seminar as dissemination of news about sulfoxime and dioxychlor would have an adverse effect on antibiotic sales.

There may not be a single physician in the United States who knows that umckaloabo is a highly effective safe herbal therapy for advanced tuberculosis.

Veterinarians in the United States have learned that treating animals prior to conception with vitamins, minerals and nutrients nearly completely eliminates congenital anomalies. This biologic concept would almost certainly work in humans but may never be introduced because it would eliminate too many profitable diseases.

The future for natural products appears to lie with the continuing education of the general public about the virtue of natural approaches to health problems. Word of mouth about successful results can be a powerful factor promoting change. As this proceeds the revenue of drug companies will fall. Many pharmaceutical firms are already positioning themselves for these changes by buying natural health product companies. Unfortunately this certain progress in medicine will, of necessity, come without the benefit of the medical profession and medical schools which will probably be unable to shed their strong bondage to the pharmaceutical industry. The pharmaceutical approach to medicine, with the exception of antibiotics, does not prevent or cure diseases.

## What Is The Status Of U.S. Medical Research?

The status of research in the U.S. is just as grim as the health status of the U.S. population. Enormous amounts of money are expended on research projects by the U.S. government and large corporations. Projects that look for evidence in support of new ideas do not get funded. Projects that find new information could endanger the earlier research by members of the committees who disseminate the grants. In this manner, the system perpetuates itself with mediocrity. Most research ends up being aimed at getting an income rather than seriously trying to uncover new knowledge. Considerable time is wasted trying to find grant money. The creative innovative thinker could be a risk to established researchers and does not get funded. Dr. Donald Goodwin, chairman of psychiatry at the University of Kansas remarked, "If it's trivial you can probably study it. If it's important, you probably can't."

This huge influx of grant money has led to the incorrect assumption that the best teacher is the best researcher. The end result of this process was the conversion of medical schools into a kennel of researchers who secondarily teach medical students. To survive in this academic milieu one must "publish or perish." Naturally, the quality of most of these publications is mediocre or worse and much fraudulent research is yet to be uncovered.

Many researchers receive money from pharmaceutical firms. This, of course, colors their results. Even the highly respected *New England Journal of Medicine* has become contaminated. They have established a policy that they will only accept papers from authors who are receiving less than $10,000 annually from a pharmaceutical firm. Naturally, a researcher getting only $9,999 would not be tempted to alter his research to please the drug firm. Incidentally, I am also guilty of taking money from drug companies having attended wonderful meals, golf tournaments, received medical bags, etc. at the expense of pharmaceutical companies.

## What Public Health Measures Need To Be Instituted?

Serious efforts to improve public health must begin with stopping the sale of disease-causing margarine and trans fats, removing fluoride and chlorine from drinking water, ending the use of mercury for dental amalgams, encouraging grazing of cattle instead of feedlots, banning irradiated and genetically modified foods and ending hormone injections in cattle. A massive education campaign to warn the public about the danger of sugar excesses, aluminum and processed foods is needed. All these steps will be vigorously resisted by powerful, entrenched, special interest groups. Physicians who offer the public alternative health therapies need to be protected from harassment by governmental agencies.

## Medicine and Its Dangers

Medicine is the study of death and illness. It is not based on life and health. We must carefully consider the dangers of traditional medicine, as our society tends to assume it is the most effective way to treat health problems.

When we are sick, doctors prescribe drugs to treat our symptoms. Doctors rarely identify the root cause of our problems. The media also programs us to take medicine for whatever ails us. When our symptoms disappear, we're healthy again.

We've been programmed to recognize health as the absence of symptoms. Of course, pharmaceutical drugs enable us to live as we always have, without making any changes in our lifestyle. We disregard the laws of good health. We continue to live our lives without making any changes in the way we eat, think, move and breathe.

Each year, we spend hundreds of dollars to eliminate symptoms rather than addressing the root cause of our health problems. What is commonly called a disease is caused by toxins in your body. You are sick because you haven't eliminated the toxins that are caused by stress, nutritional deficiencies, lack of water and oxygen and mismanaged emotions.

The real reason that people get sick is because they violate the basic laws of health. Prescription drugs only cover up the symptoms. In reality, the illness is still at work in the body. After a few years of taking drugs (and more drugs for the side effects) your body is so impaired that it is vulnerable to more serious illnesses.

**Here are the ten worst beliefs that people have about their doctor:**

**Belief # 1:** "If I'm sick, I need to go to the doctor as fast as I possibly can to get my problem under control. The medicine he prescribes me will help me to recover in no time."

**The Truth:** Doctors treat the symptoms of disease rather cure than the root cause. This is not an effective way to treat illness. Your symptoms are temporarily covered up and blocked, yet the real problem remains or becomes worse. Most pharmaceutical drugs are mind altering. For instance, if you take medicine for back pain, the drugs will trick your mind into thinking the pain is gone. In reality, your back still hurts and your health problem remains. The pain and discomfort is a red flag from your body telling you that something is wrong. You just covered up the symptoms with drugs. Nothing has been done to correct the problem. If you are sick, consult a certified alternative health practitioner. Most illness and disease can be safely treated without drugs or surgery.

**Belief #2:** "If I take medicine, my condition will improve. I'll be myself in no time."

**The Truth:** Traditional medicine kills more people than it saves. Prescription drugs are the fourth leading cause of death.

Disease is caused by the accumulation of toxins in the body due to stress, lack of energy, poor nutrition, mismanaged emotions, lack of elimination, low self-esteem, lack of oxygen and lack of exercise. If you want to recover from illness, you need to take care of yourself. You need to start eating more nutritious food, drink extracted juice and take vitamin supplements. Of course, you need to do all the other things mentioned in this book. If you need help with a specific health problem, talk to an alternative health practitioner.

**Belief #3**: "I trust my doctor completely and never question his authority. If he recommends drugs or surgery, I should follow his orders."

**The Truth**: Your doctor is not correct 100% of the time. Always think for yourself, and carefully consider your doctor's advice, recommendations for drugs, or surgery. Don't be naïve. If you engage in passive behavior, you are not taking full responsibility for your health. Ultimately, you will be taken advantage of and manipulated. Always use common sense, explore your options, and research your health problem using the internet or library. Talk to a qualified alternative health practitioner.

**Belief #4**: "My doctor has my best interests at heart. That's why he practices medicine; he really wants to help people."

**The Truth**: If you think this way, you are embracing the myth of objectivity. No one is completely objective. We all have mixed motives. Unfortunately, your doctor may not have your best interests at heart. He has a limited frame of reference, based on what he was taught in medical school. Your doctor is probably ignorant about nutritional physiology. Most doctors are, as they don't teach nutritional physiology in medical school. Your doctor is trained to treat the symptoms of your disease with drugs or surgery. Don't expect anything else.

**Belief # 5**: I need to comply with my doctor's orders, because he is a lot smarter and better educated than I am.

**The Truth**: When you visit the doctor, you are a customer and he is providing you with a service. You are very much in control of the situation. Don't be intimidated by your doctor's credentials. It's wonderful that he got an education and worked so hard to get where he is today. You have different gifts and abilities. There is no need to think of yourself as less worthy or less intelligent than your doctor. Use that computer between your ears (your brain) and think for yourself. Carefully consider whatever your doctor has to say, but don't comply with his recommendations on the basis of his authority alone.

**Belief # 6**: "If vitamins and healthy eating would help me to recover, then my doctor would tell me about it."

**The Truth**: Your doctor probably doesn't know anything about nutrition. That is not his area of expertise. Your doctor knows about drugs and surgery. You can't expect your doctor to tell you about vitamins when it is outside his frame of reference.

**Belief # 7**: "When my doctor tells me something, I take his word for it. End of discussion!"

**The Truth**: Your doctor's recommendation should be the beginning of the discussion, not the end of it. You're in a dangerous situation when you allow someone else to make your decisions and do your thinking for you.

**Belief # 8**: "My family has a history of colon problems. This means that I need to get my colon checked once a year. Hereditary dispositions make me susceptible to colon cancer."

**The Truth**: Illness is not caused by heredity, but by bad choices. Health is the result of the right choices in life. Your genes or family history don't make you sick. This is a major misconception of the medical industry.

**Belief #9**: "There is no known remedy for my illness. That is why I am incurable! My doctor told me there was nothing I could do but accept my condition, take medicine and learn to live with pain."

**The Truth**: Medicine does not have a remedy for your illness, but nature does! No disease is incurable. When my mother was diagnosed with liver cancer, the doctors gave her a maximum of two years to live. The doctors insisted that no one could recover from her advanced stage of cancer. Today, my mother is 70 years old, and has completely recovered. You can do the same. In my professional practice, I've seen thousands of people recover from terminal or incurable disease.

**Belief # 10**: "My doctor insists that I must have surgery immediately, or my tumor will explode, and I'll surely die."

**The Truth**: Don't let the fear of dying scare you into surgery. When your doctor diagnoses your health problem, you are hearing about it for the first time. However, your condition has probably been in your system for years. It has taken time to accumulate and grow. You are afraid of what might happen next, or that things will inevitably get worse. It is rare that surgery is needed immediately. In fact, surgery may worsen your condition. I write this from personal and professional experience. My mother suffered for years from a botched gallbladder operation. A second operation revealed that only half of her gallbladder had been removed, and that a new stone was lodged in the remaining portion of the gallbladder, blocking the passageways and poisoning the liver. Consequently, everything in that part of her body was poisoned and destroyed. Professionally, I've met thousands of people whose condition became worse after surgery. I urge you to get a second opinion and consult a certified alternative health practitioner before getting surgery.

### Is illness induced by doctors?

Each year, 250,000 people die from iatrogenic causes, according to Dr. Barbara Starfield of the Johns Hopkins School of Hygiene and Public Health. In a landmark article published by the Journal of the American Medical Association (JAMA), Dr. Starfield describes how the U.S. health care system may contribute to poor health. A quarter million people die each year from iatrogenic causes!

What does iatrogenic mean? It refers to doctor-induced disease or medical complications caused by a physician. The practitioner need not be a physician. It could be a nurse, technician or healthcare worker.

Dr. Starfield says that doctors are the third leading cause of death in the United States. The first and second top causes of death are heart disease and cancer. Dr. Starfield concluded that 4% to 18% of patients experience negative effects in outpatient settings resulting in:

- 116 million extra physician visits
- 77 million extra prescriptions
- 17 million emergency department visits
- 8 million hospitalizations
- 3 million long-term admissions
- 199,000 additional deaths
- $77 billion in extra costs

The high cost of health care seems to be tolerated under the assumption that better health results from more expensive care. However, Dr. Starfield uncovered evidence that as many as 20% to 30% of patients receive inappropriate medical care.

## Intervention Versus Prevention

There is a difference between intervention and prevention. Intervention refers to surgery and emergency medical treatment, which are often necessary. For instance, if you break a leg or arm, you need a cast or perhaps surgery to reconstruct your broken bones. When necessary, reconstructive surgery and physical therapy can produce outstanding results. Competent diagnostics, tests, procedures and medical intervention are all vital to healthcare.

America has the best emergency healthcare in the world. When it comes to intervention, medical doctors are effective at saving lives. However, only a small percentage of all health cases involve trauma. The majority of health problems are treated with drugs, which is a major cause of our healthcare crisis.

When it comes to prevention, traditional medicine rarely prevents illness. Doctors cannot cure illness. Medicine is more based on pharmacy than science. In contrast, alternative medicine treats the root cause of the disease. It internally cleanses the body and removes toxins. It also provides the necessary tools to heal and restore the body, maintain health and prevent future malfunction.

## Conventional Medicine Offers No Guarantees

Have you ever tried to get a definite answer from your doctor? Ask him or her how long therapy takes. Are the results guaranteed? Where exactly does my illness or problem come from? What causes cancer? In the rare case that you get an answer, they probably won't give it to you in writing. Later, they may even later deny that they made certain statements.

Conventional medicine is nothing more than the accumulation of ideas, theories and opinions regarding the cause and treatment of illness. Everything is based on symptom suppression. By treating the symptoms, doctors hope that your body heals itself. You may think that medication cured you, but really it just masked the symptoms while your body heals itself

Have you ever asked your doctor for a money-back guarantee? Can your doctor guarantee that the medical treatment will cure you? Your doctor won't make that promise. The medical profession uses antibiotics, penicillin, pain killers and chemical narcotics which contain toxins. Medicine is based on the study of death and illness rather than health and longevity.

If you get an infection, doctors may give you an antibiotic and hope the body cures itself. They probably won't tell you that your lack of energy— caused by emotional stress, nutritional deficiencies, lack of exercise or lack of water— caused your immune system to break down, resulting in an infection. They probably won't tell you to change your lifestyle because it's making you sick and susceptible to infection. Instead, they tell you a virus or bacteria made you sick. In reality, only an already toxic or acidic body can be harmed by germs. Bacteria and viruses can only live in toxic environments. These bacteria and viruses eat dead tissue and dead cells.

## Media Manipulation is Hazardous to Your Health

Do you realize that the media has programmed you to utilize doctors and medicine, and consider them scientific and authoritative? Whenever a doctor is interviewed on TV, he is positioned as a health expert who has all the answers. We've been conditioned to think of doctors as efficient, well-educated and wise. We've been told that so long that we believe it.

Whenever we watch TV, we're bombarded with advertisements for pharmaceutical drugs which claim to be safe and effective. It is rare that any investigative program looks into their claims and questions the safety and effectiveness of medicine. The media programs want us to be passive, rather than think for ourselves.

Reliance upon conventional medicine is a conditioned, automatic response. Like Pavlov's dogs who drooled when a bell was rung, we are conditioned to use drugs to alleviate sickness. As soon as we get sick, our subconscious pulls up the information we've seen on TV programs, news and commercials. This information influences the way we think and react. Without thinking twice about it, we seek medical treatment and get our prescription filled. That's the way the media conditions us to respond to health challenges.

Of course, this means we aren't taking responsibility for our health. We blame our illness upon hereditary factors or being in the wrong place at the wrong time. We believe that we picked up a germ, when actually our bodies are toxic and acidic and too weak to resist infection. We may read something about nutrition here or there, but the media always brings us back to their agenda.

When it comes right down to it, we've been brainwashed. The media has programmed us with misinformation, distorted facts and biased viewpoints. Our perspective about health is wrong, because our programming is wrong.

Part of the solution is reading this book. I encourage you to put this material into practice, and make it a part of your life. Think for yourself and take charge of your health. As you do so, you'll be programming yourself for optimum health and energy. You'll be erasing destructive habits and old ways of thinking. Instead of doctors, drugs and surgery, you will focus on simple, all-natural tools and technology that enable the body to heal itself. By activating your body's natural healing powers, you can recover from virtually any disease.

## The Agenda Setting Power of the Media

The media sets our agenda by programming our minds about doctors, drugs and surgery. Like anyone else, the media has mixed motives. The only way that a TV program can afford airtime (and make it profitable) is by securing advertisers. Obviously, TV will do everything possible to make sure their advertising clients are happy so they can maintain their business relationship and generate income. They usually aren't selective when it comes to advertisers. They're not going to stand up and say, "Let's not work with that drug manufacturer because their product isn't safe or effective." That line of reasoning is the furthest thing from their mind. They aren't asking for documentation or evidence to support their advertiser's claims. The only thing that TV programs care about is revenue, which they generate with advertising. The credibility of their advertisers doesn't matter. TV programs assume no liability for the products advertised in their commercials. That is why you can't trust advertising. Their objective is to sell you something. Commercials often use flashy images, music and slogans to grab your attention and program your mind. The effect is almost hypnotic, as you remember the commercial long after it's over.

Where do the media get their information from? Most of the time, the media is educated by the pharmaceutical companies and medical industry. After all, pharmaceutical companies purchase the majority amount of advertising time.

Commercials advertise plenty of pharmaceutical drugs. Due to the revenue and business relationships involved, drug companies influence the agenda of news broadcasts and investigative reports. It's no wonder that the media has a pro-drug and pro-medicine perspective.

When medical doctors conduct studies, the media presents their findings as genuine scientific proof. It is rare that the media reports on medical research objectively. A lot of information is so guarded that it isn't reported unless it promotes the interests of doctors and pharmaceutical companies.

The medical profession is trained and educated by a group of business people that want to sell their product. Pharmaceutical manufacturers make over $1.5 trillion a year on drugs, illness care and the treatment of symptoms. Lots of jobs, products and facilities are on the line. The industry generates tremendous revenue when the public takes prescription drugs. It is in their best interest for you to stay sick. They want life- long customers. If they had a cure, they would experience a huge loss of revenue. Everything focuses on their bottom line.

Chills run up my spine when I think about the pharmaceutical industry programming our doctors as well as the TV, radio and print media. We've been programmed to swallow their bitter pill, and now we have a society that is dependent upon conventional medicine.

## Advanced technology or dangerous experiment?

We often hear about medical advancements. The media tells us about new and improved diagnostic, surgical and therapeutic measures. Does new technology enable doctors to be more effective and their patients to recover faster? The media seems to think so.

We hear about medical advancement, but are also confronted with medical catastrophe. We hear about assessment, drugs and treatment which are found to be dangerous or even deadly, after they've been on the market for years. We hear about medication that was once widely administered and is now considered lethal. Sometimes we hear about the adverse reactions to vaccinations, but these incidences are discounted as rare. After all, the remedy was the best solution at the time. Progressively, scientists and medical researchers develop more effective solutions, drugs and treatment to meet the needs of our rapidly changing society.

The media insists that technology is quickly advancing conventional medicine. We are programmed to believe that this is a step in the right direction. We completely miss the obvious. Conventional medicine conducts itself like an experiment. New medical advancements aren't necessarily safe or effective. Sure, they've tested it, but they can't ensure that their product works for everyone. Of course, their motives aren't pure either. They're driven by profit, greed and the pressure to generate new products as quickly and inexpensively as possible. When the medical field makes mistakes, people suffer or even die from it. By the time they take a product off the market, thousands of people have already paid the price with their livelihood or even their life.

Whenever the media reports on death or disability caused by medical mistakes, prescription drug use or adverse reactions to immunizations, they imply that it's a small price to pay for medical advancements that could possibly save millions of lives. Realistically, medical mistakes and oversight cannot be reasonably explained away as a necessary sacrifice for the benefit of a disease-free society.

Conventional medicine is widely accepted, but it's also dangerous. It is not scientific when it makes mistakes and recalls drugs that are already on the market. Conventional medicine is not objective when its bottom line is profit. It is not valid when doctors want to treat symptoms rather than the root cause. It is not reliable when doctors want you to take drugs for the rest of your life. Conventional medicine doesn't have your best interests at heart. It wants to drain your bank account. Conventional medicine will devour you with dangerous drugs and unnecessary surgery. It will chew the flesh off your bones and spit you out when there is nothing left.

Remember the story of my father, Lothar? Don't let that happen to you! I hope that it isn't too late. I hope that drugs and surgery haven't destroyed your mind and body to the point of no return.

This is your wake up call. Take a deep breath and hold your head high. Refuse to be deceived any longer. You are behind the wheel of the car now. You are in control. Decide which way you want to go. Don't ignore the red flags of conventional medicine. You should have seen this deception a mile away. Of course, the media clouded your vision. You didn't see things clearly before. You let your doctor take responsibility for your health. You were programmed to endorse conventional medicine. You're aware of the landmines now. Stay clear of them, and you will reach your destination in one piece.

# Chapter: 3

## *Dangers of Pharmaceutical Drugs*

Lest you think this chapter is about doom and gloom, let's begin by reflecting upon the wonderful benefits of taking prescription drugs. They are a quick and easy fix. All you have to do is ask, and your doctor will prescribe whatever drugs you want. If you have insurance, you only pay the deductible, which isn't that much. When you take drugs, your symptoms go away. Instant relief! You can continue to live as you always have, without making any changes. You don't have to think about nutrition, exercise or mental hygiene.

Come to think of it, drugs enable you to live in a state of ignorant bliss. Depending on the type of medication you take, you may have the privilege of turning into a zombie.

Have you ever been to a nursing home and seen these catatonic people who are all drugged up, with their eyes glazed over, staring straight ahead? Physically, they're alive but mentally, they're somewhere else. That's what I mean by zombie.

Are you a zombie? This can be fun at Halloween. If you have enough strength to answer the doorbell for Trick or Treat, the kids will be frightened out of their wits! Your catatonic state isn't a kooky costume or makeup; it's the real thing! Wait a minute; you don't have any treats to hand out. Your bowl is empty. There is no money left for treats. You've spent all of your hard earned cash at the pharmacist, which literally means "poisoner".

Did you know that the word pharmacy comes from the Greek word pharmacia, which means sorcery or witchcraft? Well, you don't have treats but you are living proof that pharmaceutical drugs work. If every day was Halloween, then you could enjoy it more. As you look in the mirror, you realize that your creepy appearance is no longer funny. Your skin is purple blue and covered with red bumps. Your hair is falling out. You are a living eye sore. What's next? Maybe a visit to the plastic surgeon is in order. Oh, that's right, there is no money left. Back to square one.

Seriously, is this the kind of "positive" results that you want from drugs?

## Ten reasons why you should consider not taking pharmaceutical drugs:

**1.** Drugs mask symptoms rather than curing or eliminating disease. Your symptoms may be a runny nose, earache, sore throat, diarrhea, vomiting, excessive perspiration, gas, fever, etc. These are symptoms rather than the cause of your problem. These symptoms are your body's way of cleansing itself of toxins. In other words, your body is attempting to eliminate the garbage from your body. This is a good thing, because your body is attempting to heal itself. If you take drugs, you may stop these symptoms, but you will also stop the cleansing process of the body. The toxins have no place to go, so they remain in your body. If you have a high fever, remember that your body is attempting to the kill the virus inside you. It is rare that you need to stop a fever.

**2.** Drugs clog, rather than cleanse. If you use drugs to stop symptoms, then you stop the cleansing process and clog the immune system. This should be obvious from reading the label of your prescription bottle. If it says, "side effects include dry mouth" that means it will dehydrate you. Dry mouth is an understatement. Your body is initiating a drought management system as it seeks to conserve water. Remember that water plays an important part in nearly every body function. If you don't get enough water, then your cells become weak and vulnerable to disease. Your brain is made up of 85% water. If the brain is dehydrated, then you will feel confused, tired, dizzy, moody and irritable. Another common side effect is constipation. Obviously, not going to the bathroom is a sign that your body is clogged. Removing waste and toxins may be your body's greatest challenge.

3. Drugs don't cure disease. No drug will cure you; it will only relocate the disease and mask the symptoms. Self-healing takes place in your immune system. The only one who can cure your body is you. If you're sick, it is caused by stress and a lack of energy.

4. Drugs are unnatural and are foreign to the body. Drugs work by altering the body's natural biochemistry to suppress symptoms. Even with suppressed symptoms, the true cause of the problem may grow worse as the body's natural healing mechanisms are compromised by the drugs. By interfering with normal cell function, drugs cause a cellular malfunction which is the same as causing disease.

5. Drugs cause disease. When drugs cause disease, we have been trained not to call it disease. Instead we use the deceptive term, "side effects". In 1984, the drug industry attempted to obtain a legal exemption from the liability laws that apply to virtually all manufacturers. Why? Because even the people who make the drugs know they are not safe.

6. All drugs have side effects. These may be worse then disease itself. Medication causes anxiety, depression, high blood pressure, constipation, dehydration, etc. Drugs create toxicity and severe nutritional deficiencies by depleting the body of essential nutrients. Antibiotics, anti-inflammatory meds and steroids all damage the human digestive system by impairing the ability of the body to digest food and absorb nutrients.

7. Drugs are addictive. Prescription drugs are harder to withdraw from than street drugs. If you take prescription

medication for an extended time, your body may also build up immunity, so that you need something stronger to get the same results.

**8.** Drugs create dependency. You need to go back to the doctor for follow-up visits. Then, you return to the pharmacist to have your prescription refilled. This is time consuming, expensive and creates a dependency. You are dependent upon doctors and drugs for healthcare. It is easy to let conventional medicine make your decisions, rather than thinking for yourself and taking care of your body.

**9.** Drugs are expensive. Even if you have insurance, the cost of prescriptions, doctor's visits, tests and surgery can add up to hundreds or even thousands of dollars each year. Many elderly people with limited income must choose between putting food on the table and paying for their prescription.

**10.** Drugs may be in your doctor's best interest, rather than your health. Your doctor may be prescribing drugs in order to receive a kickback or incentive from the pharmaceutical manufacturer.

## Is Drug Promotion Ethical?

Every year, the pharmaceutical industry generates $122 billion dollars in sales.

In 2004, pharmaceutical companies spent over $2.5 billion on "direct-to-consumer" advertising on TV and in magazines. This kind of drug advertising is profitable for pharmaceutical companies, as prescriptions written for the top 50 most heavily advertised drugs rose 24.6 %, compared to 4.3 % for all other drugs combined in 2000.

Advertising equals increased sales, more profits and healthier bottom line. However, the issue of a health industry driven by profit raises serious ethical questions.

Opponents of DTC advertising maintain that it is wrong to increase consumer demand for medicine with ads for newer, higher priced drugs. They argue that increased consumer demand leads to higher prescription drug use and contributes to the shift in higher priced medicines, which both play key roles in the continuing increase in prescription drug spending. Opponents have also suggested that the ads cause patients to have unrealistic expectations.

How influential are those DTC ads? According to a survey conducted by the Kaiser Family Foundation, one in three adults have talked to a doctor, and one in eight has received a prescription, in response to a seeing an ad for a prescription drug on TV or in magazines.

Be aware that drug advertising is an attempt to persuade you to use drugs and stay on them the rest of your life. Let's face it, these drug companies aren't advertising to educate the public or to promote healthcare. They certainly aren't advertising because they want you to get better. They aren't interested in eliminating disease or preventing it. They have billions of dollars at stake. They want to create lifetime customers. It is obvious that pharmaceutical companies are motivated by profit rather than patient welfare.

## Eradication of Disease

Sometimes we're led to believe that doctors and pharmaceutical companies want to eradicate disease. Isn't that why they're in business, to help people recover from disease? Wouldn't it be wonderful if a cure for cancer, diabetes, multiple sclerosis or other terminal diseases were found?

Of course, a cure would be wonderful for the victims involved. It's a different issue for the drug companies and doctors, who would suffer a major loss of revenue. Pharmaceutical medicine would lose billions of their investment dollars. They would be stuck with a surplus of drugs that the public no longer wants. The expense and loss would be devastating. Doctors and healthcare specialists would have empty waiting rooms, and there would be no need for their expensive diagnostic tests and advanced treatment. There would be no more demand for medical services or hospitalization. Doctors would be forced to close shop. A successful cure could wipe out the entire medical industry.

## Who Really Educates Your Doctor?

There are over 8,000 prescription drugs on the market. For the majority of doctors, 70% of all prescription drugs were not around when they went to medical school. How do doctors educate themselves about new drugs and pharmaceutical alternatives? Do they stay abreast by reading medical journals and scientific literature? Or, do they get their information from pharmaceutical companies attempting to peddle their goods?

Evidently, drug companies have a greater influence on doctors than anything else. The pharmaceutical industry is more influential than scientific journals, medical associations or even their medical school education. "The education of American physicians about drugs…has relegated to drug companies by default," charges Dr. Jerry Avon, a physician and associate professor at Harvard Medical School who has studied the influence of pharmaceutical marketing. "As a result, pharmacological solutions are thought of first, rather than non-pharmacological approaches that could be just as effective and safer."

## Advertising at the Doctor's Office

Have you ever noticed the abundance of advertising at the doctor's office? As you sign in, you notice the clipboard is decorated with drug logos. The pen you use has a drug name on it. As you plop down in a chair and wait for your name to be called, you notice the TV. It's playing advertisements for drugs and pharmaceutical products in a continuous loop. By the time you go in to see the doctor, you've watched the whole thing twice. As the receptionist shows you to the examining room, your vision is saturated with messages and images from drug manufacturers. The wall is covered with drug posters and glossy propaganda.

According to the Massachusetts Medical Society, "'these items would not be so readily produced if they were not an effective form of advertising."

## Hermetical Incentives for Doctors

Before the law changed, drug companies spent billions of dollars on incentives and promotions to entice doctors to prescribe their products, and these dollars are tax deductible. They gave doctors free meals, stereos, watches, jewelry, concert tickets, tickets to sporting events and all-expense paid vacation trips.

Most doctors receive incentives worth $15,000 or more from pharmaceutical companies every year. These kickbacks induce doctors to prescribe drugs for their own financial and material gain rather than the patient's best interest.

Not only are drug incentives unethical, but they could also be considered illegal. By allowing tax deductions for gifts to doctors, current tax law actually encourages this potentially illegal practice.

In 2004, Pfizer, the world's largest pharmaceutical company, plead guilty and agreed to pay $430 million to resolve criminal and civil charges that it bribed thousands of doctors to prescribe its epilepsy drug, Neurontin, to patients with ailments that the drug was not federally approved to treat.

The company encouraged doctors to prescribe Neurontin for patients with bipolar disorder, even though a study had shown that the medicine was no better than a placebo in treating the disorder. Other disorders for which the company illegally promoted Neurontin included Lou Gehrig's disease, attention deficit disorder, restless leg syndrome, and drug and alcohol withdrawal seizures. Although doctors are free to prescribe any federally approved drug for whatever use they choose, pharmaceutical companies are not allowed to promote drugs for non-approved purposes.

Public interest can only be served when drug promotion is "free of the insidious effects of kickbacks and related financial conflicts of interest" which artificially inflate sales and prices, said Michael Sullivan, a Boston attorney involved in the case. In other words, tax-deductible dollars contribute to the rising prices of prescription drugs.

The Pharmaceutical Research and Manufacturers of America (PhRMA) pretended to discourage improper marketing ploys by issuing conflict-of-interest guidelines in April 2002. After announcing the guidelines with fanfare, they then paid the American Medical Association to "educate" their members on these guidelines. In other words, they gave doctors financial incentives to promote ethical guidelines that called for an end to financial incentives. It is obvious that PhRMA is not serious about ending the practice of pharmaceutical incentives for doctors.

Congressman Pete Stark maintains that clever marketing ploys that influence physicians' prescribing habits don't save lives, but do much to increase drug prices and corporate profits. He introduced the Prescription Drug Safety and Affordability Act. This bill would eliminate the tax-deduction that pharmaceutical companies currently receive for the gifts they give to physicians.

## Doctors Financial Ties to the Drug Industry

The *New York Times* reported that nearly 9 out of 10 doctors involved in clinical trial protocols had financial ties to the pharmaceutical industry (such as research funding, travel or consulting fees or personal stock investment). Six out of 10 doctors had financial ties to companies whose drugs were either considered or recommended in the clinical trial guidelines they wrote.

Obviously, this situation constitutes a conflict of interest. Objectivity goes out the window and research becomes nothing more than propaganda to further selfish interests.

Beware when the media reports on research findings about pharmaceutical drugs. They may not be telling you the truth. We can't trust research that is tainted by physicians biased by ulterior motives. These types of studies are not reliable, valid or even scientific. What pharmaceutical companies present as documented evidence might be nothing more than a slick public relations ploy to influence your buying decisions. Only 15% of all medical advice is based on science.

## Name Brand vs. Generic Drugs

Has your pharmacist ever told you that your insurance plan will not cover a generic drug? You end up getting the name brand drug, which is more expensive. Pharmaceutical companies routinely make payments to insurance plans to increase the use of their products, to expand market share and to be added to the list of recommended drugs. Drug companies also reward doctors and pharmacists for switching patients from one brand of drug to another.

Sometimes pharmacy benefit managers send letters to doctors recommending that they shift Medicaid patients from generic drugs to brand-name medicines, says Eric J. Wexler, general counsel of the Great Lakes HMO plan in Michigan. In many cases, the brand-name drugs cost more and are less effective, says Mr. Wexler.

For each letter sent to a doctor, Mr. Wexler said, "the pharmacy benefit manager receives an administrative fee, and the pharmacy may get additional remuneration for converting patients from one drug to another."

AdvancePCS, a pharmacy benefit manager based in Irving, Tex., confirmed that it received payments from drug companies for letters sent to doctors and patients urging them to use particular drugs.

AdvancePCS justified the payments — typically a flat fee for each letter — as an educational service that could help control drug spending. It's also convenient to deduct these "educational services" from their taxes as legitimate business expenses. Critics would argue that this kickback is unethical and possibly illegal.

**Side F-X**

Aside from bureaucracy and pharmaceutical manipulation, there are plenty of other problems with prescription drugs. Accidental death from prescription drugs, even when they are correctly given, is now the fourth leading cause of death. Before you take another prescription pill, think carefully. Just because your doctor prescribed it is no guarantee you'll benefit from it or even emerge unscathed from the experience. Your prescription medicine could be hazardous to your health and life.

Adverse reactions to prescription drugs are a major cause of death in the U.S. An estimated 106,000 hospital patients die each year from adverse reaction, making adverse drug reactions the fourth most frequent cause of death.

A 2000 study in the Archives of Internal Medicine stated that drug-related morbidity and mortality costs are $136 billion a year more than the cost of cardiovascular disease, the leading cause of death in the United States.

According to the National Council on Patient Information and Education, over 50% of all prescriptions are used incorrectly. Misuse or noncompliance is a major health problem in the United States, resulting in 218,000 deaths and the hospitalization of 1 million individuals annually. The total cost to the economy is approximately $177 billion annually.

Not all adverse reactions to new drugs can be anticipated or avoided under the present system, according to medical experts. "It is simply not possible to identify all the adverse effects of drugs before they are marketed," according to a study in the *New England Journal of Medicine*. In fact, "Overall, 51% of approved drugs have serious side effects not detected prior to approval."

Side effects from new drugs cannot be anticipated for two main reasons: (1) Individuals vary greatly in their reactions to chemical substances; and (2) drugs are tested where side effects may not appear in such a small group but may become painfully obvious when millions of people start taking the drug.

Americans consume over 15 tons of aspirin a day, or 34 billion aspirin tablets per year. Non-Steroidal Anti-Inflammatory Drugs (NSAIDS) which include drugs like aspirin, ibuprofen and acetaminophen, are thought to be harmless drugs, but in an average year they will cause:

- 200,000 cases of gastrointestinal bleeding
- Between 107,000 and 120,000 deaths.
- Kidney malfunction (NSAIDS causes fluid retention, high blood pressure and reduced kidney function)
- Stomach ulcers, toxicity, headaches and Reye's syndrome in children

The elderly are especially likely to be medicated. Their average prescription rate is 13 per patient per year. Elderly Americans spend over $3 billion a year on prescription medications. Adverse drug reactions especially trouble the elderly because they are more likely to have multiple underlying health problems and also tend to have a weakened liver and kidneys, which break down and eliminate medications.

Public Citizens Health Research Group reports the following prescription drug induced conditions per year for people over the age of 60.

- A million adverse reactions to prescription drugs.
- 243,000 hospitalized due to prescription drugs.
- 163,000 mentally impaired due to prescription drugs.
- 2 million addicted to prescription drugs.

Young or old, we should all think twice about taking prescription or over-the-counter medication. It is not proven that drugs can cure illness, however they do suppress symptoms. Most drugs will never address the cause of illness. The side effects can also be hazardous to your health.

Illness is a sign of imbalance. You may suffer from nutritional imbalance, emotional imbalance, stress overload, dehydration, acidity, or lack of oxygen. Detoxification will balance your tires and get you back on the road to wellness. Are you sitting behind the wheel? Is your vehicle energized, loaded with fuel and ready to go? Then drive as if your life depended on it.

# Chapter: 4

*Vaccinations and Why You Should Educate Yourself*

## Dangers of Vaccinations

The purpose of vaccination is to produce immunity. A strong immune system is one where antibodies attack viruses and bacteria, stop them from multiplying and prevent infection from developing.

Antibodies are specific to each individual disease. Having antibodies to measles does not protect you from catching mumps or rubella.

Traditional medicine claims that injecting either a killed or a "modified" live virus (a vaccination) sensitizes the immune system to that particular virus. If you're further exposed to that particular virus or disease, then your antibodies will be able to kill and attack it, and prevent infection from developing.

## It Sounds Amazing, Doesn't It?

The American medical community, government and public school system believe that all children should be vaccinated, starting at birth. In fact, daycare centers and public schools won't admit your child unless they have up-to-date immunization records. Legal alternatives are rarely mentioned, although they are available. This is not based on scientific research, but in my opinion it is the money that keeps them pushing this issue in schools, etc. Immunizations are not necessary, in fact, it is the childhood diseases which build and strengthen the immune system.

## Vaccination Challenge

Dr Viera Scheibner challenged Simon Chapman (a pro-vaccination advocate and university professor) to appear on television and allow himself to be injected with all the baby vaccines, adjusted to his body weight.

Dr. Scheibner suggested the vaccines to be administered according to the timetable of traditional medicine:

- Diphtheria, tetanus, pertussis (or DTaP)  3 doses within 4 months
- Hepatitis B: 3 doses within 4 months
- Polio: 3 doses within 4 months
- Haemophilus influenzae type b: 3 doses within 1 month of each other.

"There isn't a better way to demonstrate that vaccines are safe and effective than by Simon taking his own medicine," wrote Dr. Scheibner, in a challenge that was published in the Medical Observer newspaper[6].

"If Simon does not agree to this easy and safe demonstration, then it will show us all that vaccinators are dishonest and are afraid of their own medicine. In other words: Put up or shut up."

Simon Chapman had no comment.

## Are Vaccines Safe and Effective?

We've always been told that vaccines prevent the spread of infectious disease. In reality, the opposite is true. Vaccines cause disease. Massive amounts of scientific, documented evidence clearly show that vaccines are neither safe, reliable

---

[6] Scheibner, V. (1999) "The Vaccination Challenge." Medical Observer. Waverton, Australia. February 19 edition. http://www.vaccination.inoz.com/vaccchallenge.html

nor effective. This is not unsubstantiated heresy. For over 100 years, doctors, scientists and researchers have documented adverse reactions, including permanent disability and death. There is a tremendous amount of literature that exposes the serious flaws in immunization theory and practice.

The malfunction of vaccines is documented by government statistics in reports from the Center for Disease Control (CDC), Food and Drug Administration (FDA) and credible research scientists around the world.

## Aren't Vaccines Responsible for the Eradication of Polio?

We have been told that vaccination saved the world from polio. Let's look at the facts. By the time the polio vaccine was introduced in 1956, the disease was already on the decline. It was no longer a serious threat to society. For this reason, the polio vaccine cannot be credited for wiping out the disease. After the vaccine was introduced, the incidence and deaths from polio increased, which was a major problem.

You may be wondering what eliminated polio. According to research scientist and author Dr. Viera Scheibner, 90% of polio cases were eliminated from statistics when health authorities redefined the disease[7]. Restrictive diagnostic criteria caused the number of "polio" cases to plummet, while the other diseases skyrocketed such as viral meningitis" and cerebral palsy. Up to 75% of these cases could still be diagnosed as polio. Many vaccines (DPT, MMR, Hib, polio, etc.) continue to induce polio, but the term "polio" is very rarely used.

The current polio vaccine has been associated with hundreds of adverse reactions, including 83 deaths in the US from 1991-1998. If anything, the polio vaccine temporarily reversed disease declines that were underway before the vaccine was introduced.

Another problem is that children are routinely vaccinated for diseases which are practically nonexistent in the United

Hancock, B. (2004) "But What About Polio?"
http://www.vaccination.inoz.com/polio.html

States. Are vaccines responsible for the eradication of these diseases? Truthfully, most diseases have been eradicated by hygiene, sanitation and clean drinking water.

## Five Reasons Vaccines Don't Work:

**1.** Vaccines don't work because they don't remove the root cause of infection. Unfortunately, the public has been conditioned to adopt a "germ theory" concept of disease that validates vaccinations. In other words, germs are the cause of disease, and germ-killing drugs are the solution.

Natural medicine contends that the injection of viruses – both the human and animal contaminants – deep into the body past the outer levels of defense is a dangerous practice. The body often has no way to eliminate the virus. Trapped inside the body, the virus slowly grows or remains dormant for years, and then causes a brain tumor (in the case of the SV40 monkey virus) or neurological problems such as autism (which has been reported with DTP,) and so on.

Traditional medicine contends that vaccinations encourage the body to build up antibodies. The problem is that toxins never strengthen the body; they only weaken it. Vaccinations place the virus directly into the bloodstream, and give it free and immediate access to the major immune organs and tissues, without any obvious way to get rid of it. Rather than prevent disease, vaccinations cause disease.

**2.** Vaccinations don't work because they cause disease. When we are sick, the symptoms that we experience (runny nose, flu, sore throat, etc.) are our body's attempt to rid itself of toxins. By masking these symptoms with pharmaceutical drugs or vaccines, the body does not eliminate the original toxins (or the additional ones). Instead, these toxins are forced deeper into our tissues where they cause infections capable of developing into chronic illnesses.

The toxic residue of vaccines circulates in our bodies— along with malnutrition, dehydration, stress and lack of elimination— to create an internal environment that is similar to a mosquito-infested swamp. If the immune system is polluted and stagnant then germs will thrive. If your immune system is toxic then it is conducive to the development of cancer, asthma, AIDS, multiple sclerosis and other autoimmune diseases.

If you read vaccination literature, check out the statistics. Often the risk of adverse reaction is often greater than the possibility of contracting the disease. The Oral Polio Vaccine (OPV) was routinely administered to millions, yet was discontinued in 2001 because children were contracting polio from it. The rotavirus vaccine was taken off the market after thousands of children got bowel obstructions from it. Incredibly, the CDC and FDA knew about this "side effect" prior to licensing the vaccine, but still gave their unanimous approval.

3. Vaccinations don't work because they contain toxic ingredients. It is no secret that vaccines contain diseased animal tissue, formaldehyde (embalming fluid,) phenol, ammonium sulfate, mercury derivatives (such as Thimersol and ethyl mercury,) aluminum phosphate, and phenoxyethanol (commonly known as antifreeze). These ingredients are toxic and carcinogenic. Even in small doses, these ingredients can cause serious harm. Remember that toxins never strengthen the body; they only weaken it.

Vaccines have been linked to autism, epilepsy, ADD, ADHD, minimal to serious brain damage, learning disorders, arthritis, diabetes, Guillain-Barre Syndrome, encephalitis, anaphylactic shock and various other serious conditions.

When children are vaccinated, they often receive two to four vaccines in one doctor's visit. This means that they are injected with 60 times the safe allowable limit of mercury, the most toxic non-radioactive substance known to man.

4. Vaccinations don't work because they cause death and disability.

The federal government created the Vaccine Adverse Events Reporting System (VAERS) in 1986. Every year, it receives about 11,000 reports of serious adverse reactions to vaccinations, which include as many as one to two hundred deaths and several times that number of permanent disabilities.

The National Vaccine Information Center (NVIC) is a grassroots organization founded by parents of vaccine-injured victims. Their independent research suggests that VAERS numbers are low because many adverse reactions to vaccines go unreported. According to NVIC, only one out of 40 doctor's offices confirmed that they reported a death or injury following vaccination.

In other words, 97.5% of vaccine related deaths and disabilities go unreported. These findings suggest that vaccine-related deaths and serious injuries may be from 10 to 100 times greater than the number reported[8].

When you factor in underreporting, the vaccine may be 100 times more deadly than the disease.

Since 1988, the federal government's National Vaccine Injury Compensation Program (NVICP) has paid out over $1.2 billion to the families of children injured and killed by vaccines. Evidently, this money comes from a tax on vaccines that vaccine recipients pay.

5. Vaccinations don't work because it isn't based upon scientific theory and practice.

It has never been scientifically proven that vaccinations are an effective means of immunization. "The medical community's gold standard, the double blind, placebo-controlled study, has not been used to compare vaccinated and unvaccinated people, and so the practice remains unscientifically proven," says Alan Phillips, a lawyer and Director of Citizens for Healthcare Freedom.

The main proponent of germ theory, Louis Pasteur, retracted on his death bed, with his famous words: "The seed is nothing, the soil is everything." That is, isolated germs don't cause disease. For a germ to take root, it must find toxic soil to thrive in. Pasteur recognized that the terrain on which the

---

Phillips, A. (2001) "Dispelling Vaccination Myths." Citizens for Healthcare Freedom. http://www.citizensforhealthcarefreedom.org/Vaccinations/DISPELLING%20VACCINA TION%20MYTHS.pdf

disease appears is the root cause of the illness, not the micro organism itself.

A healthy person with a strong immune system is able to resist disease, even when exposed to pathogens. However, this does not mean that injecting pusses and poisons into the body produces antibodies. The only true antibodies are ones that you naturally possess. Vaccinations are an attempt to trigger something that the body does naturally.

The human body has an incredible capacity for regeneration. It can heal itself by replacing or repairing injured tissue or cells. Also, healthy cells take over the function of damaged cells, either indefinitely or until the damage has been repaired. In this way, the body naturally immunizes itself. This natural immunization cannot be replicated by the artificial stimulation of antibodies.

Conventional medicine correlates antibody response with protection. If the body produces antibodies (or proteins) which bind to vaccine components, then the vaccine is assumed to be effective and safe. According to Dr. John B. March, a scientist who develops animal vaccines, antibody levels and protection are totally unconnected. Dr. March insists that antibody response is generally a poor measure of protection and no indicator at all of safety. When it comes to viral diseases, the body's cellular immune response is much more significant.

The fallacy of antibody theory was exposed over 50 years ago. In 1950, a study published by the British Medical Council during a diphtheria epidemic concluded that there was no relationship between antibody count and disease incidence. Researchers found resistant people with extremely low antibody counts and infected people with high antibody counts.

"Antibodies are as useful as a black eye in protecting the victim from further attacks," says Lionel Dole, an organic research scientist and author. Ultimately, a healthy lifestyle is the best immunization against germs and disease.

## Legal Alternatives to Vaccination

Vaccination is a multi-billion dollar industry. Every man, woman and child is a potential recipient of vaccination. With this potential customer base, it is no wonder that conventional medicine, the pharmaceutical industry and government is eager to fill the void.

Parents are told that their children must be vaccinated in order to attend school. School enrollment forms demand that children have the necessary paperwork from their doctor, and "no exceptions will be made."

There is a legal exemption, or way to get around the system. Go to your local health department (or DHHS) and ask for a "Religious Immunity Form" or "Philosophical Immunity Form." This is a simple, one-page sheet that must be officially notarized. Of course, you can obtain a free notary seal and signature at your local bank, as well as your auto insurance office.

These forms are a legal alternative to vaccination and must be accepted by schools. Another alternative is a "Medical Immunity Form," but these are more difficult to obtain. Ask your doctor if he has these forms and if he will authorize it for you.

Be prepared for some opposition about vaccinations. You might be told that you're putting your child at risk, or endangering the other kids in the class. You might be told that your child will be sent home, without an excuse, in case of an outbreak. Stand firm, and hold fast to your convictions. Don't let anyone make you feel guilty about whether or not you vaccinate your child.

## The Four Postulates of the Germ Theory

Dr. Robert Koch, a prominent figure in the controversy over the germ theory, set down four postulates which are still the law of basic science:

"If germs cause disease, then in any germ-caused disease, definite, specific unique germs must be:

1. Found in every case of the disease.

   This is absolutely not the case! It is a well-known fact that so-called "infectious diseases" may arise in the absence of the so-called pathogenic (disease-causing) germs that are supposed to cause them, proving germs do not cause disease. A germ cannot be a cause if it does not accompany the condition it is supposed to cause. A causeless effect is not possible.

2. Every time you find this germ you will find this disease.

   The best works on bacteriology declare that the germs of diphtheria, pneumonia, tuberculosis, etc. (the alleged "causes" of those conditions) are often found in perfectly healthy people who do not have, have not had, and do not subsequently develop the disease. A germ cannot be a cause if, when present in the body, the condition it is supposed to cause never develops. An effect-less cause is not possible.

3. Same germ, same disease.

   Never has a culture been made with normal, healthy living tissue. Medical theory declares that germs "attack and destroy" healthy tissue within the body; however, no germ has ever been known to multiply in normal tissues or normal secretions in the laboratory. Bacteriologists use "dead food", not living tissue, to grow their cultures, clearly demonstrating the natural function of bacteria, namely, to decompose once-living tissue into the original elements (gases, minerals, etc.) of which it was formed. They do not multiply on nothing. They will multiply only as long as their food is provided, which is decomposing waste, not living tissue.

**4.** Germs should be able to destroy healthy cells.

The U.S. government bulletin, Hygienic Laboratory, No. 123, February 1921, reported the results of experiments using 62 volunteer Navy personnel. The experimenters attempted to "cause" a contagion of influenza using every possible method-subcutaneous injections of blood from active influenza cases, direct transfer of secretions from nose to throat, spraying so-called infectious germs into the volunteers' throats and on their food. The results were: "NO APPRECIABLE REACTIONS!" The government never made these findings public. If specific germs cause specific diseases, then they should cause those diseases, and only those diseases, every time they are injected into the body. A cause must be constant and specific in its influence, or it is not a cause.

**Conclusion**

Vaccination is a seriously flawed concept and potentially fatal practice. It is a cruel experiment on innocent babies, children and adults. Immunity cannot be achieved by injecting the body with needles filled with pusses and poisons. Toxins never strengthen the body; they only weaken it

Conventional medicine is a legalized drug pusher who thinks he has outwitted Mother Nature. It is high time that the public be given full disclosure of the risks and dangers of vaccinations. Everyone is free to choose their own pathway to health. We must use our mind, heart and intuition to make informed choice about any vaccinations and any other medical intervention that carries a risk of injury or death.

Many scientists believe that vaccination is the sole or major component of multiple sclerosis, arthritis, Parkinson's disease, and many more health issues.

## Who Really Educates the Doctor?

There are over 8,000 prescription drugs on the market and for the majority of doctors, 70% of all prescription drugs were not around when they went to medical school.

The U.S. market for prescription drugs is the world's largest, valued at $30 billion annually. Drugstores dispensed 1.61 billion prescriptions in 1987.

Robert Mendelsohn, M.D., pediatrician, medical historian, author of *Confessions of a Medical Heretic*, and outspoken critic of current medical practices, discusses the examples of Diethylstilbestrol (DES), which was known in advance to be highly toxic, but was still widely prescribed to prevent miscarriages.

"DES was a substance that early on in the studies was shown to be capable of causing congenital malformations. The doctors knew about it, but they kept on giving it anyway. Diethylstilbestrol was given to six million women in this country between 1940 and 1980."

Eli Lilly was the first manufacturer then there were a number of manufacturers after Lilly. The control studies were completed at the University of Chicago in 1952. These studies showed that DES did not work, but it didn't make any difference: they kept on using it. Now we have a generation of DES daughters with cancer of the vagina, DES sons with tumors of the testes. The women who took DES have an increased incidence of cancer eight times higher than normal."

"I'm pretty sure that the individual doctors did not know that it didn't work, but the company knew and the leading researchers knew. That is why the lawsuits are coming up.

## The Brainwashed M.D.

A licensed doctor can never be outstanding or a healer in any way because he is brainwashed in exactly the same way as all other doctors and he is bound by law to follow the guidelines for specific illnesses. He cannot be different because they are trained to be the same. That is the reason why it is true that all major changes and positive developments in medicine are always made by an outsider and never by a brainwashed M.D.

I have witnessed a very strange phenomenon, the fact that people are brainwashed to believe only trained experts. Doctors can easily manipulate the public by discounting other experts who are not doctors; saying they have no right or authority to make any kind of qualified statements. That is really wrong. The true and non-manipulated statements always come from outsiders. People who think research and study for themselves.

What is a university degree: just reading, and listening and talking and researching material? You can do it yourself without being manipulated. Only the establishment wants you to believe that they have the only answers. A degree just means the person is successfully manipulated by the brainwashers that want control over others and their money. You only hear the truth from independent people or alternative groups. The others just tell you what they are paid to say.

The medical profession with all its glory was created by John D. Rockefeller to create salespeople for the chemicals he created. He created the entire medical curriculum for the entire world. All you get from them is a sales pitch for expensive, mostly unnecessary, diagnostic techniques with expensive technology. Even if you know what's wrong, they cannot fix it anyway. They sell you expensive, lifelong medication and treatments as well as senseless surgeries.

Do you know that if you go under full anesthesia three times you may have memory problems for life? That you get cancer from x- rays and chemotherapy? That the medical profession is responsible for more deaths than all wars? That you have a much larger chance of contracting a deadly infection in a hospital then anywhere else? Your chance of lifelong damage or dying from treatments and diagnostics is countless times higher than if you would not do anything.

I and many others believe that early detection of cancer is a guarantee that you die earlier and under horrible circumstances. There is absolutely no proof that early detection has any positive affects — least of all on your life expectancy or quality of life.

Have you ever seen that the government does anything right? Why do you believe they have the right or competence to tell you what is good for your health?

Politicians are usually lawyers manipulated by big business. The brainwashed greedy doctors tell them what is right for the public and the politicians believe it. They, in turn, pass senseless and dangerous laws controlling your health. Many of my friends believe mandatory vaccination is an assault with a deadly weapon and to make a law that holds the pharmaceutical industry harmless for vaccination damage is criminal in my opinion.

It is criminal to limit lawsuits against medical doctors. They should learn not to mess up so often and if they mess up they should have to pay for it. Many fraudulent lawsuits are filed and there needs to be protection for the doctor. Pass a logical law: the person who loses the lawsuit pays all the legal costs for both parties. That is the way it is in Europe. If someone files a fraudulent lawsuit he goes to jail – that is a very simple solution.

You can go to a doctor just don't trust him or her. Act like you would if you were giving a financial expert all your hard-earned money. Ask questions, get second and third opinions and ask for references, etc. Ask until you are satisfied. You would act in this way if you were trusting someone with your money. Why don't you act this way if you are trusting someone with your life?

All medical doctors are brainwashed and trained as salespeople for John D. Rockefeller's chemicals and his successors and there poisons.

## Side Effects

The United States has the most extensive health care system in the world. Americans pay more for health care than citizens of any other country. In 2002, we spent more than $1.5 trillion, an average of $5,300 for every man, woman and child. Yet, the United States ranks as one of the least healthy nations in the developed world. Our infant mortality rate is worse than 20 other nations. People live longer on average in 25 other countries. We are in the top five for incidents of cancer, heart disease, diabetes and autoimmune disorders.

What has gone wrong? Why are U.S. health care costs rising faster than any other country even as our overall health declines? It is important to note that the United States has the best emergency health care system in the world. Medical doctors are very successful at saving lives. But these types of trauma cases represent a very small percentage of all health problems.

The majority of health problems are treated with drugs, which is a major cause of our health care crisis.

- There are currently 25,000 prescriptions and 200,000 over the counter drugs on the market.
- 3.05 billion prescriptions are written each year.
- The average family has 29 different drugs in their medicine cabinet.
- Americans consume 68% of all the drugs in the world at a rate of 25 million pills each hour, 24-hours-a-day.

Drugs are foreign to the body. Drugs work by altering the body's natural biochemistry in order to suppress symptoms. Even with suppressed symptoms, the true cause of the problem may grow worse with the body's natural healing mechanism compromised. In fact, by interfering with normal cell function, drugs cause a cellular malfunction which is the same as causing disease.

In addition to toxicity, drugs also cause severe nutritional deficiencies by depleting the body of essential nutrients. Antibiotics, anti-inflammatory and steroids all damage the human digestive system by impairing the ability of the body to digest food and absorb nutrients.

*"There is no healing force outside of the human body."*
-- Dr. Issac Jennings

Healing only occurs from within the body, never from the outside. Symptoms such as coughing, sneezing, fever, vomiting, diarrhea, and pain are methods that the body uses to eliminate germs and other foreign materials. When drugs are given for relief, the body's natural healing process is interrupted and this can cause even more health problems.

"Symptoms represent the body's best efforts to heal itself. By treating symptoms, you are suppressing the body's natural response and inhibiting the healing process. Instead of treating symptoms, doctors should stimulate the body's defense to allow for completion of the healing process.

## Just How Serious is This?

"Adverse reactions to prescription drugs are a major cause of death in the U.S. An estimated 106,000 patients in hospitals die each year from adverse reactions, making adverse drug reactions the fourth most frequent cause of death.

A 2000 study in the *Archives of Internal Medicine* stated that drug-related morbidity and mortality costs are $136 billion a year— that is more than the cost of cardiovascular disease which is the leading cause of death in the United States.

According to the National Council on Patient Information and Education, over 50% of all prescriptions are used incorrectly. Misuse or noncompliance is a major health problem in the United States, resulting in 218,000 deaths and the hospitalization of 1 million individuals annually. The total cost to the economy is approximately $177 billion annually.

A 1994 study in the *Journal of the National Cancer Institute* and the *Journal of the Federation of Experimental Biology* warned that antihistamines and anti-depressant drugs (including Prozac) contain chemicals known to accelerate tumor growth. While these drugs do not directly cause cancer, they can speed its growth.

Not all adverse reactions to new drugs can be anticipated or avoided under the present system, according to medical experts, "It is simply not possible to identify all the adverse effects of drugs before they are marketed," according to a study in the *New England Journal of Medicine.* In fact, "Overall, 51% of approved drugs have serious side effects not detected prior to approval."

Side effects from new drugs cannot be anticipated for two main reasons: (1) Individuals vary greatly in their reactions to chemical substances; and (2) drugs are tested where side effects may not appear in such a small group but may become painfully obvious when millions of people start taking the drug.

Americans consume over 15 tons of aspirin a day, 34 billion aspirin tablets per year. NSAIDS, which include drugs like aspirin, ibuprofen and acetaminophen, are thought to be harmless drugs, but in an average year they will:

- Be responsible for over 200,000 cases of gastrointestinal bleeding, 107,000 and 20,000 deaths.
- Be the leading cause of kidney disease.
- Cause stomach ulcers, toxic, headaches, and Reye's syndrome in children.

The elderly are especially likely to be medicated. Their average prescription rate is 13 per patient per year. Elderly Americans spend over three billion dollars a year on prescription medications. Adverse drug reactions especially trouble the elderly because they are more likely to have multiple underlying health problems and also tend to have a weakened liver and kidneys, which break down and eliminate medications.

Public Citizens Health Research Group reports the following prescription drug induced conditions per year for people over the age of 60.

- A million adverse reactions to prescription drugs.

- 243,000 hospitalized due to prescription drugs.
- 163,000 mentally impaired due to prescription drugs.
- 2 million addicted to prescription drugs.

## Why Have Drugs Become Such a Big Part of our Society?

The drug industry has been able to heavily influence our health care system. Fifty thousand pharmacies and 700,000 outlets for drugs add up to a $125 billion a year industry, which has the highest profitability margin of any business in the United States. In 2002, drug companies had the greatest return on revenues of any industry, reporting a profit of 18.5 cents for every $1 of sales. That was eight times higher than the median for all Fortune 500 industries easily surpassing the next most profitable industry, which was commercial banking with a 13.5% return on revenue. The top 10 drug companies reported profits averaging about 30 percent of revenues – a stunning margin.

## Is Their Bottom Line Health or Profits?

In 2002, drug companies spent over $5 billion (more than $13 million a day) to persuade customers to buy their products. One third of all television commercials are advertisements for drugs. The average 18 year old has been exposed to 20,000 hours of pharmaceutical advertising. Articles touting new wonder drugs are usually press kits sent out by drug companies. "Expert" physicians are normally paid company spokesmen. Many newscast segments about prescription drugs are nothing more than canned promotions called "video news releases" put together by the drug companies for promotional purposes. These segments rarely warn consumers that the drugs are potent agents that can cause severe, even life threatening, reactions.

Drug companies spend an average of $10,000 per year on each and every medical doctor to persuade them to use their drugs. In addition to free samples, TIME magazine reported that:

- Wyeth-Ayerst Labs gives medical doctors 1,000 points on American Airlines frequent flyer programs for each patient they put on the hypertension drug Inderal LA.
- Roche pays medical doctors $1,200 for every 20 patients for whom they prescribe Roecephin. Roche makes more than $11,000 on 20 patients treated for only 10 days.
- Ciba-Geigy offers free Caribbean vacations to doctors in return for their sitting in on a few lectures about Estraderm, an estrogen patch.

Drug companies also sponsor continuing medical education courses. Doctors who attended these classes altered their prescription habits to the products sold by the sponsoring company, according to a Time magazine article.

## Misleading Drug Ads

The journal *Lancet* reported that nearly <u>half of all drug advertisements published in medical journals cite studies or other evidence that does not support their promotional claims.</u> As part of their research, co-author Dr. Salvador Piero and colleagues with the Valencia School for Health Studies reviewed 102 promotional claims made in numerous medical journal advertisements. According to the study's findings, references in advertisements did not support promotional claims 44% of the time.

## Doctors and the Pharmaceutical Companies

Different doctors recommend different treatments however; a 1991 article in the *British Medical Journal* revealed that less than 15% of all the treatments prescribed by doctors are based on solid scientific evidence. Hardly a month goes by where I do not receive a letter that states that a drug currently on the market is now getting taken off the market. Disturbingly, a month earlier this drug was considered a wonder drug. What usually happens is side effects that were not disclosed when the drug was approved start to show up in the public and physicians start to notice them and find them hazardous to the patient's health. People can often die because of this fraudulent behavior. Reports of side effects should be filed immediately to protect users.

We would like to continue our normal unhealthy habits and have a doctor cure us with a pill. However, drugs will never cure what is wrong with you. Cancer is a deficiency of health and a strong immune system, not of radiation and chemotherapy. If you want to be well again then you must make yourself well. All of the steps you can take to cure yourself are completely free except for the food, but you have to buy that anyway. You do not have to be afraid of cancer anymore.

Conventional treatments for cancer are taught to our doctors and they are methods such as radiation and chemotherapy. Your doctor wants you to get well, they do care. However, they just do not know how to cure you. All doctors are taught to do is to burn or cut out the cancer. These methods will never cure cancer. There are people who do survive cancer after these treatments, but it is in spite of the treatment not because of it. At first the chemotherapy seems to work. The tumor does get smaller, this is true, but it will not cure it. Street drugs feel good at first, but eventually you will pay a terrible price. It is the same with radiation and chemotherapy and you often pay for it with your life.

Here is why conventional treatments never cure cancer. The only way that you can cure cancer or any other disease is to understand what causes it. If you can find the cause you have the cure because the cure lies in reversing the cause of the disease. The doctors think that they do not know what the cause of cancer is, but they do.

Dr. Leonard Coldwell

Why is this information not taught to people? The pharmaceutical companies want to sell drugs; they do not want to fund natural ways of treating cancer. You cannot make money by telling someone that they need more sleep or need to drink more water. Sunlight, fresh air, water and sleep are all free things. This is just one of many examples.

Pharmaceutical companies provide large, expensive research studies. They control much of what is taught to doctors about how to treat diseases. The cause of disease is termed by companies as *ideology*. They used to list this in all the textbooks under every disease, but now it is almost completely removed. The medical textbooks do not even mention this because they admit that they do not know the cause of cancer and many other diseases. The treatment of cancer with radiation, chemotherapy or surgery really does not make any sense in the grand scheme of things. Cancer is not caused by deficiencies of any of these things and both chemotherapy and radiation cause cancer. Some people get very angry when they hear this.

If the doctors do not prescribe these kinds of treatments to you they could loose their license to practice medicine, because this is what they have been taught to do for you. In California, it is against the law for a doctor to treat you with anything other than chemotherapy, radiation or surgery. I was handed a booklet by one of my doctors that said that a doctor could refuse to treat a cancer patient if they refused to take radiation, chemotherapy or surgery.

Science can be very dangerous. Doctors are becoming agents of death. In the United States medical doctors are 9,000 times more likely to cause an accidental death than guns. There are a lot of people trying to ban guns, but no one is trying to ban doctors! New information has revealed that the new laser surgery that is being done all over the U.S. is ruining peoples' eyes. Patients are rarely warned of the damages.

Science can be naive. They only look at one variable at a time, for example, for the cause of cancer they look at vitamin deficiencies. They then make two research groups and give

134

them pills that look the same. One actually has the vitamin and the other has nothing. Here is the flaw, because cancer is not only because of vitamin deficiencies, there is so much more. You need to correct each of the problems, not just one. Someone might have cancer because of the stress in his life. Cancer is unique to every person. Research will never give you any kind of conclusion or answers. This kind of research can be useless and is expensive and they never come up with any answers. This is why they never heal.

True science is always simple and easy to understand. Cancer is cancer and it all results from the immune system not working properly. All someone with cancer needs to do is rebuild the immune system properly. The way we eat and the way we live is what develops cancer. We must treat our bodies like we would treat a garden. We must give it ample amounts of water, sunlight, nourishment, fresh air and an environment free of stress. If any of these factors are off we need to fix them.

Medical professionals are often under the control of these pharmaceutical companies. For example, a cancer center in New York that is one of the most influential cancer centers in the world is controlled and managed by a board of trusties, who are more often than not linked to various pharmaceutical companies. Frequently, they are executives of corporations that have the greatest interest in the cancer industry and the treatment of cancer patients. The major players that control the cancer industry, including the control of the information that you and your physician are allowed to know are the following: The Cancer Center in New York, the American Cancer Society, the National Cancer Institute and the FDA.

In the 1880's the wealthy Ashter family who made their money from fur trading and tenant properties provided the initial funding for the New York Cancer Hospital which later became the Memorial Sloan Cancer Center. With their large contributions they demanded control. They dictated who would occupy the leading positions of the board of directors and who would be the medical director of the hospital. In the 1920s, the

Rockefellers who controlled Standard Oil of New Jersey signed an extensive agreement with a German pharmaceutical company called IG Fargan. After this partnership was established, the standard oil Rockefeller Empire suddenly developed a great interest in the worldwide pharmaceutical industry. The Rockefellers then began their systematic contributions to Memorial Hospitals and in a few years a vice president of Standard Oil was invited to join the Memorial Hospitals Board of Managers. He was made chairman of the newly organized research committee. When World War II began, Cornelius Rose, who was involved in the beginning research of chemotherapy, became Chief of Research for the Chemical Warfare Service of the United States Military. His official purpose was to carry out studies on the effects of poisonous gas. These studies were also being done on cancer patients under the cover of military secrecy. Nitrogen mustard and chemical warfare, killing agents and the grandfather of chemotherapy, is still used on cancer patients today. They use names like alcalan or lucoran. Nitrogen mustard is used to kill people and it frequently does this job very well when given to cancer patients.

In the 1960's the leaders of hospitals where individuals who could loose or gain a great deal of money depending on how cancer was treated. Individuals like Lawrence Rockefeller and Ben Schmit of Werthington Biochemical Company who was chairmen of the board of directors. By 1988, over a third of the entire board of directors had ties to the medical industry whose corporations produce a wide range of known or suspected carcinogens. For example, Exxon is one of the world's largest producers of benzene, a major cancer causing substance. General Motors is responsible for about 1/3 of the nation's air pollution. These are only the direct cooperate links. If you look at the other boards you will find asbestos manufacturers, allied chemical companies and other producers of life threatening chemicals. How ironic is it that those who are making millions by mass producing cancer causing substances are now making money on the other end, first by controlling the types of cancer treatment allowed and then by producing the treatments of cancer. These directors use the same philosophy at the hospital that they use in their business and financial activities. They want to make money. The result of this is that research is directed away from prevention, away from natural, inexpensive remedies and toward more profitable treatments.

Why don't we hear this information through the media? Let's look at the media ties on the board of directors for the cancer centers. In 1988, two board members were directors of the New York Times Corporation, two members were executives at Readers Digest, one member was president of Warner Communication and one was director of CBS. When a story of a promising alternative treatment of cancer was dropped from United Press International and Associated Press, the two news wire services, investigative journalists asked why? They were told that, "all cancer stories had to be cleared through the science editing department of the Associated Press in New York". So, the story did not run. All the stories had to run through the board of directors who control everything, even all the treatments have to be approved. If you think that was an isolated incident, here are a few more illustrations documenting how the media is controlled. John Swenson was one of America's best loved newspaper men and former chief- of-staff for the *New York Times*. He was called the dean of his profession by his peers. In 1953, he was asked to give a toast before the New York Press Club. After listening to numerous hypocritical toasts to our American free press John spoke candidly to his colleagues. This is what he said:

> "There is no such thing to this date in the world's history in America as an independent press, you know it and I know it. If I allowed my honest opinions to appear in even one issue of my paper before 24 hours my occupation would be gone. The business of the journalist is to destroy the truth, to lie outright, to pervert, to

vilify and to sell his country and his race for his daily bread. You know it and I know it and what folly is this toasting an independent press. We are tools for the rich man behind the scene. We are the jumping jacks, they pull the strings and we dance. Our talent, possibilities and our lives are all the property of other men. We are intellectual prostitutes."

Richard Salnic, former president of CBS news stated, "Our job is to give people not what they want, but what we decide they ought to have." People know that there is a media monopoly in the hands of a few families and global corporations. Cancer is big business and they are sacrificing your life in the process.

How about the American Cancer Society? This is one of the nation's largest volunteer health organizations. It collects over $400 million a year, yet not a single breakthrough has resulted from this colossal collection of money. Obviously the American Cancer Society benefits from the intense concern from the public about cancer. Even though cardiovascular disease is responsible for twice as many deaths as cancer the American Heart Association receives far less in donations and research funds than the cancer establishment. Why, because the American Cancer Society does a splendid job of keeping the public very conscious of cancer. Hardly a day goes by without a newspaper article on cancer. The deaths from cancer of Hubert Humphrey, Yule Brenner, John Wayne, Jacqueline Kennedy and other celebrities become a national drama which the public follows with fascination.

The American Cancer Society was originally founded as The New York Harvard Club in 1913 by none other than John Rockefeller Jr. and his friend. Rockefeller even provided the funds for this founding. From the start the society's role was to be a shaper of public opinion. The main goal was to urge the general public to consult their general physicians at their very first suspicion of cancer. In the early 1940s, a group of very wealthy individuals began to plan a reorganization of the American Cancer Society. Key figures among the new leaders were Elmer Boast, president of Hoffman Laroch Drug Company and Albert Lasker a prominent advertising man whose greatest advertising triumph was for the American tobacco companies. His slogan "reach for a lucky instead of a sweet" convinced thousands of women to start smoking in the 1930s and 1940s. (again follow the money). Lasker first made money by encouraging women to smoke and then made even more money through the American Cancer Society by directing fund raising supposedly for research and treatment of the very cancers his advertising encouraged. Boast and Lasker introduced the most advanced Madison Avenue techniques in the cancer fund raising and dollars flooded in to the society. In 1978, journalist Barry Chelka investigated the American Cancer Society and found that this nonprofit agency was hording and investing many millions of dollars contributed by the public to fight cancer. While at the same time, they were claiming that vital research was not being done because of a lack of funds. Of the money that the American Cancer Society spends to supposedly fight cancer, 61% goes to staff salaries, executive travel, office supplies and other expenses. Less than 5% is allocated to assisting patients.

The American Cancer Society is not interested in a cure; it would go out of business. The following incident illustrates this point. In 1952, a county chapter of the IOWA Cancer Society ran a full page add in the local paper asking for the American Cancer Society parent organization to investigate claims of four new possible cancer cures. The chapter was promptly expelled from the American Cancer Society. The chairman of the expelled chapter was astonished and said that they did not understand the crime that they had committed; they just wanted to help conquer cancer. Has the American Cancer Society another motive? The underlying motive is revealed in an article that appeared in *Harpers* magazine stating: "The American Cancer Society was designated by charter as an emergency organization that must disband the day a cure is found." Why would the American Cancer Society ever admit that a cancer cure exists? They would have to disband and give up the $400 million a year.

The National Cancer Institute is a government research agency that has the primary responsibility of funding the so-called war on cancer. It hands out billions of your tax dollars in research funds in support of science at various institutions. Both the American Cancer Society and the New York Hospital guide the direction of these funds and studies. In 1971, the National Cancer Act was passed which began the war on cancer. Before that in the late 1960s Congress established a national panel of consultants to study the conquest of cancer. It was this committee that ultimately recommended the war on cancer to Congress. Of the 26 panel members who proposed the war on cancer ten were officers of the American Cancer Society and several others were from chemical and pharmaceutical companies.

This is the way that the National Cancer Institute works: A researcher applies for research funds, this grant request must be approved by a wide variety of scientist, bureaucrats and businessmen. It must be approved by these many individuals. Almost by definition such an application must be well within the bounds of conventional science. These constraints make it almost impossible for radically new ideas to be approved by the National Cancer Institute. That is why the National Cancer Institute will never fund the investigation of natural treatments of cancer or any other disease. The recently formed branch of alternative medicine at the NCI has been nothing but a sham to appease Congress and especially to appease the public. Furthermore, the public pays for chemotherapy drugs to be developed with their tax money. Then the public pays again, this time at monopoly prices, to purchase these same drugs from private companies who patent them for their own gain. They charge you an astronomical price for something that your tax dollars already paid to develop.

The Federal Drug Administration is a government agency staffed by civil servants and political appointees. Theoretically, its role is to prevent harmful or useless methods of treating cancer from entering the marketplace. Yet they strongly endorse radiation and chemotherapy, both of which are extremely harmful treatments. In 1974, eleven FDA scientists testified in a Senate hearing that their own agency was a pawn that pharmaceutical industries were trying to control. They testify that they were harassed by agency officials whenever they recommended against the approval of marketing some new drug. In 1976, the *New England Journal of Medicine* commented on this state of affairs at the FDA saying, "There was open drunkenness by several employees that went on for months, there was intimidation internally by people, division directors and their staff would engage in the kind of behavior that invited insubordination. I am describing physicians, people who would slouch in their chair and moan and groan. I have never seen this kind of behavior in any other institution and I am a grown man. One author said that this behavior seems more characteristic of an insane asylum than that of a top government agency. These are the people that ridicule natural healing methods as quackery.

In addition, there is a revolving door between pharmaceutical companies and the FDA. Certain FDA members push hard to get a certain drug approved and then, surprise, they suddenly quit their job at the FDA and go to work for that very drug company. Everyone just pretends that this is all legal. The American Cancer Society, the National Cancer Institute and the FDA are all in bed together. They are working for themselves, not for you.

Now let's discuss cure rates. Your doctor may give you statistics on rates of cure with different types of therapies. What does your doctor mean by cure? For years, the ACS maintained a peculiar definition of a cancer cure as a five year survival after diagnosis. In 1979, a *New York Times* reporter asked for a definition of the word cure and an embarrassed ACS spokesperson admitted: "I have never gone to a dictionary to look up the definition of cure; we really don't know what we mean by cure." Doctors rarely use the term cure when they talk with one another because they know that the conventional methods of treatment really do not cure cancer. In recent years, however, the ACS definition of cure has become even hazier. Among the two million cured cancer victims in the United States, the ACS admitted that they had included people who still had evidence of cancer. This means that a man, who has cancer, is treated and then later shows more signs, but is still listed as being cured. It does not make any sense.

You will hear much from your doctor about the impressive statistics of survival after treatment of cancer. Let's look at how those figures are derived. In his book *The Cancer Industry,* author Ralph Moss magnificently details the fraud and deceit of the statistics associated with cancer. Here is an illustration: Dr. Hardon Jones, the professor of medical physics at University of California Berkley and an expert on statistics, aging and the effects of drugs on aging said, "The notion that patients treated with conventional therapies live longer than those who are untreated is biased by the methods of defining the groups. If a person in the untreated category of a study dies at any time during the study this is recorded as a failure of the no treatment approach. However, if someone in the treated group dies before the treatment is completed their records disappear completely. To the researchers they are not considered treated because they died before they had the chance to complete the treatment."

So a person who dies on day 89 on a prescribed 90 day course of chemotherapy would just disappear from the list of treated patients and would not be listed as a failure. If this bias effect is taken out then studies would show a remarkable similar death rate whether treated or untreated according to Dr. Jones.

Also, there is no proof that early detection affects survival. New techniques are able to detect cancer about six months earlier. What does this do? It converts a six month survival rate to a five year survival rate, which is what they call a cure. Nothing has changed on the survival graph except for the beginning point from which they chose to measure. Naturally, the earlier the detection the longer the survival from that point and the more time they have to give you expensive painful treatment. However, the real survival rate is not affected at all. It is also obvious that conventional treatments have not been able to stop the rise in cancer mortality. There has been a steady rise in the cancer death rate in the U.S. in this and the previous century. In the 1900s, cancer caused one in 27 deaths. In the 1920s it rose to one in 16 deaths; one in 12 in the 1930s; one in nine in the 1940s, one in seven in the 1950s, one in six in the 1960s and the death rate continues to climb. It may appear that we are living longer and that cancer is a disease of the old and middle aged but this is not the only reason for the increase. These figures are already age adjusted and have already taken into consideration the shifts in population. In the 1980s, the standard figures for cancer cures— five year survival — was around 33%. Then, suddenly, the ACS was proclaiming that 49% would still be alive five years after diagnosis. At first glance, this seems like a remarkable improvement. How did this happen? The cancer industry had developed a new standard to announce to the public. This was called a variant on the five year survival statistic which they named the "relative survival rate". According to cancer officials, relative survival rate is considered a more accurate yard stick for measuring cancer progress. It takes into account the expected mortality figures. This means that if a person had not died of cancer they might have been run over by a truck and that must be factored into the equation. With the use of this fraudulent yard stick they now say that 49% of the cancer patients will be alive five years after cancer treatment. This is the basis for the 50% cure rate. That is called lying with statistics.

Another serious flaw in the NCI number was that it chose to use only the figures for white people. Statistics show that the cancer rate and the death rate are higher for blacks than they are for whites. So, the NCI chose to present the figures for whites as the norm. These claims of great progress were exposed as a fraud when an article appeared in the *New*

*England Journal of Medicine* revealing that these figures did not include the death rates for black people or for lung cancer patients. They excluded these numbers because they were higher. There are books available that provide these fraudulent statistics, but you probably will not find any in your local book stores. The book, *Betrayers of the Truth*, shows how science really works and how they distort statistics. The government and the medical profession suppress the natural ways of treatment.

The FDA and the pharmaceutical advertisement council, known as PAC, which represents some 35 major drug companies have formed an organization called the National Council Against Health Fraud. Reportedly they are paying large sums of money to doctors and public health specialists to discredit all nontraditional therapy, particularly those that are proven to have the most promise and present the greatest threat to the pharmaceutical companies. Yet, the FDA regularly approves dangerous often lethal drugs. When one of these wonder drugs fails or causes serious injury or death in either one person or thousands of people, no one in the pharmaceutical profession or medical profession is held accountable. At most, the drug is quietly removed from the market. Chemotherapy and radiation, both of which cause cancer and both of which have been responsible for hundreds of thousands if not millions of deaths, are the only therapies that the government endorses and approves. These therapies, reportedly introduced as new approaches, promise that in the near future we will have a cure for cancer. Yet the so- called alternative therapies are consistently accused of offering false hope. On the contrary, the government has proven to provide the largest amount of false hope the country has ever known.

When the statistics are eliminated the long term survival rate of cancer patients using conventional therapies remains abysmal at about 3%. This statement was noted in the prestigious medical journal *Lancet* in 1996. The cost of care for these millions of Americans with cancer is estimated to be between $4 and $7 trillion over the last 20 years. That is a frightening amount of money flowing into the hands of the medical and pharmaceutical industries. Is it any wonder that they will not admit that cancer can be cured by natural methods? Dr. Benjamin Wrech, a signer of the Declaration of Independence, had great insight 200 years ago. He said:

> "Unless we put medical freedom into the Constitution the time will come when medicine will organize into an undercover dictatorship. To restrict the art of healing to one class of men and deny equal privileges to others will constitute the Castile of medical science. All such laws are un-American. They are fragments of monarchy and have no place in a republic. The Constitution of this Republic should make previsions for medical freedom as well as religious freedom."

Dr. Wrech was absolutely correct. Everyday that passes that our medical freedom is still in the hands of doctors just out for money, is just another day closer to when conventional medicine will only be available to the rich and famous. Our Constitution should have set some guidelines for this corrupt behavior.

## Prescription Drugs

The drugs that your doctor prescribes to you can cause major problems. Anti-inflammatory drugs can cause depression, confusion, paranoia and can have toxic effects on your kidneys. Even antibiotics have lots of side effects. Antibiotics do not even cure the disease and they clear out the good bacteria in your colon. These bacteria are needed for you body to digest food. When you take a drug you may relieve the symptom of the disease, but will never cure it. They only change the form or location of the disease. Your immune system is the only system that can cure you from your illness.

When you put drugs into your body it has an adverse effect on your body. What you need to do is learn to eat right and eliminate the medications in our bodies. The most important thing to remember is to discontinue the use of prescription drugs gradually.

Here are some of the admitted side effects of Prozac given by the pharmaceutical company. Prozac is prescribed to patients who are suffering from depression and anxiety. However, the number one side effect is anxiety. Other side effects include nausea, nervousness, tremors, dizziness, anorexia, insomnia, sweating, hemorrhage, and high blood pressure, loss of strength, cardiac arrest, heart failure, amnesia, paranoia, delusions and coma. These are just for Prozac, think of all the other medications. In 1992, it was found that women who use anti-depressant drugs are 17 times more likely to have a heart attack. The definition of a drug by a true follower of the word is this- a drug is anything you use to remove the effects of transgression without requiring obedience.

**Anti-Estrogen Drugs and Phytoxin**

Many people do not realize that anti-estrogen drugs are also a form of chemotherapy. The anti-estrogen drug that doctors do not classify as chemotherapy is Alimadex. This causes numbness, chest pain, vomiting, high blood pressure, anxiety and blood clots. Tramostapin is prescribed to people who simply have a history of breast cancer. They do not currently have it, so why continue poisoning their bodies? This can cause uterus cancer, increased tumors, blood clots and vision problems.

Phytoxin is one of the oldest drugs used for chemotherapy. We first used this drug to kill our enemies in World War II. When the war was over, there was leftover phytoxin so they decided they would try to use it to kill cancer. However, chemotherapy causes cancer. Chemotherapy causes bleeding around the heart and in the urinary tract. It also causes hair loss. The warnings for phytoxin say that deaths could occur and that allergic reactions are fatal. Phytoxin is a deadly drug.

## Diabetes

There have been people that have recovered completely from diabetes. However, the best thing to do is to prevent it. Your doctor will even tell you that you can prevent type- two diabetes by eating a healthy diet and getting plenty of exercise. To prevent this horrible disease you need a diet rich in vitamins and enzymes. There is evidence that diabetes in adolescents is caused by cows' milk. These people suffer from many problems. The best thing to do is to eliminate dairy. Another way to prevent diabetes is to stay away from refined sugar. This causes your insulin levels to rise which can lead to hypoglycemia.

## Joint Problems and Our Immune Systems

Joint and tissue problems are a huge problem in Americans. Doctors will tell you that you are having problems because your immune system is too strong. This is not possible; you cannot be too healthy. When your immune system is working properly you will not have medical problems or get diseases. Diseases are from nutritional deficiencies. Doctors treat joint and tissue problems with cortisone. However, cortisone causes ulcers, bone problems, mental disturbances, degeneration of the nerves, acne, facial hair growth in women, diabetes, metabolism difficulties along with a tremendous appetite. Cortisone can also lead to cancer. For arthritis, a doctor will often put a patient on a high dosage of aspirin. However, aspirin can cause ulcers and bleeding in your intestines. These are side effects that could ultimately kill you. It is possible to cure yourself with the proper nutrition. Eat lots of healthy raw foods and exercise and you will see that your condition will improve drastically.

## Genetics and Cancer

The medical profession continues to look solely in one place to find the root of cancer. They look at genetics, but cancer is not genetic. This can be proven very easily. Since the early 1900s, the incidents of breast cancer have continued to rise dramatically. All the experts and national medical associations agree. In the early 1900s, it was older women (grandmothers) who got breast cancer.  Now, the young women (grandchildren) get breast cancer. Grandmothers back then had a very low incidence of breast cancer compared to the young granddaughters of today. This means it is not possible for it to be genetic. If it were genetic then there would be a high incidence of cancer in the grandmothers who then pass it down, but this is not the case. It is the reverse. Look at the women in Japan, they eat a lot of rice and fish and the breast cancer rate is very low.  Take those same women, bring them to America and feed them what we eat. You will see that their rate of cancer will increase to the same rate as the American women.  Even the women in Japan who do not eat well are developing cancer.  We see the same patterns with diabetes, autoimmune disease and many other diseases.  They are not genetic; it is our lifestyle.

You may say you inherited your illness. However, the truth is that only about 1% of diseases are inherited. The fact that all women in your family had or have breast cancer does not necessarily mean that you will have breast cancer. However, with this in mind, you should change the way in which you eat and handle stress. This is how it is passed down. Unless you address the underlying cause, which in most cases is lifestyle, you will not solve the problem.

## Sunlight and Cancer

If you are not eating enough good nutritious food you will lose your barriers from the sun.  At Bayer University they did a study with two groups of experimental animals. They gave a

148

standard American diet, with too much fat, protein and sugar to one group. They gave the other group a highly nutritious diet. They then exposed both of them to the ultraviolet rays of the sun. In the group with the standard American diet, 25% tested positive for skin cancer. In the other group, not one of them was positive.

Sunlight lowers blood pressure and cholesterol. It turns your cholesterol into vitamin D in your skin. It enhances the immune system and kills bacteria. Sunlight also causes your nervous system to calm down. This is why you fall asleep in the sun. It increases oxygen in the blood and decreases your heart rate and your stress level. Yet, doctors are telling their patients to stay out of the sun.

Can you grow a garden with out sunlight? No. You cannot grow a healthy human without sunlight either. Just think of the things that a plant needs. A plant needs proper nutrition, water, sunlight, fresh air and freedom from toxins. All of these things are what a human being needs as well. You do not want to give a bunch of drugs to a plant, yet so many people are given drugs all of the time.

The fresh air taken in from the outdoors is essential for good health. In fact, cancerous tumors grow twice as fast if you are breathing indoor air compared to outdoor air. If you are being treated for your illness in a hospital you are continuously breathing in the exhaled air of every other person in the hospital. Hospitals often have the windows shut all the time. This will harm the patient more than help them.

**Something to think about**

The leading causes of death in the 1900s were pneumonia (11%), tuberculosis (11%), diarrhea (8%), heart disease (8%), injury (4%), cancer (3.7%) and diphtheria (2.3%). The leading causes of death in 1994 were heart disease (32%), cancer (24%), injury (3.9%), and suicide which was not even on the 1900 list. What has happened during this time? In 1909, the average American ate 300 lbs of grain a year and 200 lbs of potatoes. By 1994, the amount of grains fell to half. The amount of milk and meat consumed had doubled. Cancer also increased from one out of 33 people to one out of three. Stress was also more prevalent. Everyone also drinks more sodas and caffeine than they did back then. People back then may have smoked and had a few drinks, but they didn't have meat with hormones in it and fast food places everywhere. Families cared about each other. They usually raised their own produce. The healthiest Americans lived during World War II. This was because all of the doctors were in the Army. Sugar and meat were rationed and everyone had a vegetable garden. We think that we have made progress, but we have not. We have gone downhill. One out of two people will develop cancer. By the year 2020, everyone will have cancer at some point in their life. You should be frightened enough to take these things into consideration.

Diabetes is now an epidemic. Type one diabetes appears in children and type two in adults. Now, children are starting to get type two. The difference is that in type one the cells in the pancreas are actually destroyed or appear to be destroyed. With type two they are there, but they are not functioning. The number one cause of juvenile onset diabetes is caused by drinking milk. We are the only animals that drink milk from another animal once we are weaned. We don't need milk. We have all bought the lie. How would you feel if you were the reason why your child has blindness or possibly amputation? Children do not need milk past weaning. The dairy farmers have sold you this lie. There are close to 50 different kinds of hormones found in milk. It also causes early puberty in children. The government allows 10 million bacteria per teaspoon of milk. Most of these bacteria are fecal or puss. If you want an alternative you can buy rice milk. Children who have diabetes and are on insulin should eat the best diet possible and exercise regularly. Adult onset diabetes is also an epidemic. Most are not told by their doctors that it can be reversed by diet and exercise. The diabetes drugs are awful. One is called Lipotrol; it increases the risk of cardiac disease. It can cause heart attack and death. They even teach you in med school that it can be reversed with diet and exercise. The reason why they don't tell you is because the doctor doesn't want to take the time to explain it to you and patients want a pill to fix their problem. When you eat too much sugar or too much fat your body has to produce so much insulin that the cells get fatigued and the fat makes the cells resistant to the insulin so your body is pouring out all the insulin. Those cells just stop. They will start again if you eat the right food and exercise. Exercise is critical to all diseases. Do not exercise too much if you are wearing yourself out.

What is a drug? A drug is anything you use to remove the effects of transgression without requiring obedience. If you are lazy you can get a drug to fix what is wrong with you. There is a tremendous occurrence of homicide with the use of Prozac. We want to modify our behavior with drugs. Every day 26 million people die from heart disease. That is the equivalent of 10 jumbo jet crashes a day. You would be upset with that wouldn't you? If you have cancer be glad that you didn't have a heart attack, because you have time. With a heart attack the first symptom is sudden death. Ninety percent of all heart attacks are preventable with lifestyle changes.

When we get upset and angry our stomach contracts so that we cannot digest our food, our intestines stop so we can't eliminate waste and our adrenal glands produce all kinds of hormones. One minute of anger suppresses your immune system for six hours. One minute of laughter boosts your immune system for 24 hours. Our attitude makes a huge difference in our health. When you have sudden stress you have the fight or flight response. This response is natural if we are in true danger and need to act quickly. However, people are living under constant stress and are in this state all the time which destroys your immune system. The fight or flight response causes an increase in blood pressure, increase in heart rate, an increase in the contractions of the heart and increase in mental activity. Your body ends up in debt because you have drawn on your reserves and you now need to rest and regenerate. When people are under chronic stress their bodies never regenerate.

Children laugh an average of 400 times a day; adults laugh maybe once a day. We are too burdened by life. It is the everyday events that drag us down. Worry is a major stressor. We try to do too much. Sugar makes stress worse and so does dehydration. Exercise increases your ability to handle stress. Sunlight decreases stress. Noise will cause a major increase in your stress level (such as young peoples' music). Ongoing stress is what causes diseases. Some signs of stress are confusion, forgetfulness, anxiety, panic, tension, frustration and depression. Anger can trigger high blood pressure and heart disease.

The AMS says that heart disease is the number one cause of death in America. When people have artery bypass surgery it is never a permanent solution. This is a quick fix but you need to change your diet and lifestyle in order to keep it from happening again. In the hospital, they feed you the very food that will ensure your return. The doctor also gives you drugs that have horrible side effects. When a drug goes on the market, doctors will give them to their patients as tests. They have never really tested these drugs on people, yet still give them to you.

Nitroglycerin can cause many problems including heart pain. If you have high cholesterol then you need to stop eating animal fat. You won't have high cholesterol if you don't eat this. Cholesterol in some levels is healthy. There is good cholesterol and bad cholesterol. The complexity of the body is actually very simple to maintain. If you had to sit here and remember to breath, some of you would forget and die. The body knows what to do. If you have chest pain and heart pain it is because the body is not getting the good nutrients to build good new cells. You also need to exercise and drink lots of water and get sunlight. You need to remove all harmful chemicals from your diet. You also need fresh air. Proper rest at the proper time of the night is also vital.

Trust nature. Nature is the way to health. A quick fix is not the answer. Your attitude makes a huge difference on your health. If you are unhappy, you will inevitably get sick. You need to have joy in your life. Happiness is momentary, but joy is lifelong.

*Joy is*

*Lifelong*

# Chapter 5

## Facts That May Make You Think

### General Information

The American Medical Association concluded in a recent study that the suicide rate for the USA's 461,000 physicians is at least double – and maybe triple – the national suicide rate of 12.7 per 100,000 people.

Suicide rates for dentists and psychiatrists are even higher, reports medical anthropologist John-Henry Pfifferling, co-director of the Center for the Well-Being of Health Professionals in Durham, North Carolina. Pfifferling estimates that as many as 15% of the nation's doctors may suffer from alcohol or drug abuse, which often impairs their practice.

Part of the problem, he says, is that health professionals – and physicians especially —face tremendous stresses trying to "maintain a façade of superiority." Copyright, USA TODAY, Mar 3, 1984. -- (Printed with permission)

Chicago Tribune – July 17, 1987 Reports Say Diagnostic Errors Can Be Fatal

The article states that one out of ten hospital deaths may be caused by misdiagnosed diseases that could have been treated, an autopsy study involving 32 hospitals around the country has disclosed. The author of the article concludes that in some small hospitals, the rate of unnecessary deaths from erroneous diagnoses may be more than one in five, the study found.

The report states the autopsies, which are conducted to discover the cause of death and the nature of disease, showed that overall there was a major discrepancy between the diagnoses before death and the autopsy findings afterwards in 34%of the cases.

Dr. Robert Anderson, a member of the study team and chief of pathology at the University of New Mexico Medical School says "These are serious discrepancies." The findings are reported in the current issue of the Journal of the American Medical Association.

"Even more significant is that more than 10 percent of all autopsies showed that a better diagnosis may have resulted in a better outcome," he said in a telephone interview. "If the correct diagnosis had been made before death and the appropriate treatment instituted, the patient would be alive"

The study also shows that the most commonly misdiagnosed disorder was blood clots in the lungs, followed by infections and bleeding. Typical examples include diagnosing diverticulitis, a treatable bowel infection, as an inoperable tumor or misdiagnosing a lung blood clot as a heart attack.

Dr. George Lundberg, Journal editor, said "The findings point out a serious crisis in quality assurance in medicine caused by a dramatic decline in autopsies, which has fallen bellow 5 percent in some hospitals."

"I'm very concerned about the quality of care of any hospital with a very low autopsy rate," he said, "Less than 20 percent is low and less than 5 percent is abysmally low." So says Dr. George Lundberg

"They are missing diagnoses often and they don't even seem to care. How can they possibly be interested in quality when they aren't assessing the quality of care given to the people who die – their sickest people?"

The study findings, which include 2,067 autopsies, showed that small community hospitals, which tend to perform the fewest autopsies, had the highest rates of diagnostic errors while university hospitals, which do the most autopsies, had the lowest error rate. You see that there are a lot of ways to manipulate statistics.

Anderson said: among two small hospitals in the study that had fewer than 249 beds, there were 71 major diagnostic errors, which meant that as many as 24 percent of the people who died in those hospitals may have had their lives prolonged with a proper diagnosis and subsequent treatment.

Among five large university hospitals, on the other hand 23% of the cases were misdiagnosed, which means that only 8% of the deaths may have been unnecessary, claims Anderson.

"The findings are saying that medicine is an inexact science and that we physicians tend to forget that" he said.

Autopsies have traditionally served as the last word in determining the cause of death, and the chief means of allowing doctors to learn form their mistakes. But the medical profession has turned away from autopsies in the last two decades, he said. And we all can see why.

"This is an issue that is a societal concern, not just a medical concern," Anderson said. "We spend billions of dollars on trying to keep accurate records on what kinds of illnesses people have and why they die. Obviously if you don't know these records are recording information that's not very good."

Anderson is convinced that one of the prime reasons for the near demise of the autopsy is modern medical technology. Such things as CAT scanners and magnetic resonance imaging are seen by many doctors as a replacement for the diagnostic accuracy of autopsies, but they only exchange one type of error for another.

The AMA's Council of Scientific Affairs came to the same conclusion, and is saying: "With the introduction of new technology, the types of errors in diagnosis have shifted but mistakes continue, practically in complex cases."

One could also conclude that the other reasons for the decline of the autopsy are costs, de-emphasis in medical school and fear of malpractice suits, Anderson said. Many experts also place a significant share of the blame on the Joint Commission of Accreditation of Hospitals that dropped its recommendation that all hospitals perform a minimum of 20 to 25 % autopsies in 1970.

Common sense tells us that there is no way a physician can be right 100 percent of the time. We need the information on disease and the cause of death, and at the moment we are burying much of that information underground.

The Tribune article also stated that in Chicago, autopsies plummeted from a high of 51 percent of all hospital deaths in 1965 to 17 percent last year. The figures are similar for the country. Of 83 hospitals in the Chicago area, 57 of them had an autopsy rate of less than 20 percent in recent years. Of these, 37 had autopsy rates below 10 percent and eight were under 5 percent.

"The hospitals that need to be worried about it the most are the ones that have an autopsy rate under 5% and maybe the ones under 10%," Lundberg said. "It has to make one worry about how much they care about what kind of job they are doing."

Rightfully fearing that autopsies have been abandoned as a quality control measure, the AMA's policy-making House of Delegates last December called for new programs to promote an increase in the use of autopsies and it endorsed the efforts of the Institute of Medicine to establish a national autopsy policy.

**Interesting medical facts:**

**Prozac**
- The use of Prozac is responsible for a loss of 60% of all serotonin receptors in the brain. An animal experiment showed this clearly.
- Anti -acid drugs cause massive damage.
- Xanax and Zoloft cause all symptoms of depression, they do not cure it. Antibiotics can do the same thing.
- Prozac does nothing but prolong the existence of serotonin in the body.

- Prozac has 575 known side effects. This did not include suicide.
- Before Prozac was approved for use by the FDA there were 76 cases of death that were not reported to the FDA.
- The FDA has 1,800 suicides recorded from Prozac and 1,300 deaths registered.
- Only 1% of all side effects that occur are actually reported to the FDA. This means that 2,800 complaints times 100 is 280,000 side effects or complaints that really exists for Prozac.
- In the Physicians Desk Reference the known side effects of Prozac are anxiety, nervousness, tremor, dizziness, heart attacks, personality disorders, cardiac arrest, delusion, coma, etc.
- Medication causes anxiety, high blood pressure and depression.
- Heart medication can cause depression.

**Stress**
- Asthma is not a disease it is a symptom of dehydration usually caused by stress. Asthma can also stunt the growth process in children.
- Chronic fatigue, a shortened attention span, depression, irritability and feelings of rejection are also symptoms of dehydration caused by stress and/or water and salt deficiencies. The body needs to be lightly alkaline to be healthy.
- Stress causes lack of oxygen, water and nutrition.
- Most back pain is caused by stress.
- Stress causes dehydration which prevents water replacement with leads to toxemia and acidosis in the body.
- Diabetes can be caused by chronic dehydration.

- Stress is a dehydrating state in the body and instead of treating it with stress reduction and water we treat it with dangerous drugs.
- The only way to concur or eliminate stress in certain parts of your life depends on a stable self-confidence and self-esteem based on your own individual value system with a strong instinct-based decision making process. You need to value your life. Stress can only be conquered by the person themselves.

## Dehydration

- Sixty percent of illnesses could be cured with stress reduction and water consumption.
- Water is needed for hydroelectricity. The neurotransmitters in the body can only be transmitted properly if there is enough water.
- Calcium and water make energy. If there is no water it releases more and more calcium from the bones and will cause osteoporosis.
- Proven DNA damage has been shown from dehydration.
- A good way to tell how acidic you are is to look at your urine; the more yellow it is the more acidic you are.
- Dehydration makes the system acidic.
- Dehydration can mimic symptoms of other illnesses.
- Dehydration causes degenerative diseases such as cancer.
- The hydration of cells goes down from 1.1 to 0.8 between the ages of 20-70.
- Aging is the dehydration of cells.
- Treating hypertension with diuretics is a crime.
- The reverse osmosis system is the filter system of the body.
- The heart will try to compensate for the lack of water pressure with higher blood pressure in the system.

- We have two water oceans in our bodies that need to remain under the same pressure inside and outside the cell. If there is not enough pressure the blood pressure will go up.
- Dehydration can be caused by stress and can lead to depression. Three glasses of water and a good 20 minutes of relaxation can do wonders for your stress level.
- Water and nutritional deficiencies can lead to depression, schizophrenia and suicidal thoughts. They are caused by stress.
- If you have to drink tap water you should let it sit for 30 minutes to let the chlorine disappear.

## Dehydration and Stress

- The body is 75% water and the brain is 85% water.
- Allergies are also caused by stress which caused dehydration and water management disorders caused by histamines.
- Asthma is not a disease it is a symptom of dehydration and is based on stress.
- 17 million people in America suffer from asthma.
- Strokes and heart attacks are caused by dehydration which is caused by stress.
- Joint pain is caused by dehydration. There are two bags of water surrounding the joint, if they are dried out this causes pain and damage.
- Obesity and back problems can, in many cases, be fixed with rest and water.
- The body produces histamines when it feels dehydrated.
- Constipation is caused by dehydration. Usually two glasses of water will fix this.
- Heart burn is a side effect of dehydration. You can usually cure this with a lot of water, salt and rest.

- Allergies, asthma, back pain, obesity, head aches, Alzheimer's, strokes, arthritis and migraines can all be caused by dehydration and stress.
- Dehydration causes stress or fight or flight hormones. This has a distinctive effect on the immune system.
- Lack of water can also cause ulcers.
- Our neurotransmitters in our brains are depended on water because they won't move without water. If the brain is dehydrated the neurotransmitter will not move properly.
- Stress leads to anxiety, depression and suicide as well as every kind of illness.
- Asthma often leads to depression and suicide.
- Fibromyalgia is caused by stress, because the stress causes dehydration in the muscles and leads to a deficiency of oxygen.
- Chronic fatigue syndrome is caused by stress.
- Stress causes dehydration, dehydration causes stress; it is a vicious cycle.
- Water and nutritional deficiencies can lead to depression, schizophrenia and suicidal thoughts. They are caused by stress.

## Other Techniques
- Hypnotism is nothing more than brain washing. It never addresses the cause of the problem.
- Positive thinking kills people. Only people that use positive action combined with positive thinking will survive. Many people believe if they just think positive thoughts everything will turn out fine. But that is the furthest from the truth – positive thinking without positive action is guaranteed death.

## Artificial Sweeteners
- Artificial sweeteners are a major danger. Obviously, the FDA doesn't care.

161

**Alternative Therapies**
- Meditation often leads to passivity and never helps to heal the causes of life stresses.
- Clearing your mind does not fix a bad lifestyle.

**Serotonin**
- The side effect of <u>stress is a lack of Serotonin</u> because stress causes a <u>lack in vitamin B6 and zinc.</u> <u>Vitamin B6 leads to the production of serotonin</u> by removing the acid in triptophan.
- During the <u>day serotonin</u> controls all the functions of the human body and at night transforms into <u>melatonin.</u>
- <u>B6</u> and <u>zinc</u> are very important for <u>brain functions.</u>
- <u>Serotonin stabilizes calcium in the body.</u>
- <u>Serotonin and histamines</u> are responsible for <u>water functions</u> and water is important for every function in the body.

**Water**
- When <u>water enters the cell</u> it produces <u>electricity</u> (energy) which has to be stored in the cell.

**Water/Histamines**
- <u>Histamines</u> are responsible for <u>building the embryo.</u>
- Histamines are the water and immune system organizers.

**Lifestyle**
- A <u>positive</u> <u>attitude</u> has been scientifically proven to <u>enhance your immune system and functions.</u> It can keep you from getting sick.
- <u>Loud</u> <u>noises</u> are bad for our immune system. We are born with <u>two fears.</u> The fear of falling and the fear of loud noises.
- <u>Loud</u> <u>music</u> causes negative emotions like <u>anger</u> and hate.

- The best stress reduction is to find your own values and live by them.
- Learn to listen to your instincts. Depression is not caused by a chemical imbalance; a chemical imbalance is caused by stress and negative effects in your life.
- Let go of your past. *Yes*
- Let go and move on, you don't need psychotherapy or a psychiatrist.
- Feelings of helplessness and hopelessness will disappear as soon as you start to feel better about yourself.
- Exercising once a day can do a lot for your stress level and improves your immune system.
- Get sunlight because it produces vitamin D and is good for your stress level.
- Sixty percent of all health care costs could be avoided if we use our common sense.
- Exercising stimulates brain function.

## Medical
- Only 1% of all articles in medical journals are based on sound science.
- The FDA said that a mammography is not any more accurate than a diagnosis by a trained surgeon.

## Self Healing
- When people start to forgive themselves the healing process can begin.
- Rest and restful sleep is vital for your revitalization process.

## American Cancer Society
- Of all the money that the American Cancer Society receives, 61% pays employees. Less than 5% actually goes to the patients themselves.

- Remember that the <u>American Cancer Society</u> has to <u>close</u> the <u>day that a cure for cancer is found.</u>

## Drugs

- The leading <u>health problem</u> in the <u>U.S.</u> is <u>clinical depression</u> and feelings of <u>helplessness</u> and <u>hopelessness.</u>
- <u>Prescription drugs</u> are <u>harder to withdraw</u> from than <u>street drugs.</u>
- <u>Kids</u> get their <u>drugs</u> on the <u>streets</u> and <u>parents</u> get their <u>drugs</u> form their <u>doctor.</u>
- The <u>word pharmacy</u> comes from the Greek root word pharmacia, <u>which means sorcery</u> or <u>witchcraft.</u> The word <u>pharmacist</u> means <u>poisoner.</u>
- <u>Doctors</u> are only <u>taught</u> to <u>treat illnesses with drugs.</u>
- <u>Suicide</u> and <u>murder</u> is a <u>side effect</u> of people who are treated with <u>drugs for depression.</u>

## Mental Illness

- <u>Anxiety</u> and <u>depression</u> are an <u>epidemic</u> in the U.S.
- There are more hospitals in the U.S. that treat mental illnesses than there are that treat physical illnesses.
- Most people with depression are treated by a regular M.D. instead of a psychiatrist.
- <u>Depression</u> <u>means</u> <u>fear</u> and <u>knowing what you are afraid of.</u>
- <u>Anxiety means fear without knowing what you are afraid of.</u>

## Sugar

- <u>Hypoglycemia</u> has the <u>same symptoms</u> as <u>depression</u>
- Hypoglycemia causes memory loss and Alzheimer's, caused by stress.

## Diet

- Fluoride causes stiffness and pre- aging.
- Milk is indigestible because it has way too high of a protein level which is not digestible for us.
- One of the strongest glues (Elmer's glue) in the world is made from cow's milk.
- If you do not eat right or drink enough water you will not be able to think clearly.
- MSG the taste enhancer is a cyto-toxin and can lead to Parkinson's disease and seizures.
- Cooked food is dead, worthless and even toxic and acidic if it is heated over 107 degrees.
- Alcohol causes massive dehydration. Anyone who has experienced a hangover can testify to this.
- The normal American needs 40 grams of protein a day yet they eat 114 grams a day. The excess is stored as fat in the joints.
- Meat and poultry are full of drugs. They are allowed to put 1,000 different drugs into what you eat.
- This doesn't include the pesticides that are present.
- Sometimes the animals are fed dead animals. This means you are eating a diseased animal.
- The antibiotics in the animals will cause you to build up a tolerance to antibiotics that is unnecessary.
- Animals produce stress hormones when they are killed and we are eating them and being affected by them.
- This is why meat eating usually stimulates the human body.
- Smoking has the neurotoxin nicotine.
- Suicide can be caused by diet.
- Have four liters of water and half a teaspoon of salt once a day.
- Salt is vital to bone structure. A lack of salt can cause osteoporosis.
- Water loss due to exhaling can constrict the bronchioles and can lead to bronchitis.

- Stress causes acidosis and toxemia which is the cause of most illnesses. The dehydration caused by stress shuts down the metabolism and the digestive system.
- Water makes the mucus in the stomach thicker and prevents ulcers.
- Water makes it possible for the cells to stick together.
- Imagine a grape or a raisin.
- Aspartame causes brain tumors, seizures, damages your smell and your vision. It also can affect your thinking.
- Drink a huge glass of water a half an hour before you eat.
- You need enough liquid for optimum digestion.

## Allergies
- Lack of water produces histamines. Water and salt are the best histamines.

## Health
- The ph should be between 7.1 and 7.3 in the blood and 7.36 in the body.
- We live in a sick care instead of a health care world.

## Salt
- Salt is needed for the body to be able to absorb minerals.
- There are 82 elements in sea salt.

## Caffeine
- Caffeine is the bad habit glue.
- Coffee drinkers drink a lethal dose of caffeine in one day. Caffeine is a diuretic.

## Cholesterol
- Cholesterol lowering medications cause damage.

## Cancer and Other Diseases

- A biopsy can spread cancer into the entire body in some cases.
- The trauma of surgery can spread cancer throughout the entire body.
- There is a huge danger with anesthetics.
- Chemotherapy and radiation cause cancer.
- Mammograms damage the heart.
- Each mammography heightens your chance of cancer by 2%.
- Science is greedy and corrupt. yes
- Double blind studies are fraudulent because they are looking for the answer they want.
- Pharmaceutical companies train our doctors. It started with Rockefeller.
- Silicone breast implants have a serious negative effect on the immune system.
- The Aborigines have a medicine doctor who can point a bone and the person will die. Very often our medical doctors do the exact same thing when they tell patients how long they have to live.
- Patients who like their doctors die.
- Genes do not make you suicidal or more prone to illness.
- The leading cause of death is from the side effects of prescription drugs.
- It is not proven that drugs can cure, however they do suppress symptoms.
- Most of all drugs will never address the cause of any illness.
- Lifestyle, diet, stress levels, breathing, water, success and exercise are the major components for health.
- Body builders believe that protein is the key to their success. This is false, the acids and hormones in the meat can be very damaging. One million Americans die each year from heart disease.

167

- Two components affect <u>health:</u> ph<u>ysical</u> condition and <u>stress levels.</u>
- <u>Cancer</u> takes <u>years to grow</u> so don't be <u>rushed</u> into <u>surgery</u>.
- <u>Radiation</u> and <u>chemotherapy</u> cause <u>cancer</u>.
- I am sure that every doctor wants to help you but they are not taught to do so.
- <u>Doctors</u> even <u>admit</u> that they <u>do not know the cause of cancer</u>. They say that the cause of cancer is atrophied and mutated cells. These are the <u>symptoms</u> not the cause of cancer.
- <u>Doctors</u> will <u>lose</u> their <u>license</u> if they don't treat a cancer patient with surgery, chemotherapy or radiation. This is a law in California and maybe some other states by now.
- Radiation leads to disorientation, damaged skin and lethargy.
- <u>Cancer patients</u> <u>don't survive because</u> of radiation and chemotherapy; they <u>survive in spite of it.</u>
- <u>Cancer</u> is caused by a <u>compromised immune system</u>. <u>Chemotherapy kills</u> your organs and your <u>immune system</u>.
- <u>Lymph nodes</u> are the <u>filter system</u> for <u>cancer</u>. If they fight the cancer they are <u>protecting</u> the cancer <u>from spreading</u>.
- <u>Every illness</u> is caused by a <u>compromised immune system</u>. Most of these cancer <u>treatments compromise</u> the <u>immune system</u> even more.
- <u>Chemotherapy suppresses</u> the bone marrow functions and causes <u>severe pain</u> and <u>discomfort</u>. It also <u>poisons normal healthy cells.</u>
- Some <u>patients</u> have such dramatic reactions that they will start to <u>vomit</u> even if they just <u>see the nurse.</u>
- Every <u>doctor</u> advises you to <u>avoid radiation,</u> but <u>when you have cancer</u> they want to <u>fill you with radiation.</u>

- Chemotherapy causes bleeding, cardiac arrest, loss of reflexes, fertility problems and many more lasting problems because the immune system does not work anymore. You are vulnerable to everything.
- Most of the time the doctor will give you more medications to suppress the side effects of the chemotherapy; these drugs also have side effects.
- Doctors are 9,000 times more likely to cause accidental deaths than gun owners.
- Too much protein in the diet can cause osteoporosis.
- Treating eye problems with laser surgery can lead to blindness.
- To perform a bone marrow transplant they have to kill the immune system first.
- Arthritis is usually caused by nutritional deficiencies; however it is treated with drugs that have horrible side effects.
- Food additives are usually all toxic.
- Estrogen therapy can cause breast cancer.
- Protein causes acidosis.
- Diabetes type one is caused by milk.
- Diabetes type two can be fixed with the correction of the diet.
- Hypoglycemia is caused by too much sugar.
- Allergies are caused by dehydration and milk.
- You don't love your enemies and it is not worth your emotions to hate them.
- Suppression of emotions is a major cause of death.
- Chemotherapy causes cancer, bleeding of the heart and in the urinary tract.
- Cancer is not caused by genes. What are passed down are bad habits and bad diets and lifestyles.
- How children handle stress is taught to them by their parents.
- Everything we do either makes us healthier or sicker.

- You can not get cancer unless your immune system is severely depressed.
- Silicone implants cause cancer or auto immune diseases.
- If your child has chickenpox would you cut off all the sores to treat your child? If you have an inflamed foot would you cut out the swollen lymph nodes in the groins?
- Many medicines can cause caner. High blood pressure medication can cause cancer.
- Stress suppresses the immune system and causes dehydration, anxiety, depression, panic attacks and nutritional problems.
- Stress suppresses the immune system.
- Only 15% of all medical advice you hear is scientifically based.
- Drugs only cover up symptoms; they don't cure or fix anything.
- Cholesterol is not bad.
- All drugs have side effects.
- Anger raises blood pressure and kills hormones.
- Many diseases are never as bad as the drugs the doctors give you.
- Many people die from the side effects of the drugs rather than from the disease itself.
- The AMA states that 65% of all cancer could be avoided by a change in diet and lifestyle.
- Cancer is not possible if the immune system is not stressed.
- All cancers are caused by an insufficient immune system, no matter what kind of cancer.
- Stress reduction, fresh juice and a lot of water, exercise, nutrition, salt and detoxification and self esteem are the main components of health.
- Cancer does not grow well in oxygen rich environments.

- Sun, sleep and exercise lower blood pressure.
- You can only repair and heal while you are asleep or in a deep relaxation state.
- Stress takes away the bodies ability to live happily and stay healthy.
- Milk causes an acidic environment in the body and leads to many problems.
- It causes juvenile diabetes and seizures.
- For four hours after you eat sugar your immune system is paralyzed.
- Drugs don't cure the disease; they relocate the disease and mask the symptoms.
- Stay away from tap water if you can. Fluoride is a side product of aluminum which causes Alzheimer's and can cause death in children.
- If they had a solution for cancer then why do famous and rich people die of cancer?
- Lack of oxygen causes cancer cells.
- No one can cure you! No drug, doctor, system or treatment. The only one that can cure you is you! Your own immune and self- healing system will cure you.

## The Meaning of Vitamins and Minerals

Vitamins can play a significant role in the battle against illness including cancer. Some vitamins even play a part in prevention of cancer. It has been proven that 83% of the population does not get enough minerals and vitamins in their diets.

## Some information about vitamins and minerals:
- People who have a high level of vitamins live longer.
- Smoking causes a shortage of vitamin-C.
- We need magnesium for changing nutrition into energy.
- When we have a shortage of magnesium the best nutrition is useless.

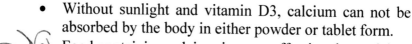
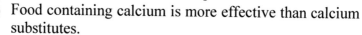

- Without sunlight and vitamin D3, calcium can not be absorbed by the body in either powder or tablet form.
- Food containing calcium is more effective than calcium substitutes.
- It is a fallacy that we can get our calcium from milk.
- The body needs twice the amount of calcium available in milk for its digestion.
- Vitamins should be fresh, so that they can be processed immediately by the body and are not made useless by preservatives.
- Vitamin C can destroy free radicals including cancer cells. We should take 12 grams as a measure of prevention every day.
- The amounts of minerals and vitamins advised by health agencies worldwide are the absolute minimum necessary for survival.
- We know that chromium is used in the building of muscle tissue and assists in breaking down the fat content of the body.
- With the aid of chromium the fat is broken down three times faster and the build up of muscle tissue is activated four times.
- Today our bodies are exposed to many outside hazards for which they are not intended. Our bodies have to cope with particles of pollution and preservatives, which are hard to process; therefore, we have to protect ourselves. Vitamin A, E and C and certain minerals like beta-carotene are necessary basic elements for continued health.

Get all the important information you need at www.instinctbasedmedicine.com

## Death by Traditional and So-called Modern Medicine

Something is wrong when regulatory agencies pretend that vitamins are dangerous, yet ignore published statistics showing that government-sanctioned medicine is the real hazard. Here are some facts:

The number of people having in-hospital, adverse reactions to prescribed drugs is estimated to be 2.2 million per year. The number of unnecessary antibiotics prescribed annually for viral infections is 20 million. The number of unnecessary medical and surgical procedures performed annually is 7.5 million. The number of people exposed to unnecessary hospitalization annually is 8.9 million.

The most stunning statistic is that the total number of deaths caused by conventional medicine is an astounding 783,936 per year. It is now evident that the American medical system is the leading cause of death and injury in the U.S. (By contrast, the number of deaths attributable to heart disease in 2001 was 699,697, while the number of deaths attributable to cancer was 553,251.[5])

The startling findings from a meticulous study by Garry Null ND and others indicate that conventional medicine is "the leading cause of death" in the United States.

Over 700,000 Americans die each year at the hands of government-sanctioned medicine, while the FDA and other government agencies pretend to protect the public by harassing those who offer safe alternatives.

A definitive review of medical peer-reviewed journals and government health statistics shows that American medicine frequently causes more harm than good.

Each year approximately 2.2 million U.S. hospital patients experience adverse drug reactions (ADRs) to prescribed medications. [1] In 1995, Dr. Richard Besser of the federal Centers for Disease Control and Prevention (CDC) estimated the number of unnecessary antibiotics prescribed annually for viral infections to be 20 million. In 2003, Dr. Besser spoke in terms of tens of millions of unnecessary antibiotics prescribed annually.[2, 2a] Approximately 7.5 million unnecessary medical and surgical procedures are performed annually in the U.S.,[3] while approximately 8.9 million Americans are hospitalized unnecessarily.[4]

As shown in the following table, the estimated total number of iatrogenic deaths—that is, deaths induced inadvertently by a physician or surgeon or by medical treatment or diagnostic procedures— in the U.S. annually is 783,936. It is evident that the American medical system is itself the leading cause of death and injury in the U.S. By comparison, approximately 699,697 Americans died of heart in 2001, while 553,251 died of cancer. (5)

Table 1: Estimated Annual Mortality and Economic Cost of Medical Intervention ( from " Death by Medicine " by Garry Null and others )

| Condition | Deaths | Cost | Author |
|---|---|---|---|
| Adverse Drug Reactions | 106,000 | $12 billion | Lazarou(1), Suh (49) |
| Medical error | 98,000 | $2 billion | IOM(6) |
| Bedsores | 115,000 | $55 billion | Xakellis(7), Barczak (8) |
| Infection | 88,000 | $5 billion | Weinstein(9), MMWR (10) |
| Malnutrition | 108,800 | ---------- | Nurses Coalition(11) |
| Outpatients | 199,000 | $77 billion | Starfield(12), Weingart(112) |
| Unnecessary Procedures | 37,136 | $122 billion | HCUP(3,13) |
| Surgery-Related | 32,000 | $9 billion | AHRQ(85) |
| Total | 783,936 | $282 billion | |

Using Leape's 1997 medical and drug error rate of 3 million[14] multiplied by the 14% fatality rate he used in 1994[16] produces an annual death rate of 420,000 for drug errors and medical errors combined. Using this number instead of Lazorou's 106,000 drug errors and the Institute of Medicine's (IOM) estimated 98,000 annual medical errors would add another 216,000 deaths, for a total of 999,936 deaths annually.

Table 2: Estimated Annual Mortality and Economic Cost of Medical Intervention ( from " Death by Medicine " by Garry Null and others )

| Condition | Deaths | Cost | Author |
|---|---|---|---|
| ADR/med error | 420,000 | $200 billion | Leape[14] |
| Bedsores | 115,000 | $55 billion | Xakellis[7], Barczak [8] |
| Infection | 88,000 | $5 billion | Weinstein[9], MMWR [10] |
| Malnutrition | 108,800 | ----------- | Nurses Coalition[11] |
| Outpatients | 199,000 | $77 billion | Starfield[12], Weingart[112] |
| Unnecessary Procedures | 37,136 | $122 billion | HCUP[3,13] |
| Surgery-Related | 32,000 | $9 billion | AHRQ[85] |
| Total | 999,936 | | |

The enumerating of unnecessary medical events is very important in our analysis. Any invasive, unnecessary medical procedure must be considered as part of the larger iatrogenic picture. Unfortunately, cause and effect go unmonitored. The figures on unnecessary events represent people who are thrust into a dangerous health care system. Each of these 16.4 million lives is being affected in ways that could have fatal consequences. Simply entering a hospital could result in the following:

In 16.4 million people, a 2.1% chance (affecting 186,000) of a serious adverse drug reaction[1]

In 16.4 million people, a 5-6% chance (affecting 489,500) of acquiring a nosocomial infection[9]

In 16.4 million people, a 4-36% chance (affecting 1.78 million) of having an iatrogenic injury (medical error and adverse drug reactions).[16]

In 16.4 million people, a 17% chance (affecting 1.3 million) of a procedure error.[40]

These statistics represent a one-year time span. Working with the most conservative figures from our statistics, we project the following 10-year death rates.

Table 3: Estimated 10-Year Death Rates from Medical Intervention ( from " Death by Medicine " by Garry Null and others )

| Condition | 10-Year Deaths | Author |
|---|---|---|
| Adverse Drug Reaction | 1.06 million | (1) |
| Medical error | 0.98 million | (6) |
| Bedsores | 1.15 million | (7,8) |
| Nosocomial Infection | 0.88 million | (9,10) |
| Malnutrition | 1.09 million | (11) |
| Outpatients | 1.99 million | (12, 112) |
| Unnecessary Procedures | 371,360 | (3,13) |
| Surgery-related | 320,000 | (85) |
| Total | 7,841,360 | |

Our estimated 10-year total of 7.8 million iatrogenic deaths is more than all the casualties from all the wars fought by the U.S. throughout its entire history.

Our projected figures for unnecessary medical events occurring over a 10-year period also are dramatic.

Table 4: Estimated 10-Year Unnecessary Medical Events ( from " Death by Medicine " by Garry Null and others )

| Unnecessary Events | 10-year Number | Iatrogenic Events |
|---|---|---|
| Hospitalization | 89 million[4] | 17 million |
| Procedures | 75 million[3] | 15 million |
| Total | 164 million | |

These figures show that an estimated 164 million people—more than half of the total U.S. population—will receive unneeded medical treatment over the course of a decade.

**Is Medicine as We Know It Working?**

U.S. health care spending reached $1.6 trillion in 2003, representing 14% of the nation's gross national product

Medicine is not taking into consideration the following critically important aspects of a healthy human organism: (a) stress and how it adversely affects the immune system and life processes; (b) insufficient exercise; (c) excessive caloric intake; (d) highly processed and denatured foods grown in denatured and chemically damaged soil; and (e) exposure to tens of thousands of environmental toxins. Instead of minimizing these disease-causing factors, we cause more illness through medical technology, diagnostic testing, overuse of medical and surgical procedures, and overuse of pharmaceutical drugs. The huge disservice of this therapeutic strategy is the result of little effort or money being spent on preventing disease.

## Underreporting of Iatrogenic Events

For example, a 2003 study found that nearly half of medical school faculty who serve on institutional review boards (IRB) to advise on clinical trial research also serve as consultants to the pharmaceutical industry As few as 5% and no more than 20% of iatrogenic acts are ever reported

## Medical Ethics and Conflict of Interest in Scientific Medicine

According to an ABC News report, pharmaceutical companies spend over $2 billion a year on over 314,000 events attended by doctors.

The ABC News report also noted that a survey of clinical trials revealed that when a drug company funds a study, there is a 90% chance that the drug will be perceived as effective whereas a non-drug-company-funded study will show favorable results only 50% of the time. It appears that money can't buy you love but it can buy any "scientific" result desired.

Cynthia Crossen, a staffer for the *Wall Street Journal*, in 1996 published *Tainted Truth: The Manipulation of Fact in America*, a book about the widespread practice of lying with statistics.(22) Commenting on the state of scientific research, she wrote: "The road to hell was paved with the flood of corporate research dollars that eagerly filled gaps left by slashed government research funding." Her data on financial involvement showed that in 1981 the drug industry "gave" $292 million to colleges and universities for research. By 1991, this figure had risen to $2.1 billion.

## The First Iatrogenic Study

Dr. Lucian L. Leape opened medicine's Pandora's box in his 1994 paper, "Error in Medicine," which appeared in the *Journal of the American Medical Association* (JAMA).(16) He found that Schimmel reported in 1964 that 20% of hospital patients suffered iatrogenic injury, with a 20% fatality rate. In 1981 Steel reported that 36% of hospitalized patients experienced iatrogenesis with a 25% fatality rate, and adverse drug reactions were involved in 50% of the injuries. In 1991, Bedell reported that 64% of acute heart attacks in one hospital were preventable and were mostly due to adverse drug reactions.

Leape focused on the "Harvard Medical Practice Study" published in 1991, (16a) which found a 4% iatrogenic injury rate for patients, with a 14% fatality rate, in 1984 in New York State. From the 98,609 patients injured and the 14% fatality rate, he estimated that in the entire U.S. 180,000 people die each year partly as a result of iatrogenic injury.

Why Leape chose to use the much lower figure of 4% injury for his analysis remains in question. Using instead the average of the rates found in the three studies he cites (36%, 20%, and 4%) would have produced a 20% medical error rate. Leape acknowledged that the literature on medical errors is sparse and represents only the tip of the iceberg, noting that when errors are specifically sought out, reported rates are "distressingly high." He cited several autopsy studies with rates as high as 35-40% of missed diagnoses causing death. He also noted that an intensive care unit reported an average of 1.7 errors per day per patient, and 29% of those errors were potentially serious or fatal.

In 1995, a JAMA report noted, "Over a million patients are injured in U.S. hospitals each year, and approximately 280,000 die annually as a result of these injuries. Therefore, the iatrogenic death rate dwarfs the annual automobile accident mortality rate of 45,000 and accounts for more deaths than all other accidents combined

The survey found that more than 100 million Americans have been affected directly or indirectly by a medical mistake. Forty-two percent were affected directly and 84% personally knew of someone who had experienced a medical mistake

At this press conference, Leape updated his 1994 statistics, noting that as of 1997, medical errors in inpatient hospital settings nationwide could be as high as 3 million and could cost as much as $200 billion. Leape used a 14% fatality rate to determine a medical error death rate of 180,000 in 1994.(16) In 1997, using Leape's base number of 3 million errors, the annual death rate could be as high as 420,000 for hospital inpatients alone.

If hospitals admitted to the actual number of errors for which they are responsible, which is about 20 times what is reported, they would come under intense scrutiny.(32) Jerry Phillips, associate director of the FDA's Office of Post Marketing Drug Risk Assessment, confirms this number. "In the broader area of adverse drug reaction data, the 250,000 reports received annually probably represent only 5% of the actual reactions that occur."(33) Dr. Jay Cohen, who has extensively researched adverse drug reactions, notes that because only 5% of adverse drug reactions are reported, there are in fact 5 million medication reactions each year

## Public Suggestions on Iatrogenesis

In a telephone survey, 1,207 adults ranked the effectiveness of the following measures in reducing preventable medical errors that result in serious harm. (36) (Following each measure is the percentage of respondents who ranked the measure as "very effective.")

- giving doctors more time to spend with patients (78%)
- requiring hospitals to develop systems to avoid medical errors (74%)
- better training of health professionals (73%)
- using only doctors specially trained in intensive care medicine on intensive care units (73%)
- requiring hospitals to report all serious medical errors to a state agency (71%)
- increasing the number of hospital nurses (69%)
- reducing the work hours of doctors in training to avoid fatigue (66%)
- encouraging hospitals to voluntarily report serious medical errors to a state agency (62%).

## Drug Iatrogenesis

Prescription drugs constitute the major treatment modality of scientific medicine. With the discovery of the "germ theory," medical scientists convinced the public that infectious organisms were the cause of illness. Finding the "cure" for these infections proved much harder than anyone imagined. From the beginning, chemical drugs promised much more than they delivered. But far beyond not working, the drugs also caused incalculable side effects. The drugs themselves, even when properly prescribed, have side effects that can be fatal, as Lazarou's study (1) showed. Human error can make the situation even worse.

## Medication Errors

A survey of a 1992 national pharmacy database found a total of 429,827 medication errors from 1,081 hospitals. Medication errors occurred in 5.22% of patients admitted to these hospitals each year. The authors concluded that at least 90,895 patients annually were harmed by medication errors in the U.S. as a whole.(37)

A 2002 study shows that 20% of hospital medications for patients had dosage errors. Nearly 40% of these errors were considered potentially harmful to the patient. In a typical 300-patient hospital, the number of errors per day was 40.(38)

Problems involving patients' medications were even higher the following year. The error rate intercepted by pharmacists in this study was 24%, making the potential minimum number of patients harmed by prescription drugs 417,908.

## Adverse Drug Reactions

In a *New England Journal of Medicine* study, an alarming one in four patients suffered observable side effects from the more than 3.34 billion prescription drugs filled in 2002.

Reuters also reported that prior research has suggested that nearly 5% of hospital admissions (over 1 million per year) are the result of drug side effects.

## How Do We Know Drugs Are Safe?

In one very telling report, the federal government's General Accounting Office "found that of the 198 drugs approved by the FDA between 1976 and 1985... 102 (or 51.5%) had serious post-approval risks... the serious post-approval risks (included) heart failure, myocardial infarction, anaphylaxis, respiratory depression and arrest, seizures, kidney and liver failure, severe blood disorders, birth defects and fetal toxicity, and blindness

The leading causes of adverse drug reactions are antibiotics (17%), cardiovascular drugs (17%), chemotherapy (15%), and analgesics and anti-inflammatory agents.

## The Problem with Antibiotics

The CDC warns that 90% of upper respiratory infections, including children's ear infections, are viral and that antibiotics do not treat viral infection. More than 40% of about 50 million prescriptions for antibiotics written each year in physicians' offices are inappropriate.(2) Using antibiotics when not needed can lead to the development of deadly strains of bacteria that are resistant to drugs and cause more than 88,000 deaths due to hospital-acquired infections.

## Drug Companies Fined

In May 2002, *The Washington Post* reported that Schering-Plough Corp., the maker of Claritin, was to pay a $500 million dollar fine to the FDA for quality-control problems at four of its factories

## Unnecessary Surgical Procedures

In 1974, 2.4 million unnecessary surgeries were performed, resulting in 11,900 deaths at a cost of $3.9 billion.(73,74) In 2001, 7.5 million unnecessary surgical procedures were performed, resulting in 37,136 deaths at a cost of $122 billion (using 1974 dollars).

In 1974, the Congressional Committee on Interstate and Foreign Commerce held hearings on unnecessary surgery. It found that 17.6% of recommendations for surgery were not confirmed by a second opinion. The House Subcommittee on Oversight and Investigations extrapolated these figures and estimated that, on a nationwide basis, there were 2.4 million unnecessary surgeries performed annually, resulting in 11,900 deaths at an annual cost of $3.9 billion.

Testifying before the Department of Veterans Affairs, they estimated that of the 250,000 back surgeries performed annually in the U.S. at a hospital cost of $11,000 per patient, the total number of unnecessary back surgeries approaches 44,000, costing as much as $484 million.

A 1987 JAMA study found the following significant levels of inappropriate surgery: 17% of coronary angiography procedures, 32% of carotid endarterectomy procedures, and 17% of upper gastrointestinal tract endoscopy procedures.(82) Based on the Healthcare Cost and Utilization Project (HCUP) statistics provided by the government for 2001, 697,675 upper gastrointestinal endoscopies (usually entailing biopsy) were performed, as were 142,401 endarterectomies and 719,949 coronary angiographies.(13) Extrapolating the JAMA study's inappropriate surgery rates to 2001 produces 118,604 unnecessary endoscopy procedures, 45,568 unnecessary endarterectomies, and 122,391 unnecessary coronary angiographies. These are all forms of medical iatrogenesis.

## Medical and Surgical Procedures

Unfortunately, allopathic medicine itself is a leading cause of death, as well as the most expensive way to die. A 1998

JAMA study[1] estimated an average of 106,000 prescription medication deaths per year.

## Surgical Errors Finally Reported

An October 2003 JAMA study from the U.S. government's Agency for Healthcare Research and Quality (AHRQ) documented 32,000 mostly surgery-related deaths costing $9 billion and accounting for 2.4 million extra hospital days in 2000.[85] Data from 20% of the nation's hospitals were analyzed for 18 different surgical complications, including postoperative infections, foreign objects left in wounds, surgical wounds reopening, and post-operative bleeding.

## Unnecessary X-Rays

A study of 700,000 children born between 1947 and 1964 in 37 major maternity hospitals compared the children of mothers who had received pelvic x-rays during pregnancy to those of mothers who did not. It found that cancer mortality was 40% higher among children whose mothers had been x-rayed.

The risk for lifetime fatal cancer due to radiation exposure is estimated to be four in one million per 1,000.

Gofman provides strong evidence that medical technology—specifically x-rays, CT scans, and mammography and fluoroscopy devices—are a contributing factor to 75% of new cancers. In a nearly 700-page report updated in 2000, "Radiation from Medical Procedures in the Pathogenesis of Cancer and Ischemic Heart Disease: Dose-Response Studies with Physicians per 100,000 Population," [90] Gofman shows that as the number of physicians increases in a geographical area along with an increase in the number of x-ray diagnostic tests performed, the rate of cancer and ischemic heart disease also increases. Gofman elaborates that it is not x-rays alone that cause the damage but a combination of health risk factors that include poor diet, smoking, abortions, and the use of birth control pills. Dr. Gofman predicts that ionizing radiation will be responsible for 100 million premature deaths over the next decade.

In his book, "Preventing Breast Cancer," Dr. Gofman notes that breast cancer is the leading cause of death among American women between the ages of 44 and 55. Because breast tissue is highly sensitive to radiation, mammograms can cause cancer

Even x-rays for back pain can lead someone into crippling surgery. Dr. John E. Sarno, a well-known New York orthopedic surgeon, found that there is not necessarily any association between back pain and spinal x-ray abnormality. He cites studies of normal people without a trace of back pain whose x-rays indicate spinal abnormalities and of people with back pain whose spines appear to be normal on x-ray.[92] People who happen to have back pain and show an abnormality on x-ray may be treated surgically, sometimes with no change in back pain, worsening of back pain, or even permanent disability.

## Unnecessary Hospitalization

Nearly 9 million (8,925,033) people were hospitalized unnecessarily in 2001.

Thirty-four percent of all hospital days were deemed inappropriate and could have been avoided.[93] The rate of inappropriate hospital admissions in 1990 was 23.5%.[94] In 1999, another study also found an inappropriate admissions rate of 24%, indicating a consistent pattern from 1986 to 1999.[95] The HCUP database indicates that the total number of patient discharges from U.S. hospitals in 2001 was 37,187,641,[13] meaning that almost 9 million people were exposed to unnecessary medical intervention in hospitals and therefore represent almost 9 million potential iatrogenic episodes.

## Women's Experience in Medicine

According to Dr. Adriane Fugh-Berman, U.S. medicine has a tradition of excessive medical and surgical interventions on women. Fugh-Berman notes that U.S. doctors eventually disabused themselves of that notion but have continued to treat women very differently than they treat men.(97) She cites the following statistics:

- Thousands of prophylactic mastectomies are performed annually.
- One-third of US women have had a hysterectomy before menopause.
- Women are prescribed drugs more frequently than are men.
- Women are given potent drugs for disease prevention, which results in disease substitution due to side effects.
- Fetal monitoring is unsupported by studies and not recommended by the CDC.(98) It confines women to a hospital bed and may result in a higher incidence of cesarean section.(99)
- Normal processes such as menopause and childbirth have been heavily "medicalized."
- Synthetic hormone replacement therapy (HRT) does not prevent heart disease or dementia, but does increase the risk of breast cancer, heart disease, stroke, and gall bladder attack

## Cesarean Section

In 2001, a cesarean section is still the most common OB/GYN surgical procedure. Approximately 4 million births occur annually, with 24% (960,000) delivered by cesarean section. In the Netherlands, only 8% of births are delivered by cesarean section. This suggests 640,000 unnecessary cesarean sections—entailing three to four times higher mortality and 20 times greater morbidity than vaginal delivery(105)—are performed annually in the U.S.

The U.S. cesarean rate rose from just 4.5% in 1965 to 24.1% in 1986. Sakala contends that an "uncontrolled pandemic of medically unnecessary cesarean births is occurring."(106) VanHam reported a cesarean section postpartum hemorrhage rate of 7%, a hematoma formation rate of 3.5%, a urinary tract infection rate of 3%, and a combined postoperative morbidity rate of 35.7% in a high-risk population undergoing cesarean section

## Adverse Drug Reactions

The Lazarou study(1) analyzed records for prescribed medications for 33 million U.S. hospital admissions in 1994. It discovered 2.2 million serious injuries due to prescribed drugs; 2.1% of inpatients experienced a serious adverse drug reaction, 4.7% of all hospital admissions were due to a serious adverse drug reaction, and fatal adverse drug reactions occurred in 0.19% of inpatients and 0.13% of admissions. The authors estimated that 106,000 deaths occur annually due to adverse drug reactions.

Serious adverse drug reactions commonly emerge after FDA approval of the drugs involved.

## Bedsores

Over one million people develop bedsores in U.S. hospitals every year. It's a tremendous burden to patients and family, and a $55 billion dollar healthcare burden. (7) Bedsores are preventable with proper nursing care. It is true that 50% of those affected are in a vulnerable age group of over 70. In the elderly, bedsores carry a fourfold increase in the rate of death. The mortality rate in hospitals for patients with bedsores is between 23% and 37%. (8) Even if we just take the 50% of people over 70 with bedsores and the lowest mortality at 23%, which gives us a death rate due to bedsores of 115,000. Critics will say that it was the disease or advanced age that killed the patient, not the bedsore, but our argument is that an early death, by denying proper care, deserves to be counted. It is only after counting these unnecessary deaths that we can then turn our attention to fixing the problem.

## Still to Be Uncovered

Results of the "Million Women Study" on HRT and breast cancer in the UK were published in the medical journal *The Lancet* in August 2003. According to lead author Prof. Valerie Beral, director of the Cancer Research UK Epidemiology Unit: "We estimate that over the past decade, use of HRT by UK women aged 50-64 has resulted in an extra 20,000 breast cancers, estrogen-progestagen (combination) therapy accounting for 15,000 of these."[151] We were unable to find statistics on breast cancer, stroke, uterine cancer, or heart disease caused by HRT used by American women. Because the U.S. population is roughly six times that of the UK, it is possible that 120,000 cases of breast cancer have been caused by HRT in the past decade.

# Chapter 6

## *Examples of Self-healing with IBMS*™

So many people have healed themselves of a severe illness during the past years with the help of my **Instinct Based Medicine System**™ **IBMS**™ that it is impossible for me to provide exact numbers. Among these cases of successful self-healing are many which occurred, because of the proper application of the self-learned training exercise technique described in my book ¹*The Unlimited Power of the Subconscious*, published by Hugendubel. Other people have, on the other hand, used my cassette program for guidance and still others have received the techniques for self-help from my seminars. In addition, there were many men and women who came to my **Instinct Based Medicine System**™ **IBMS**™ training centers in order to receive instruction from me or from one of my **IBMS**™ trainers, who were trained by me personally. Among these people were several incurable cases of which doctors had already given up but, who had refused to give up on themselves.

At this point I would like to emphasize once more that neither I, nor any of my **IBMS**™ trainers are healers. We are only an aid to your own success and to your health. It is you, who realizes the success that you desire.

However, please take note: the profession of an **IBMS**™ trainer is registered and these individuals  are trained by me alone. They are only allowed to call themselves **IBMS**™

trainers after they have received a certificate to that effect, which is signed by me personally. **IBMS™** is trademarked as a scientific concept worldwide and may only be carried out by myself and by persons who are licensed by me.

At this juncture, I will describe several self-healing cases that demonstrate how belief in an individual's infinite inner power, coupled with effective implementation of the **IBMS™** - techniques, lead to healing. This description should give you hope so that you never give up no matter how difficult the circumstances are. All of these patients were interviewed by the journalist Ulrich Grefe and published in many of his publications. These healing examples are published in my former books mainly in: *The Power of the Subconscious Mind* (Hugendubel Publishing). Some names have been changed.

## Recovery from Gout and Obesity

Klaus suffered from stomach bleeding, intestinal ulcers, acute circulation problems, and severe gout. Every day, he went to the doctor to have a substantial amount of fluid extracted from his knee. His family doctor advised him to change his diet; otherwise he could expect the worst. Klaus was overweight, and ate as much in a day as others would consume in a week.

Klaus came to me upon the recommendation of a friend, who had suffered from a "fatal" illness and was now fully healed with the help of my tools and technology. It was a good reference, but I needed to determine whether Klaus was committed to doing whatever was necessary to restore his health. When Klaus confirmed that he would cooperate wholeheartedly, we talked about the advantages of a healthy diet. We also talked about overeating, junk food, and the disadvantages of a bad diet. This would prepare his subconscious to accept the fact that a change must take place.

I explained to Klaus that his eating habits were nothing else but acquired abnormal behavior. He could easily be deprogrammed or reprogrammed for health. Klaus agreed, after a lengthy conversation, to put a massive block in his subconscious.

As we began therapy, I asked Klaus to think about a situation in which he had eaten a little bit, and immediately felt extremely satisfied. After that, I asked Klaus to imagine eating fresh fruits and vegetables, while feeling happy and energetic. We anchored this experience in his mind, so that eating healthy, fluid-rich food gave him a feeling of incredible health, vitality and energy.

I also asked Klaus to envision his future with positive mental images. With his eyes closed, Klaus pictured himself looking in the mirror and seeing his new slim and healthy body. He experienced feelings of pride and excitement. We also practiced self-healing exercises in which Klaus programmed his subconscious and mentally activated his body to heal itself of gout.

We met two more times for therapy. After the third session, Klaus' chronic pain and discomfort from the gout had disappeared. He no longer needed to visit the doctor to have fluid extracted from his knee. Ultimately, Klaus lost over 100 lbs in 19 weeks, without being hungry. The old, destructive eating habits were gone for good and so was his gout.

## Healing of Psoriasis

When Donna visited me, she looked exhausted and overwhelmed. She wore white gloves, and could barely move her arm or bend her elbow. She suffered from a horrible case of psoriasis on her elbows, hands and knees. An odor of decay emanated from her and puss oozed from her open sores. Donna had avoided public places, like restaurants, for the past 15 years because other people would lose their appetite and stop eating when they saw her hands or smelled the stench of her wounds.

When Donna took her gloves off, her hands looked pitiful. Her fingernails were rotting away and her hands were covered with puss and fresh blood. Donna's husband came with her and could not hold back his tears.

I discovered that Donna was hesitant to speak openly in the presence of her husband. For this reason, I politely asked him to leave the treatment room. When we were alone, I asked Donna if she had made any compromises in life. I was looking for something which might have poisoned her soul and made her life unbearable. Clinical tests showed that her liver was toxic and I suspected that her skin was ridding itself of toxins, stress and negative emotions.

With some hesitation, Donna blurted out the truth. Many years ago, her husband had an affair with her best girlfriend. Evidently, she found out during an argument with her girlfriend, when she triumphantly boasted about the affair. In response, Donna decided not to confront her husband about the affair. She asked her girlfriend not to tell him anything either, in order to save her otherwise good marriage.

A few weeks later, Donna's skin disorder surfaced. It gradually became worse, and after a few months the horrible infliction affected her whole body. Her joints, hands and feet were severely affected by psoriasis.

When I told Donna that stress and toxic emotions were the cause of her illness, she agreed to let her husband come back into the session to talk about this situation.

When confronted, Donna's husband collapsed and broke down in tears. He was devastated by the affair and his inner guilt and condemnation caused him to suffer from stomach ulcers. As the session progressed, I left the room so that they could talk about the problems they had both suppressed and reconcile the situation.

Overall, Donna and her husband came to see me 15 times. I taught Donna to breathe healing light into the source of her mental wounds. She learned to forgive her husband as well as her girlfriend by programming her subconscious. Over time, I helped Donna eliminate the buildup of hatred in her soul and helped her reconcile her emotions. She gradually reached the point of complete healing and recovery. Looking back, it is a miracle that Donna recovered in six weeks. Her psoriasis completely disappeared and Donna never experienced a relapse.

## Another Healing of Psoriasis

For 12 years, Janice suffered from psoriasis and puss oozing over her entire body. She was afraid to go out in public. Janice couldn't move without blood or puss coming out of her hands, elbows or knees.

Through detailed questioning, I learned that Janice's husband had forced her to eat snails at a restaurant. Janice didn't want to do it, but her husband insisted and even threatened to divorce her. In response, Janice gulped down the snails.

Three days later, Janice felt itching over her body. This condition became worse every time she ate, and eventually her body was covered with puss and scabs. Janice's joints and hands were affected the worst. She was hardly able to move because of the pain. The cause for this illness was a false neuro-association. Janice held on to feeling "those disgusting snails" (as she called them) inside her, which made her emotionally and physically sick.

I helped Janice recover by using a relaxation exercise. When Janice was completely relaxed, I helped her to destroy the false neuro-association by revisiting the day that she had been forced to eat the snails. I asked her to vomit up the snails in her mind, so that her sub-conscious would be given a symbol of liberation. After we had repeated this exercise several times and she began to feel relieved and liberated. Then we created a new neuro-association. I asked her to experience mentally, again and again, a conversation in which she told her husband that she would absolutely never eat snails again. Janice visualized herself pushing the plate away, while feeling great about her actions and standing by her decision.

Janice conducted this mental exercise several times. As she continually practiced and trained herself, the correct

193

behavior appeared more real than the previous behavior in which she ate the "disgusting" snails. Within days, Janice's inflammation diminished and the psoriasis began to disappear. After eight weeks, Janice fully recovered and was never bothered by psoriasis again.

## Healing Cancer of the Liver

I have witnessed many incredible, miraculous and spontaneous recoveries with cancer patients. Judy, who had liver cancer, was one of my most impressive patients. She was in her early forties and was referred by a physician from Göttingen, Germany, who gave her a maximum of two months to live. Judy was in the final stages of liver cancer. She attended other people's seminars, and experimented with various esoteric healing methods. Nothing seemed to improve her health, and Judy desperately wanted to recover.

I noticed immediately that Judy had no short term goals, nor a future perspective. She lived with her elderly, sick mother, who was waiting for her approaching death. Judy felt lonely and empty inside. After our first discussion, I encouraged Judy to attend a six-hour intensive course at our **IBMS ™** training center in Steinberg, Germany.

At the center, Judy developed a future perspective based upon her personality and interests. This gave her hope and confidence. Judy was encouraged to imagine herself interacting with sympathetic and compassionate people, even with a potential partner. Until now, Judy had never thought like that before. Within a short time, Judy changed drastically. Life became exciting for Judy, as she uncovered lots of new possibilities and opportunities for growth. She moved out of her mother's apartment, took up hobbies and developed new interests, including music dancing lessons. Shortly thereafter, Judy started dating and met a wonderful man to share her life with. Judy's healing was incredibly fast and spontaneous. Her physician examined her twelve days after the **IBMS™** training, and documented that Judy's cancer had already receded. After three and a half months, the doctor made the diagnosis that Judy was completely cured. Today, Judy looks radiant and energetic. Her liver cancer never resurfaced.

## Healing of Breast Cancer

I clearly remember the first time that Elaine came to my office. She was in her mid-thirties and suffered from breast cancer. The doctors removed her right breast and treated her twice with chemotherapy. Elaine was in terrible shape. Her hair was falling out. She was frightened and emotionally devastated.

After a short consultation, I learned that Elaine suffered from depression and a gripping angst. Since her early childhood, she was not able to leave the house or sleep in the dark alone. Elaine's constant fears led to an inner resignation and a decreased will to live. As she became more and more depressed, her body began to self-destruct.

Elaine was on the brink of a nervous breakdown. In therapy, we started doing relaxation exercises, which helped her, calm down and internalize a peaceful mental state. Elaine quickly learned that our feelings and emotional outlook affect our perspective on life. The quality of our life depends on our perception and what we think about is what our future will hold.

If someone can't envision the future, then healing is impossible. Before anything else, a person must believe that a bright future and optimum health is conceivable. As all religious books of the world state over and over again, that faith (or the power of belief) is the greatest force in human existence. In the final analysis, everything depends on whether you believe in your own success and healing.

With simple techniques and exercises, as I have described in my book *The Unlimited Power of the Subconscious*, we eliminated Elaine's fears. Like a beautiful flower, she began to blossom. As therapy continued, Elaine visualized her life integrated with her career and husband, who lovingly and enthusiastically stood by her side. Within a few weeks, Elaine was vibrant and full of energy. Previously, the doctors had given a life expectancy of six months. Now, she had every reason to live with passion.

Two years later, Elaine returned to the center with a large knot protruding from the scars of her former operation. She was terribly frightened, but felt hopeful because of her success two years earlier. I referred Elaine to the chief of surgery in a nearby hospital, who discovered something astonishing. The first operation was terribly botched. The cancer had been cut in two and half of it remained in Elaine's body. As any physician can confirm, this woman would have had less than three months to live because she carried a severe malignant tumor, the size of a walnut, in her body. This is the worst thing that can happen to a patient. The chief of the hospital had never seen anything like this, nor thought it possible. Half of the tumor was left in Elaine's body, but the tumor had isolated itself and had been pushed upward by the body's attempt to expel it.

Once the tumor was surgically removed, there was no need for chemotherapy. Elaine was told that she would never again be able to have children, but she quickly became pregnant. For this reason, Elaine remained under my care during pregnancy. The doctors told her that her baby would be sick, and possibly suffer from birth defects. After nine months, Elaine gave birth to a healthy child. There were no complications or difficulties during the birth. Elaine's beautiful little girl is now five years old. She is full of life, energy, health and vitality. She does not get the flu or colds, unlike her older brother and her playmates. Elaine is happy and now realizes that there is no incurable disease.

## Another Recovery from Breast Cancer

Tracy was an attractive, self-confident woman with an extremely stressful job. She had an abusive relationship with a man whom she dearly loved. Tracy could not bring herself to end the relationship, despite the fact that her dependency on this man was counterproductive and unhealthy emotionally.

When Tracy discovered a knot in her right breast, she visited a gynecologist who examined her with ultrasound. When the gynecologist wanted to X-ay Tracy, she went to another medical practitioner. He suspected that it was only a swollen lymph node, and gave her an injection. If the diagnosis was correct, the swelling would disappear.

When the knot remained, Tracy went to the hospital for an X-ray. The surgeon removed the knot as well as the surrounding tissue from the breast, and fifteen lymph nodes from her right armpit, two of which were malignant. She was told that an additional treatment with radiation and chemotherapy would prevent the cancer from spreading. When Tracy consulted her gynecologist, he recommended that she first take some time to recuperate from the stress of surgery. Intimidated and fearful, Tracy sought the advice of an alternative health practitioner, who suggested that her illness had a psychological cause. Finally, Tracy felt empowered to leave her abusive relationship with her boyfriend.

Tracy came to my center upon the referral of a friend who overcame breast cancer using my tools and techniques. Twice a week, Tracy strengthened her inner self by applying my **IBMS™** technique. Additionally, Tracy received oxygen treatments and metabolism therapy with natural additives. Shortly thereafter, Tracy found a new boyfriend, as well as a less stressful job. After three months of therapy, Tracy completely recovered from breast cancer. She wrote me recently, resolving to never again compromise her values with an abusive relationship, which would induce stress and cause severe health problems.

## Help for Breast Cancer

I'm always astonished when patients refuse to open up and identify the root cause of their illness. They seem comfortable with their condition and limitations. They don't seem to care that their illness has lessened the quality of their life.

In therapy, my patients are encouraged to adopt a new way of thinking, as they learn to identify the root cause of illness. This enables them to recognize the connection between energy-draining compromises, stressful emotions and the development of severe illnesses.

When I asked Greta, who suffered from advanced breast cancer, about the possible cause of her illness, she had no clue. Greta had a large open sore on her left breast, and was looking for an alternative to surgery.

Greta often talked about her mother and how fortunate she was to inherit furniture from her. The more Greta talked about the furniture, the more obvious it became that this old furniture continuously reminded her about horrible things in the past. Indirectly, she wanted to get rid of this old furniture and decorate her place in her own style

Once Greta realized these suppressed thoughts and emotions, her behavior changed visibly. She seemed relieved and her eyes became bright and lively.

Greta mentioned that she had a driver's license but had not driven a car in the past 13 years. I immediately recognized this disclosure as the next building block. I needed to know why she had suddenly stopped driving. I realized that her low self-esteem and self-confidence paralyzed her from driving and that she didn't have enough energy or strength to address this problem.

As therapy continued, Greta admitted that she had been married twice and suffered a miscarriage. Finally, the picture was coming together. We used the **IBMS™** technique to address her repressed emotions, as well as her feelings of fear guilt. After five days of therapy, the wound on her chest began to close and her ulcer visibly diminished. Eventually, Greta was completely healed and restored to her full health.

Greta is a textbook illustration of repressed emotions. She swallowed her feelings, (rather than dealing with them openly and honestly) and therefore could not identify the root cause of her illness.

An impending crisis is also common with **IBMS™** therapy. This happens when the patient becomes aware of problems that were previously suppressed. Confronted with these issues, the patient can't escape into his dream world. This often causes patients to become angry or frustrated with their **IBMS™** therapist.

Finally, the client is self-aware and accepts full responsibility for their health and emotions. This is an astonishing and wonderful phenomenon. Often, the patient looks ten to fifteen years younger. Their eyes sparkle, and they appear to be more relaxed. Even if the patient remains physically weak, they are now mentally balanced and optimistic about the future. Their strength and energy are visibly restored. Afterwards, healing and recovery is accelerated at high speed. In more than 90%of all cases, astounding physiological changes occur. Even doctors are amazed at how fast cancers recede or diminish.

## Healing of Bone Cancer

Gayle was a courageous woman who came to me with cancer that spread into her spine, pelvis, and hips. She was referred from a renowned cancer clinic, as her doctor saw no possibility of helping her.

Gayle was energetic and committed to fighting for her health. She met all the prerequisites for my **IBMS™** therapy. Gayle loved her life and career, had clear goals, and a healthy relationship with her children and husband. Initially, it was difficult to find a cause for what ignited this horrible cancer. The only thing I noticed was that Gayle became nervous when we discussed her previous relationships.

Gayle was so incredibly strong that it took four sessions to reach a breakthrough. She finally developed enough trust and rapport to tell me that she had been married previously. She was married to a gentleman from Turkey, who had convinced her to relocate there with vague promises and lies. Her life in Turkey was a living hell. Her mother-in-law abused and tormented her, and her husband treated her like an animal. This ordeal destroyed Gayle's personality. She started to isolate herself and withdraw. At times, Gayle was even suicidal. Her mother-in-law also tried to murder her. On a visit to Germany, Gayle visited a specialist who was supposed to examine and treat her because her condition had become life-threatening. During this visit, she successfully escaped from her husband and began a completely new life. Her health seemed to improve, but she repressed her past experiences and was filled with hatred toward her ex-mother-in-law and her former husband. She could not forget how she was abused, degraded and tortured.

Using the **IBMS™** technique, I helped Gayle erase the past. She was stricken with cancer due to feelings of hatred, despair and helplessness. After ten appointments, Gayle could finally forgive her ex-husband and her former mother-in-law. She learned to accept them as they were and finally succeeded in letting go of these two people. Gayle also let go of her nervous responses whenever the past was mentioned. She also developed a new future perspective, as well as a new way of thinking that facilitated healing and recovery. Within four months, Gayle fully recovered. Today she is working full time and is active, happy, and content with life.

## Healing of Spinal Muscular Atrophy *(severe form of Muscular Dystrophy)*

When Hans came to my office, he was in pitiful shape. He used to be an accomplished athlete and worked professionally as a building engineer. Now he was unable to climb stairs and could hardly move. Hans spent his days in a wheelchair or in bed, as he suffered from severe pain. The doctor diagnosed Hans with Spinal Muscular Atrophy.

Even though Hans was stricken with illness, I was impressed by his courage. He said, "As long as I can breathe, I will fight." Hans had heard that my techniques were effective, even in the most hopeless situations. He was determined to do whatever it took to recover and become healthy.

As we began to talk, I discovered that Hans wanted nothing less than optimum health. We began by stimulating his brain because the healing and regeneration process is initiated by the brain.

Doctors had given Hans a maximum life expectancy of 12 to 18 months. (These were opinions from experts of medical universities.) Although they offered no hope for healing or recovery, Hans courageously placed himself in my care for **IBMS™** self-healing and therapy.

I asked Hans to visualize himself at a fitness center, which was filled with symbols that facilitated healing. Because the subconscious works with symbols, Hans worked out step-by-step in his mind. He visualized himself using a variety of exercise equipment. With each mental workout, Hans strengthened every single muscle in his body. He programmed his conscious to see himself as healthy and strong. He visualized himself interacting with his children and wife as a healthy man. These mental exercises strongly motivated Hans, and enabled his subconscious to perform the powerful act of healing from this incurable illness. After four weeks, Hans was completely pain free. It was the first time in 12 years that he was pain free. His muscles substantially improved, which was also confirmed by a medical exam. After six weeks, Hans' success was clearly visible. His arms and legs, which hung previously lifeless in the joints, began to take their natural shape. After eight weeks, Hans could climb steps by himself. After eight months, he could do light physical work. Ultimately, Hans activated his self-healing power and created a new quality of life for himself.

Today, Hans is one of my best friends. Whenever I see him, he is happy and filled with zest for life. I share his story because it confirms that everyone possesses a God-given power to heal himself. Dear reader, you too can improve the quality of your life, even if you are severely ill, if you are willing to do whatever is necessary to restore your health.

## Healing of a Spastic Nerve Condition

At our **IBMS™**-training center, I noticed a painter who moved his eyes quickly back and forth, without ever looking at someone directly. His eyelids were swollen and it appeared that he was under the influence of drugs.

His name was Leon. As I began to talk to him, I discovered that Leon took painkillers for the past 15 years. The medicine affected his stomach and inner organs. Leon could hardly stand the pain, and saw a variety of doctors and specialists. One doctor gave him the option of severing the nerves in his face with surgery, so that he would no longer feel the pain. However, this surgery would paralyze half of his face, and there was no guarantee that the nerve endings wouldn't join with the other nerves, causing pain again.

I felt sorry for this industrious and talented man. I did an **IBMS™** exercise with Leon, and estimated that he could reduce his pain substantially after six months of intensive programming. To my surprise, it happened much sooner than that.

I was relocating to America and did not have enough time to concentrate on Leon. I asked my medical manager to take over using the **IBMS™** technical method. After the second session, Leon's pain, which he endured for 17 years, completely disappeared.

To our astonishment, Leon ran around in the center telling everyone (whether they wanted to hear it or not) how well he felt. Leon could not believe what had happened to him. He was now completely free of pain, and even his back pain completely disappeared.

Leon's recovery proves that you do not have to take expensive medication or undergo surgery to be liberated from illness. The power of your own mind will enable you to handle any obstacle that comes your way. It is always wise to set goals. If you don't accomplish your goals that does not mean that it is unattainable. You must look for new ways and possibilities to make things happen. When it comes to your health, you must look for ways to eliminate or reduce your pain and suffering and restore your health. Never accept limitations, or settle for less than you can be. You don't have to live with pain or illness. Don't allow your mind to dwell on negative thoughts. Keep working on improving the quality of your life and don't allow your mind to accept limitations, pain or illness.

Success is a journey. If you are on your way toward achieving your goals, then you are successful. If you focus on your health, then you're on the way towards improving or restoring it. If you don't give up, you will find a way to improve the quality of your life. I am 100% certain of that.

## Healing of Osteoporosis

Gertie was in her early fifties, but looked at least fifteen years older. She limped into my office, hunched over from pain. Gertie was in a terrible, catastrophic state, mentally as well as physically. Gertie had been married for 30 years to a well-known corporate executive. He was an alcoholic, and physically abused Gertie. He threatened to kill her, and she lived in constant fear for her life. Twice, he had thrown her down the stairs. If her husband would "lose it again" (as she called it) Gertie planned to escape by jumping through a window, into her car, which was ready to go with a full tank of gasoline. Gertie had osteoporosis in a very advanced state and her overall physical condition was that of a handicapped person. Her mental condition was catastrophic and her physical condition was not much better.

I tried to convince Gertie to leave her husband immediately. She refused to do so, but did agree to undergo **IBMS™** therapy. At first, we did several strengthening, regenerating, and relaxing exercises to stabilize her energy reserve and prevent a total collapse. After a few days, Gertie was ready for a new get- away plan. While her husband was on a two-day business trip, she called a moving company, temporarily moved in with friends, and later into her own apartment.

During this time, we continued to meet and also talked over the telephone, to prevent a mental or physical collapse. For a year, Gertie and I worked on stabilizing and building up her mental and physical condition. I also supported her during the difficult divorce procedure and visits to lawyers. After 18 months, Gertie wrote me a letter. She said that her physician discovered that her osteoporosis had disappeared, and her bone density and elasticity was comparable to that of a healthy person. I've kept this documentation for my records. Gertie's story illustrates that compromises (not standing up for yourself) can destroy your health and literally cripple your body. She was restored to full health by eliminating unhealthy compromises in her life and ending her relationship with her abusive husband. Gertie was also strengthened with relaxation exercises, which enabled her body to heal and restore itself.

## Healing of Sexual Disturbances

Katrina, age 26, came to me at the advice of her husband, who had heard of my success in treating emotional problems. Katrina loved her husband very much, but didn't want to be intimate with him. Three years ago, she had given birth to their first child and lost interest in having a physical relationship with her husband. As soon as her husband touched her, she felt repulsed, and wanted nothing to do with him. Of course, her marriage was now in danger, and something had to be done.

In therapy, the first step was identifying the root cause of the problem. Katrina's negative feelings started with her child's birth. The baby was conceived out of wedlock. They married quickly and then the baby was born. As a strict Catholic, Katrina suffered from guilt. Her guilt subconsciously manifested itself by punishing herself and her husband. This guilt made her think that sexual intimacy was dirty and disgusting.

When Katrina started **IBMS™** therapy, she learned to accept her situation. She practiced relaxation exercises and mentally returned to the past to recall a positive sexual experience with her husband. Katrina associated herself with the loving, tender feelings that she felt for her husband. She remained in this condition of association for at least ten minutes.

The next morning, Katrina and her husband both called to thank me, independently of each other. They both had a wonderful night together. It took only one session to resolve this problem. It isn't difficult to resolve such conflicts. Most of the time, it only takes a little push to get people back on track with the behavior, feelings and actions they desire.

**IBMS™** treatment is simple and easy, but never trust anyone who lacks the training, knowledge and experience that is necessary to produce results. When people come to therapy, they must be carefully trained and conditioned, so that the conflict is permanently resolved. Nothing is worse than a relapse after recovery.

## Healing of Impotence Because of Fear of Failure

Impotence is a serious problem that is rarely discussed. Like the aforementioned case, it is a sexual disturbance that can be quickly and easily resolved.

Jerry, age 52, married a woman who was 12 years younger than him. He experienced tremendous misfortune, personally as well as professionally. Jerry lost his confidence and feared that he could not satisfy his young wife. His mental block caused impotence. After 12 sessions, Jerry set clear goals and used **IBMS™** techniques to build his self-confidence. He made new plans for the future and visualized them as being real. These experiences anchored Jerry's new feelings of success. He visualized himself in depressing and frightening situations, yet was able to remain calm and level headed. He also conditioned himself to experience happiness and enthusiasm with a snap of his finger.

Jerry also programmed himself to be loving and passionate with his wife. He was able to generate feelings of confidence, energy and strength in any situation, at any time. Jerry could recall his programming and was able to develop effective goals and solutions. His impotence also disappeared and his relationship with his wife was restored.

## Finger Amputation Is No Longer Needed

My mother received a frantic phone call from her friend, Linda. The doctors told Linda that her finger needed to be amputated. My mother advised her to visit the IBMS™ center and get a second opinion. This woman had fallen down the basement steps, crushing the joints in her pinky finger. She waited six days before consulting a doctor. Apparently, the delay made the damage irreparable. Linda's finger was dark blue, extremely swollen and hurt so severely that painkillers could not help.

Two doctors, independently of each other, had advised Linda to have her finger amputated. She came to see me with little hope, but with great motivation to keep her finger.

I led Linda into a mental state where she found herself strong and confident. She visualized her finger returning to its normal size and color, with the joints tightening and healing. This mental vision was associated with feelings of self-confidence and was strengthened by her overwhelming desire to recover. Linda trained and programmed herself intensely and repeated the exercises several times throughout the day.

Surprisingly, Linda called my mother later to say that she was pain free. Her finger was regaining its normal color and shape. Today, Linda's finger is fully functional. The two doctors who advised amputation had no comment.

## Help for Multiple Sclerosis

Anna was diagnosed with multiple sclerosis. She was living in a dream world, which had nothing to do with reality.

She swayed back and forth between reality and fantasy. Her subconscious began to fight the part of the brain that was in control over discerning reality from fantasy.

When someone has multiple sclerosis, their immune system regards the brain as a foreign object. Their body begins to attack certain nerve endings, which are damaged and destroyed in the process. Anna was already paralyzed on the right side of her body. Her balance was completely destroyed, after many years of excruciating pain. In therapy, I explained to Anna that she needed a miracle, and it had to come from within. This realization enabled Anna to change her thinking and behavior with unbelievable energy and strength. Gradually, she started to accept reality. She learned to make the best of situations, which she previously was unable to do.

After two months of **IBMS**™ therapy, Anna reported that the following health problems were resolved:

- severe leg cramps & numbness;
- inability to stretch her legs;
- inability to pull her legs up close to her body without the use of her hands;
- uncontrollable nervous leg twitches;
- intense feelings of pins and needles in her legs, feet and hands;
- sensitivity to changes in the weather;
- acute sensitivity to pressure: like in the fairytale, *The Princess and the Pea*.(Every wrinkle in the bed sheets caused her pain and discomfort);
- bladder problems;
- sensitive finger tips;
- pain associated with hot and cold temperatures; and
- back pain.

## Healing of Severe Depression

When Connie visited my office, she cried uncontrollably. Her boyfriend explained that Connie was unable to work and could not be left alone. For months, she had been on sick leave from work and her condition was becoming worse.

Connie worked at the university cafeteria. One of her co-workers was domineering, controlling and verbally abusive. Connie was on the verge of a nervous breakdown. She felt weak, helpless and did not believe that she was capable of doing anything successfully.

In **IBMS™** therapy, Connie built up her energy with relaxation, visualization and breathing exercises. Connie immediately felt stronger. She promised not to make any major decisions in the upcoming month. Connie was advised to take it easy, and only do things that she wanted to do. Rest and recuperation would enable her to overcome her depression.

After the third relaxation exercise, Connie felt like herself again. She felt motivated to return to work. I was pleased with Connie's attitude, but feared that she might relapse. It is absolutely necessary to initially create a reserve of energy. After the patient's energy level is stabilized, they are equipped to deal with the unpleasant situations as they unfold. They are able to cope with their own thoughts and behavior, and never again suffer an energy depletion or imbalance.

For the next ten sessions, Connie programmed herself mentally for success at work. She imagined herself at the cafeteria, acting calmly and confidently, especially with her domineering co-worker. Connie imagined herself in stressful situations and programmed feelings of confidence, power, and security into her mental pictures.

When Connie officially returned to work, she discovered that the programming worked perfectly. She had no interpersonal problems at all, even with the bossy co-worker. For the first time, work was fun and rewarding. Her depression had disappeared, and Connie felt like herself again.

## Healing of Anxiety Resulting from Rape

Marlene was raped by her father when she was ten years old. As an adult, she was claustrophobic and feared closed spaces and staircases. Occasionally, Marlene checked into a mental hospital, but that made her condition worse. Adding insult to injury was that Marlene's rape was kept secret, and she lived together with her husband and parents under one roof. Whenever her father stepped into the room, she would sweat profusely and was unable to speak or think clearly. Marlene's anxiety led to physical problems that stumped doctors and healthcare professionals.

After an initial consultation, Marlene's feelings of helplessness turned into rage. Whenever her father was mentioned, Marlene would literally explode. She screamed about what a pig he was, and how dare he take advantage of her innocence and trust. Marlene's outbursts ended with tears, which brought her relief. Afterwards, she would talk freely about feelings that were previously repressed.

Marlene and I did an **IBMS™** programming exercise in which she attempted to forgive her father on a mental level. This was not easy for her, but after three exercises, Marlene was finally able to let go and forgive.

Fortunately, Marlene's rape was an isolated incident. The rape must have been an impulsive act, or perhaps her father was under the influence of alcohol or drugs. I suggested that Marlene confront her father, and talk openly about what had happened. When she did this, her father remembered almost nothing about the incident. He was aware that something had happened, but remembered only vaguely that he suffered a nervous breakdown and had gotten drunk at a bar.

After Marlene confronted her father, she was able to come to grips with the situation and finally, put this incident behind her. Marlene was liberated from her fear and paranoia.

During **IBMS™** therapy, I helped Marlene create an anchor which enabled her to summon feelings of euphoria and happiness whenever she needed them. Marlene imagined herself climbing stairs and entering small, closed-in spaces. I anchored these mental images with happy and euphoric feelings. Ultimately, Marlene established a new neuro-association in her mind, which enabled her to climb stairs and stay in tight, closed-in places without anxiety or apprehension.

Previously, Marlene had been in psychotherapy for more than 18 years. She had been treated for psychosomatic illness and also been hospitalized in the psychiatric ward. With the help of **IBMS™** therapy, Marlene was able to change her neuro associations, identify the root cause of her anxiety, forgive, and let go of the past. Her recovery took only five weeks, and Marlene's anxiety was gone for good.

## Healing of Uncontrollable Fear

One of my colleagues told me that a crying woman was standing outside of the **IBMS™** center, but refused to come inside. Jane, age 26, appeared devastated. Hot tears stung her eyes and she folded her arms over her chest to keep her body from trembling. As I normally do in such cases, I interrupted Jane's behavior pattern. I acted as if she was invisible. I spoke to her husband about his drive to the center and how long it had taken him to get there. After chatting for a few minutes, I asked Jane's husband if he wanted to come into the center. As we stepped inside, Jane quietly asked me what was wrong with her. I simply told her that she could join us if she wished.

Obviously, I responded to Jane differently than what she expected. This interrupted her behavior pattern. My casual attitude caught her off guard, and enabled her to get a grip on her emotions. After Jane had taken a few steps, I took her arm and pointed out some pictures in the waiting room. As we walked to my office, I talked to Jane about her future plans, as well as her wishes and dreams. This kept her mind focused, so that she would not lose control emotionally again.

In my office, I asked Jane to sit down. However, I instructed her to sit straight and upright, and speak to me loudly and as fast as she possibly could. Immediately, she experienced a change in her awareness. I asked Jane to jump up, punch the air with her fist, and shout loudly, "Yes, I live!" Jane thought this was awkward and funny, but she did it. After doing it 15 times, she had enough energy to address her problems.

Evidently, Jane thought of herself as a failure after a miscarriage. It was partially her fault and Jane's husband wouldn't let her forget it. Condemnation and self-blame caused Jane to lose confidence in herself. She was afraid of doing anything, for fear of messing up. Caught up in a negative spiral, Jane lacked the energy to break free. She was paralyzed with fear, and unable to live a normal life.

In our session, it took only a few minutes for Jane to break through her fears. For at least five minutes, she felt carefree and comfortable. As we talked, Jane and her husband began to understand that the miscarriage was not her fault, as their physician had told them previously.

With **IBMS™** therapy, Jane began to eliminate the negative neuro-associations that tormented her. We talked about setting goals and creating a future, including the possibility of getting pregnant again and having a baby. As we talked about these things, we walked around my office with our heads held high and shoulders back. I asked Jane to express herself loud and clear, with self-confidence. We anchored these positive feelings over and over again by snapping our fingers, so that this feeling could be recalled at any time, should she slip into an emotional crisis. Ultimately, Jane recovered from her uncontrollable fears. She now has the courage to live life to the fullest.

## The Non-Acceptance of a Hip Implant

Bert was an intelligent, well-educated man who wanted to commit suicide. He suffered from excruciating hip pain as a result of a childhood accident (which his parents ignored.) Bert received a hip implant, and the surgery was successful according to the doctors. When Bert was back on his feet, however, his hip constantly jumped out of the joint, which made walking nearly impossible.

Plagued with pain, Bert tried to repress or ignore the pain. This only made the problem worse. During a short session, I discovered that Bert hated himself because of his physical limitations. Emotionally and intellectually, he was not willing to accept his physical handicap.

Bert repeatedly mentioned being separated from his wife, but that he would take good care of her and their children. Bert repeated this statement so many times that I suspected something else was wrong. To challenge Bert, I praised him for being an excellent father, and how sensible it was that he had separated from his wife, after he recognized that his marriage was doomed from the beginning.

All of a sudden, Bert shouted, "That's not true at all! My wife separated from me. She did not know who she was dealing with, or who I really was. My life was going no where, and she couldn't bear my self-pity any longer!"

That was the turning point. Bert identified the root cause of his problem. His hip was out of joint because mind and body rejected it. He also needed to develop clear goals, future perspectives, value systems and rules. We dealt with these things through continuous mental programming. As Bert began to develop feelings of self-confidence and self-esteem, his perspective started to change.

After talking to his wife, Bert was hopeful that the relationship could be restored. He began to set new goals and develop a clear value system, so that he could accept himself again. He stopped feeling sorry for himself. After a short time, the tension and disjointed feeling in his hip was gone. Stress had caused the hip to jump out of its joints. The initial good work by the orthopedic surgeons could now be amplified and enforced. Bert was a new man, with a fresh outlook on life.

**Concluding Remarks**

Although many of my clients say Dr. Leonard Coldwell healed me, this is not correct. It was not I who healed them; they healed themselves. That I contributed to their healing is the development of trust in themselves and in their own self-healing powers through explanation, training and demonstration. I am the one who knows how it should be done and I can relay what everybody must do himself.

I am not able to heal you, you must heal yourself. The **IBMS™-** System is a tool for self-healing. I can show you how to use this tool and can put this tool into your hands, however, in the final analysis you must use this tool.

Of course, some of the people, whose amazing cases of self-healing have been described by me here, had occasional doubts, apparent relapses and fears during periods of stagnation in the healing process.

That is, of course, part of the maturation process in every human being. What brought these people finally to the point of healing was the unwillingness to give up the will to live; they were determined to become and remain healthy.

I call those people victorious, because they changed their inactivity, their doubts and their behavior and their false thinking patterns. I respect the way they took control of their lives. They changed their diet and did everything necessary to regain their health.

These people are the true victors because they conquered their illness. The harvest they reaped was a new quality of life and the knowledge that they will be able to handle any problem that confronts them. Those people now know how to come to terms with difficulties.

I would like to say once more, success gained with **IBMS™-** training is produced and maintained by the clients themselves. We are only teachers, trainers and confidants who help to resolve emotional problems and conflicts and who search jointly for solutions to these problems and conflicts. We help to develop clear plans and strategies and to carry these plans through. Sometimes we provide care for our **IBMS™** clients beyond the initial treatment and give advice for checkups and renewal appointments to reinforce new behavior patterns and techniques.

Sometimes, we also work together with the family members so that they will know exactly how they should conduct themselves toward their loved ones in order to help them overcome their limitations, conquer their illness and maintain their health.

We must all work together toward the realization of a total therapy in which physicians, consultants, natural healers, psychologists, psychiatrists and **IBMS™** -trainers, health researchers and all other persons, who concern themselves with the health of people, share their thoughts and ideas and develop an increasingly improved concept of total health. Only in this way can humanity benefit and we, as responsible health providers, have the obligation to ensure that in a few years the exploding costs in the health industry will be reduced and that the statistics, that show that 87% of all people are frequently ill, become obsolete.

It would be wonderful for me, if you would be one of these miracle cases, one of the victors, whose successes I can describe in my next book. Should you be ill, be prepared that you will not only hear about miracles in reference to other people, but that you can become the subject of a miracle story. The healing lies in your own hands and the tool, the possibilities and the potential you possess is already within you.

I hope that you have learned from the above examples of self-healing.

There is always a way and you are the only person, who can really set your healing in motion; you alone are responsible for your life, your future and your health. If you have learned this, I will have accomplished a lot with this short venture into **IBMS™** - technology.

The above described healings are, of course, only a few of the many from my practice. I chose these stories to encourage other people, who may have similar problems, to take problems into their own hands and fight for a better quality of life.

I would be pleased to hear your comments and questions in respect to my book. I would also be interested in your personal experiences with my **IBMS™**-system. It could help others to make their own lives more successful and beautiful. If you are very successful in your profession, your health, or your relationships and could help other people to build up their courage and ability to persevere, or if you have overcome an illness which was considered incurable, then please write to:

Dr. Leonard Coldwell, 1150 Hungryneck Blvd., Suite C 379, Mount Pleasant, South Carolina 29464 or email: dr.leonardcoldwell@gmail.com and visit the websites www.instinctbasedmedicine.com and www.drleonardcoldwell.com. Your reports of success can encourage others.

# Section 2

## The root cause of all illness: Stress the silent killer

### Using the Instinct Based Medicine System™ (IBMS™ The Dr Coldwell System)

**How to conquer the root cause of all illness**

**Introduction**

If stress is at the core of all illness and discontent in life why is it not at the core of all attempts to heal? Why is a pill seen as a solution when the cause...stress...is left unattended? Dr. Coldwell understands the far-reaching effects of stress and in Stress the Silent Killer provides the missing link that allows you to avoid illness in the first place.

The famous Austrian neurosurgeon, Hans Selye, noted in his landmark book *Stress Without Distress* that *stress* is to be alive while *distress* destroys the person. Dr. Coldwell tells us in easy to read and understandable words how and why stress occurs, why it is so damaging, why it is so pervasive and why

217

*it does not need to be* ... even in this 21st century world so full of stressful circumstances, terrorism, blaring TV advertisements and even dysfunctional families. He also understands that while the written word helps us to grasp the importance of each point, it is not enough by itself to triumph over the harmful habits and conditioned responses our hyperactive world foists upon us everyday.

That is why he created the CDs that accompany his book. These are a masterpiece of science and sensitivity calculated to help you overcome the stresses in your life and create a healthier, happier lifestyle. Played through earphones, you are transported to a place of your own, true, inner calm that permits his message of countering the stress in your life to break through the demands of each day and restore the strength, confidence and good health you know you have within you.

These CDs will become your daily friend as they start you on a less stressful, healthier and more productive life while the book will become a handy reference for you and other members of your family as each of you finds your own, new source of power within and as you learn how to deal with stress the ultimate de-motivator and *Stress the Silent Killer.*

Carson E. Beadle
Chairman, The Health Project

## Disclaimer

The techniques presented in this part of the book are powerful, natural stress reducing methods, but they are not a substitute for medical care from a physician. Results will vary for each person, but these methods are so powerful that their use is occasionally capable of relieving pain from serious underlying disease processes. We offer this information for your use in stress reduction, but do not neglect taking care of what is causing the stress. Remember, stress is a signal from your body that tells you when something is wrong. Consult a doctor if you are injured or if you suffer from medical conditions. This publication presents only the author's opinions which are based on his knowledge, experience and beliefs. The techniques and theories offered here do not represent a scientific consensus in stress alleviation or prevention. Results will be based on an individual's specific situation and will vary for each individual. Dr. Coldwell's stress reduction will not work for everyone. This program is solely an educational help to self help system.

## Legal Notices

This part of the book is designed to provide information about the subject matter covered. While all attempts have been made to verify the information provided in this publication, neither the author nor the publisher assumes any responsibility for errors, omissions or contrary interpretation of the subject matter.

This publication is sold with the understanding that the publisher and author are not engaged in rendering medical professional services. If you have a medical condition you should seek the services of a competent medical professional. The purchaser or reader of this publication assumes responsibility for the use of these materials and information. Adherence to all applicable laws and regulations, federal, state and local, governing professional licensing, business practices, advertising and all other aspects of doing business in the United States or any other jurisdiction is the sole responsibility of the purchaser or reader. The author and publisher assume no responsibility or liability whatsoever on the behalf of any purchaser or reader of these materials.

The purpose of this part of the book is to educate. Any perceived affront to a specific individual or organization is unintentional.

# Preface

In spite of all the latest information available, the "health sector" still primarily revolves around illness. Conventional orthodox medicine does not leave room to address anything but the symptoms of illness in spite of the fact that there is much evidence to show that these symptoms are rooted in a deeper source. Unfortunately, patients continue to expect doctors to simply help them by fighting to eliminate only the symptoms not the root cause of the illness.

Dr. Leonard Coldwell is a health researcher who has spent his career addressing the root cause of disease/illness and how to help patients get rid of the cause of the illness. He discovered that the only way to help his patients was to help them to help themselves, which led him to be known as the "health coach." He does not care about the symptoms of disease/illness because he only addresses the root cause of the illness. If the root cause goes away then naturally the symptoms follow suit. His way of thinking is radical as he believes in health not disease. He believes in help to self-help. He believes in preventing health breakdowns, and he believes that sick people make themselves sick so only they can make themselves well.

I have personally known and worked with Dr. Leonard Coldwell for over 15 years. In that time, he has not only taught me a lot, but I have also watched his patients achieve, by doctors' standards, "miracle" results. In this book, he provides every reader with the information necessary to achieve and maintain health! In addition, as a natural side effect, the quality of your life will dramatically improve if you follow his regimen. Dr. Coldwell shares his insights, teaches and offers real solutions to heretofore unsolved health problems. If you want to stay and maintain health for years to come and achieve your dreams, this book is an invaluable tool! This is the best educational self-help systems in the world!

Spring 2008
Dr. med. Holger Crone, M.D.
Hanover, Germany

# The Coldwell Promise

Dear Reader,

**Health is not a coincidence! Health is the logical consequence of healthful decisions and healthful behavior.**

"Health is the perfect function of all biological systems."

Why do most heart attacks happen on Monday between eight and nine in the morning? No other day of the week, or time of day, comes even close. It occurs when a victim is getting ready for a job that they dread a job that gives them a feeling of being suffocated emotionally, spiritually and physically. They are literally overcome by the stress of just thinking about going back to work, and it affects their physical heart to the extent that they go into sudden cardiac arrest. They are literally being taken by stress, the silent killer. This book has been written to help you to avoid this fate!

I wrote this book to offer people a second chance, a chance to start over. No matter where you are in your life, I wrote this book for you. My book teaches you how to cope intelligently with pressure, stress and anxiety, and to no longer be overcome by it. You will also learn how to enjoy more and more of the behaviors that lengthen your life, not shorten it. I will show you how to have a lifestyle that is uniquely yours, full of success and love, one that allows you to enjoy life and all that it has to offer.

In this book you will find the means to live your life in the very best of health for many years to come. I will suggest to you in this book that the "normal" lifespan of a human being is 140-160 years. Yes! This has been proven scientifically time and again, yet there is no reason why we all don't live that long.

**This 2nd part of this book provides the foundation for you to get the most from life... starting with excellent health.**

I believe that every individual has the power to control both their physical and emotional well-being. The system I describe in this book can help you to produce dramatic results in a short time by both internally and externally activating your nervous system and your brain. Simultaneously, you will enable your immune system to function at the highest level and allow your body to produce all the bioelectrical and neuro-chemical changes necessary for optimum health, happiness, vitality and a successful life with the longest life span possible.

My **IBMS™** system is based on the premise that every human being has a conscious or unconscious ability to stimulate their nervous system to create every bioelectrical and neuro-chemical change they desire. Every human being can be healthy, happy and successful in life as long as they live according to their unique personality, following their personal desires and dreams, while constantly growing and developing themselves as human beings.

The book explains my system, which is completely based on following the natural course of neurological brain functions without any form of manipulation whatsoever. In other words, my system does not try to change you in any way, its sole purpose is to get you back to yourself, the healthy, happy you. While reading this book, you will notice direct and indirect repetitions of the subject matter; this is done on purpose as it helps you to understand, learn and apply the new information better, faster and more easily.

In addition, I want you to know that I have written this book using the latest breakthrough medical and scientific data available regarding the brain and neurological functions. To help you actually experience what you are about to learn, I have incorporated the latest developments and findings, techniques and tools being used by the most successful professional health coaches in the field.

This book is the tool you need to develop your personal goals based on your needs, desires and dreams. In it you will find your personal recipe for health using your own abilities to achieve optimum health.

I developed and perfected this method for individual health from thirty years of research, development and working with over 35,000 patients, from my experiences with over two million seminar attendees, and with the caring input from over seven million readers. Now I want to make available to you the result of my work, a self-help philosophy for your personal and individual use.

I am assuming that you chose this book because you want to learn how to reduce your stress and improve your health! You expect to discover ways to achieve a happier, healthier and more successful life, a life full of enthusiasm, vitality and strength; a life that matches your true potential.

I want you to know that this is all possible as long as you take responsibility for your outcome. If you follow the advice and do all that is necessary, you will succeed. I will show you the way, but you must do the work as you are in control of your results.

Avoid lethargy, self-doubt, hesitation or procrastination that stand in the way of your happiness! Start today by broadening your horizons. You were born to be healthy! You were born to be happy and to have fun! You were born to live a long life! Learn how to expand and develop your potential!

I see myself as your coach and friend. I chose the word "coach" on purpose because a coach does not always teach new things; instead he pushes you to strive to achieve your full potential with what you have. In my case, I press you to make use of what you already consciously and subconsciously know to get the most from life. I thoroughly believe that the only person that can make us sick is us; therefore, the only person that can heal us is ourselves!

I wish you a happy, long, healthy and successful life.

-- Dr. Leonard Coldwell

# Dedication

I dedicate this part of the book to every person who will not settle for anything less than he/she can be, achieve and own, and for optimum quality of life and vibrant health.

I specifically dedicate this part of my book to Congressman Joe Wilson, who represents the 2nd Congressional District of South Carolina. Congressman Wilson is the most impressive and honest politician that I have ever met. In my opinion, Congressman Wilson is not only a role model, but he also emulates all the values a politician should stand for. I thank my valuable friend, Congressman Wilson for his support and friendship.

# Introduction

## Your Path to Better Health

Today everyone runs the risk of suffering from stress related health problems. Many people pay such a high toll for life's demands because our modern lifestyle requires so much energy, strength, time and emotional input that their health is considerably taxed. The results can lead to stomach ulcers, intestinal problems, migraine, chronic back or circulation problems, cancer, stroke, heart attack or early death.

From the experience I have gained in my research and from working with my patients, especially for those of you who deal with everyday challenges, I created a self-help system that can assist you in the building of a healthy and vital future despite your coping with sometimes-harsh conflicts and challenges in life. This system makes it possible for you to enjoy a future with an abundance of health, fitness, energy, and quality of life, no matter what the extreme demands of your life are.

The potential lifespan of human beings is about 140-160 years (Cambridge University study) which we should be able to reach in good health. Worldwide statistics show that, alas, eighty-six percent of all people suffer from some degree of chronic illness and most of us reach less than two-thirds of our potential age.

Never before have the numbers been as high as they are today for people in need of medical care due to chronic illness, or for those who have died a premature death. The death rate from cancer and heart disease is constantly rising. The reason for this is that our bodies have not yet learned to deal with the stress and demands that diminish our energy, and affect our health in a way that has neither been known nor seen before.

We must all be prepared to accept a greater responsibility for our own health and for the health of those we love. We can no longer depend on other people, including therapists and politicians.

It is only logical that there is a cause for every illness and every symptom. The causes lie in our environments, in the way we live, in what we eat and in the way we think and feel, including the compromises we make, etc. All of these factors can lead to dis-stress and dis-ease that can take energy away from us that we need in order to stay healthy. With a lack of energy our body doesn't have the necessary power that it needs to function, much less at an optimum level. If too much energy is missing, or if energy is missing too long, the result is a logical malfunction in our biological system.

*We must take responsibility for our own lives by taking charge of our health and creating a future full of vitality, strength, energy and enthusiasm.*

This book is written to give you the opportunity to change your unhealthy behavioral patterns by using new information and techniques, some of which you know and have probably consciously or unconsciously already used. This book will help you to lay down the foundation for a long, healthy, happy and successful life. My **IBMS™** – Dr. Coldwell System™ is an amalgamation of the essence of all known, useful and result-producing systems with my thirty or more years of experience in health research and life coaching.

But let me warn you - this is not a book of positive thinking, it is a book of positive actions. This is a book that can help you to take charge of your life, your health and your fate, but only if you are willing to practice what you learn. Often laziness and/or ignorance are the reason that we get sick. The only way for us to recover and become healthy again is to take charge and make a positive change.

I assume that you are a winner, a doer, one of many who want to turn their dreams and goals into reality, even though you may not yet have reached that point at this time, but you will succeed because you are willing to do all that is necessary.

You would not have bought this book, if you were not one of ten percent of the people who take life in their own hands. You are not someone who counts on the government's dole, or waits for their ship to come in; you are not someone who waits to win the lottery, or waits for a sugar daddy to come take care of you. You are a doer and are willing to do what is necessary. I assume that this is not your first self-help book, and it won't be your last.

This book is written for people who are willing to put in the time, ideas, energy and perseverance needed, who are already using their skills and talents successfully, and who are ready to make a change to produce better health. You certainly deserve to remain fit and healthy so that you can become old enough to enjoy the pleasures you have earned from your hard life's work and you certainly deserve to see your grand and great-grandchildren grow up.

Successful people will not let other people, their surroundings or the weather influence their feelings or behavior; they create and develop their own rules for life, and they are willing to do whatever it takes to ensure their good health, happiness, and success.

*To be successful means that you set goals in every area of your life whether you have already reached a goal or not, and you are following a path by which you can reach and fulfill your wishes and dreams.*

We can excuse our failures as long as we want; we can blame others for our bad luck and for all the negative situations in our lives, but no matter who gets the blame, it does not change the final result. Looking for someone to blame will not help in any way.

Before you waste time looking for faults or excuses, it is better to quit vacillating. Draw a line over your past and previous mistakes, over the past mistakes and misdeeds of others, over your own pattern of hesitation, laziness, and omissions. Start over, take charge and take the responsibility for your future – it is truly in your own hands. Remove the whining and self-pity from your life, it will not move you forward - it only holds you back.

In this book, I offer you a complete, understandable, easy to learn health concept that will rapidly bring you positive results. In just a short amount of time you will be able to start laying the first stone towards a long, fulfilled and healthy life.

We often hear that someone who was only thirty or thirty-five years old died of a heart attack while running or playing tennis, or we learn that business-men or women in their fifties have a nervous breakdowns or simply crash from exhaustion. These situations beg the question, "What are we doing wrong, what do we need to do to live a healthy life, and what should we do so that we can enjoy finally the success for which we have worked so hard?"

*Only when you are completely healthy can you fully enjoy life and aspire to achieve optimum success. Don't settle for somewhat healthy!*

Health means the complete function of all mechanisms in an emotionally, mentally and physically successful person. Illness is an imbalance of these elements, caused by lack of energy. This shortness of energy can be triggered by environmental stress, negative behavior or thought patterns, or from deficiencies in almost any area of life.

Fitness is not the same as health; fitness is the ability to perform athletically, which does not necessarily mean that a person is healthy. People need to strive for complete health as a permanent condition, and that means a holistic sense of health, not just fitness.

Health has nothing to do with luck or misfortune, nor does it have to do with genes or inheritance. It is not a punishment to become ill, nor is health a favor. Health is the logical result of our personal conduct, the natural response of our bodies to nutrition, movement and breathing habits, including the way we cope with emotional, mental and physical stress, fear, worry and anxiety.

If we cannot handle our stress it will eventually affect our health. These factors and many others play an essential role in the developmental process of our health. If you are sick, you need to do, 100 percent, the right thing to get mentally, physically and emotionally healthy or you will stay sick. Being healthy is like being pregnant, you can't be a little pregnant - either you are or you aren't pregnant. The same is true with your health, you are either healthy or you are not!

Through modern research, we know that headaches, circulatory problems and intestinal difficulties, including other physical, emotional and mental problems, are only symptoms of illness or disease. It is not enough to treat the symptoms, you have to simultaneously look for the cause of the symptoms. If you eliminate the cause of illness, the symptoms disappear on their own.

For example, if you spend more money than you have, you must get rid of what is causing you to spend in order to stop the spending; you must find ways to prevent further spending - only then will the symptoms of the monetary shortage be removed. Therefore, you must find the cause for your illness or limited health, and get rid of the cause before you are able to enjoy optimum health.

If somebody has a headache, he can of course take one of the many headache pills on the market and hope that the headache goes away. But headaches can be the result of

233

different causes, negative emotions such as anxiety or anger, muscle tension, poison by unhealthy food, a shortage of oxygen, poor circulation, blocked nerve passages, dehydration, and much more.

If a nerve passage is blocked and you suffer continuously from pain in your neck and shoulders, you may find that your spinal column has been drawn out of its normal alignment. Stress from your work may even be the cause of a slipped disk. In these instances, you can swallow a ton of pills without the slightest chance that the disease will disappear. In other words, you can numb the pain for a limited time, but you will not achieve any long-term change without fixing the cause of the pain.

If your finger is caught in the door, it would be foolish to take pain pills while your finger is still caught in a door. Just as you must open the door and free your finger, so it is that you must remove the cause of every illness. You are responsible for your complete cure and continued health. Only you can make the necessary changes in your physical and emotional condition. Only you can relieve the symptoms by taking away the cause.

Dear reader, this book is not going to tell you that you can become healthy with positive thinking. This book is written for doers, for those who act. In the psychology of success, we distinguish between the two different types of people - those who act and those who simply talk about acting.

This book is written for positive doers. Your health does not just happen, just as money does not fall from the sky. You put extra effort into your work and your career, so you must strive for a healthy mind and body. This is the only sure way to produce and enjoy perfect health. You have to create and keep your health!

*Could you imagine yourself as successful if you were suffering from pain and in need of nursing and medical attention? I don't think so!*

My definition of success encompasses total all-around success. Success must be built in every area of our life – this means health, financial success, partnerships, contentment, happiness and love. We must recognize that for emotional and physical health, we need the same basic components for happiness and success.

Success is a feeling, not something tangible. We all have a different understanding of what success means to us. To be successful and healthy, you have to feel successful! Every individual has their own frame of reference for what will make them feel successful. Only you know what success means for you.

I am giving you a set of instructions to enable you to be completely independent from that of other people, circumstances, genetic makeup, the full moon, bio-rhythms or even your horoscope; a possibility to take full charge of your physiological, emotional and mental health. You will never be the victim of circumstances or fate; rather you will be the creator of your own future if you apply what you learn. You will be responsible for your own life, your level of health, and your success.

To avoid areas of conflict or the causes of unwanted behavior, limitations and undesired results, we must first recognize, define and understand them. Only then can we find solutions to cope with these challenges. Living in denial or delusions will not make anything better. You have to adjust to problems, limitations, etc. in order to change them.

I have written down all the information you need. I will be your health and stress reduction coach, so that you can become completely healthy and fully successful in life. I hope that this book will make it possible for you to use more of your unlimited potential, so that you can help yourself and others to recognize your talents, so that, together, you will not only reach the summit, but also stay there, and proclaim your own personal success in life and in health.

Our health is a lifelong gift that we can only experience and enjoy when we are happy, content, well balanced and satisfied in every area of our life. Most people know what they must do to change and how they should go about it – but they do nothing. Not knowing, but acting on your knowledge is the difference between health and illness, success and failure. It is not always the complex or the difficult that makes the difference between health and illness. Often a thousand little things, obvious facts, laziness, comfort, cowardice or ignorance that make the difference, whether we live and enjoy our life on the highest level ... or not.

People often believe that easy or pleasant things cannot be good. If medicine tastes good, it will probably not work. This is usually not true. It is, however, true that there are no isolated tricks or secrets that promise lifelong health, vitality and the expectation of longevity. There are no magic pills that can cure the common cold; five-day miracle diets do not work, nor do promises to be fit, slim and beautiful in three days. Health, like illness, is a slow process, the logical consequence of correct or poor behavior in many areas of life.

As your personal wellness and health coach, I want to show you how to quickly and successfully improve the quality of your life. If you are willing to practice a few basic essential elements, which are necessary, easily applied and executed, your quality of life will rapidly improve.

*"Solutions are always simple, until someone needlessly complicates them to sell you an expensive solution!"*

After many years of researching and testing people who work in stressful environments, it is now possible to identify and define the causes of chronic and even death-threatening illnesses. Only decades ago, we were convinced that health problems resulted from our genetic makeup, fate or bad luck. Today this has changed as we now are aware that every person has the possibility to live a healthy life, no matter what their genetic makeup.

If you do not reach your lifespan potential of 140-160 years, it is only due to emotional, mental and physiological stress, inferior nutrition, lack of exercise, poor breathing, and/or immune system breakdowns. You can avoid many of these health problems simply by learning how to cope with fear, worry and doubt.

You may have heard news about genetics and gene therapy, but I have these words of advice for you, *"Do not believe that genes predetermine whether or not you will get sick in your lifetime."* Studies of identical twins have proven, this is not so! Genetic predisposition does not mean that you will or will not get a disease. You are in control of your health; now is the time to take action and do something about it.

# The Instinct Based Medicine System™
# IBMS™

## *Your Individual Manual for Personal Success*

### What is IBMS™ The Dr. Coldwell's System™?

The **IBMS™** is a holistic self-help training, educational and coaching system. The system is based on the premise that every human being has a conscious or unconscious ability to stimulate their nervous system to create every bioelectrical and neuro-chemical change they could possibly desire and everyone has the ability to condition their nervous system for any level of health they wish to attain. The **IBMS™** is also based on the fact that every person already has the solutions to solve all their life challenges and that they have the power to achieve all their goals and that power is readily within their grasp.

The system's belief is that every human being can be healthy, happy and successful in life as long as they live according to their unique personality, following their personal desires and dreams, while constantly growing and developing themselves as human beings.

The **IBMS™** is a help to self-help system for people that want to take charge of their life to be the best that they can be, both in health and success in life.

239

Every individual has the power to control both their physical and emotional well being. The **IBMS™** can help produce dramatic results in a short time by both internally and externally stimulating the nervous system and the brain to create new ways of functioning that bring better health. Simultaneously, the **IBMS™** activates the immune system to function properly and enables the body to produce all bioelectrical and neuro-chemical changes necessary for optimum health, happiness, vitality for a long, successful life - with the longest life span possible.

Since there is a measurable and known neuro-chemical response for any emotion, and since that neuro-chemical response can be found in the circulation of our blood and throughout every cell in our body, we can significantly and positively influence our nervous system by stimulating the neurophysiology of our health through enthusiasm, passion, contentment, harmony and love.

The **IBMS™** is a "help to self-help system" that I will expand into a "teaching method for unlimited personal success and excellent health" later in this book. All this, however, is nothing more than a manual that teaches you how to stimulate and program your brain so that when needed, you can make full use of your physiological and mental potential.

Because we know scientifically that a strong stimulus can activate internal neuro-chemical reactions at a predetermined time and rate, I discovered that human beings could install stimuli in the nervous system simply by activating one of the five senses. By doing so, the stimuli would release a specific neuro-chemical reaction in the body. This makes it possible for every person to assume control of their health, energy, and emotional and physiological states.

*Through all of this research, I made the most important discovery - the only real help for people is helping them to help themselves.*

The **IBMS™** can only work if you are willing to modify the suggestions to suit your personal needs, imagination, dreams, wishes and goals, so that you create your unique personal success system and turn your life into the masterpiece it is meant to be. It is only when you live your own individual life and faithfully follow your dreams that you can be happy, healthy and successful in life.

## How did the IBMS™ Develop?

The **IBMS™** was originally like many other systems - a hypothesis. The **IBMS™** is a vision, motivated by the need to overcome helplessness and a desire to take control. A system designed to help people help themselves.

In my own life, I was driven to understand holistic health and the root causes of disease because my mother, in the final stages of cancer that was caused by cirrhosis of the liver due to gallbladder surgery that went wrong, was given two years to live by her physician. During the period of fighting to keep my mother alive, I continuously searched for different alternative ways to help her, but in the end, I realized that the solution to every human problem lies within the person. My mother is still alive and well today more than thirty years later.

Research at the University of California concluded with certainty that the brain can be stimulated to produce a large amount of interferon to fight cancer. From that research and similar other scientific results, I was encouraged to search for new and more effective ways to help people to heal and regenerate.

As I experienced successful results with my patients, many of whom had "miraculous healings" similar to my mother's, I was encouraged to figure out how to apply this knowledge to every other area of life.

When I documented my research scientifically proving that it was possible to consciously stimulate the bioelectric and neuro-chemical processes in the body through internal and external stimuli of the senses, I found that I had attracted the attention of the entire medical profession, which in turn, provided me with the opportunity for more extensive study and research. This enabled me to perfect and broaden my hypothesis and its application

## How does the IBMS™ Work?

Given today's typical lifestyle, we are constantly stimulating and often over stimulating our nervous system and brain, but because we are only aware of a small percentage of our abilities, possibilities and strengths, we utilize our capabilities inefficiently and get irregular and random results. Albert Einstein believed we only use ten percent of our brain capacity - modern science believes that it is only one percent.

With this system, you have the opportunity to take conscious control over your internal and external stimulus, as well as your visualization and thought processes. When you learn that you can control your emotions, you find that this allows you to control your energy level. You want to learn to control your emotional, mental and physiological behavior with internal and external skills of communication so that you can realize the results you want to produce in your life.

The **IBMS™**, therefore, offers you the possibility to take complete control of your health and life. The system is based on natural neuro-chemical and bioelectrical functions and on every individual person's inherent skills, talents and possibilities.

Using this system, I have been able to help patients with chronic illnesses, including cancer, muscular dystrophy, rheumatism, gout, asthma, ulcers, multiple sclerosis, Parkinson's, Alzheimer's, chronic pain, obesity, cardio vascular disease, psoriasis, depression, anxiety, phobias, ulcers, migraine, cirrhosis of the liver and basically every other illness you can think of. I have also worked with many athletes, helping them to reach the top in the sport, in their country and even the world. I have also trained Europe's largest companies extremely successfully with my system. My system works also for military, police and firefighters very successfully.

Because there is no standard solution for human beings, you must individualize, apply and modify what you learn from the **IBMS™** to fit your personal needs. You have to make it your own. Only you and you alone can change your life because you are the only one that knows what you want in life.

Each and every individual person alone has the ability to create and maintain a life with minimized stress for themselves that is effective, productive, filled with love, harmony and success. Because of this, my system offers easily adaptable methods that everybody can modify and apply to all aspects of their life. The key is to develop your own personalized system for your health and for your success.

You are a miracle of nature with unlimited possibilities, and the **IBMS™** helps you to realize all that you could ever want to achieve. In other words, nature provides us with the equipment to create success and health, while the **IBMS™** provides the means to recognize and use your full potential!

## Why "Managing" Stress or Stress "Management" is Dangerous and Wrong!

I often hear of programs that are really stress *management* systems and techniques instead of stress *reduction* systems and techniques. Managing stress is basically telling the brain that the bad stress is acceptable, let's just manage it. It is no different than pretending that you can manage poisons or cancer in your body.

It is important instead to learn to minimize or reduce the existing stress in your neurological system, which is why only stress reduction techniques and systems are helpful to your life and health. The goal should always be to prevent or reduce stress, not to manage it! This is because the more you manage stress, the more pressure builds inside the nervous system, which will inevitably lead to a catastrophe damaging your health.

Many people do not know that many relaxation techniques that get you and keep you in the alpha state can be damaging to your health. In the alpha state, a person's brain functions on a state of diminished alertness and limited critical thinking. Hypnotism and meditation techniques that keep you in the alpha state where you can supposedly reprogram or recondition a behavior do not generally produce lasting results because the brain does not accept information that you have not consciously agreed to accept before, during, and after the sessions. Moreover, the obvious manipulation through hypnotism can make you do the exact opposite of what you intend or can make you dependent, schizophrenic and can cause lack of self-esteem.

In order to effect a lasting change in one's life, a person must make a conscious decision using "free will" otherwise it cannot be a permanent change. If a person does not want to stop smoking for themselves, but instead quits for another person, then they will most likely go back to smoking. With hypnosis, a bigger problem arises when a person develops obsessive compulsive behavior due to the "hypnotized" foreign artificially created behavior!

Once a problem is acknowledged, it is possible to make a conscious decision to change, but this type of decision does not last when it is made in an *alpha* state of the brain. My scientific research shows that conscious decisions in the beta state are a major and very important part of the positive changes in the natural neuro-chemical and bioelectrical functions of the body and brain. Only when combined with this component can successful neurological changes be made.

To achieve a lasting change in the nervous system, your brain needs to switch frequencies in a very specific order. In other words, your brain needs to move between frequencies delta (0-2 MHz), theta (3-6 MHz), alpha (7-13 MHz), and beta (14-30 MHz) in a specific sequence. When in an alpha state, there is no way to make a conscious decision; you have to switch to beta at exactly the right time when you are making a decision to change a behavior otherwise it cannot be effective over the long term. Then you have to switch into lower states in the right frequency to build dendrites (new microchips) in your brain for effective long term results. This is the natural way of brain function. It is only when you use the natural way that we are intended to function that you can achieve healthy and long term results.

The only system I know to continuously produce lasting results over and over again is the **IBMS™** programs. This is due to the combination of the specially created music along with the newest technology of brain function, working together to effortlessly help to create the exact state of mind required to produce lasting results.

*The* **IBMS™** *uses the decoded language of the brain to produce optimum results.*

The reason that hypnotherapy can be addictive and lead to schizophrenia is because it is a manipulation of the self as the therapist is making decisions for you during the process. These decisions are called "suggestions." This can happen directly or indirectly, and too often, unknowingly. If you do not desire a clear outcome and develop a natural way to achieve this goal, the brain gets irritated.

In comparison, a **IBMS™** session is completely different because it uses open generic symbols which each person fills with their individual picture thereby personalizing the suggestions to fit with their unique experience. There is no manipulation of any kind as each person is in complete control of all of their decisions as they personalize them to their own individual self.

I believe that any form of manipulation is a crime against humanity, which is also the reason that I no longer work with hypnotherapy as a part of my treatments. When I discovered all the negative aspects to hypnosis, I immediately stopped using hypnotism in any form.

Meditation is scientifically proven to relax you, but the effect can be short lived and meditation does not eliminate or address the root of problems. Additionally, meditation can lead to inactivity and eventually feelings of failure or depression. It is a passive technique that in my experience does not achieve long-term results for active change. It is more a tool for short-term relaxation and in my opinion is a waste of time.

More potentially damaging than these are NLP techniques, Neuro-Linguistic Programming techniques. NLP can suppress emotions and cause people to act in a way that is contrary to their normal behavior. This can lead to multiple personality disorder and even illness in some cases. NLP techniques can ultimately drain people of energy and can lead to feelings of failure and depression. NLP can also set off internal conflicts that can be a major chronic stress factor. This is my personal opinion that is shared by many scientists and therapists.

It is not possible to achieve a long-term positive result that does not emanate from a person's own individual personality. In other words, the type of system that could bring about a lasting result would be a system that uses the unique personality of each person and is fundamentally based on their personal goals and desires. The **IBMS™** is the only system I know that is designed so that each person achieves their specific goals according to their personal wants and needs.

One of the side effects of massage, meditation and hypnotherapy is that people often feel tired after a session. Scientifically, we know that if a person is relaxed for more than seven minutes, the body produces sleep hormones which if you don't use them up by actually sleeping, can cause you to feel tired or even exhausted for the rest of the day. The **IBMS™**, on the other hand, relaxes you, but you remain alert and awake; after each session you generally feel regenerated as though you just had hours of restful sleep.

Remark: Some people will fall asleep during the first few sessions which often means that they are in much need of rest in order to regenerate and heal. This is a rare possible side effect that is not bad, it is simply the result of exhaustion and will disappear after the first few sessions. It actually shows you just how badly you are in need of rest and regeneration. Some people may cry during or after the first session; this is not bad and is the result of finally being able to let go of all the tension and pressure they have been holding on to in their lives. This is a sign of release and is good!

## Understanding the IBMS™

**IBMS™ session 1** is the basic component of the **IBMS™**, the worlds most advanced scientifically grounded, self-help training system that represents the amalgamation of years of study and self-help applications proven to target and eliminate the root causes of mental and emotional stress. Mental and emotional stress is the root cause of all illness.

When you use this system you will be training your brain from the ground up, and you will discover that what you are experiencing is nothing less than a total rehabilitation of your brain's cognitive functions. These applications have been scientifically proven to:

- Eliminate the root causes of mental and emotional stress that inevitably leads to illness.
- Facilitate active stress reduction and regeneration of the entire nervous system.
- Enable your body to utilize its maximum level of oxygen, a crucial component for optimizing your health and energy level.
- Boost your determination, self-esteem, confidence, and power to act.

In addition:

- Most people feel a sense of calm with more energy and lucidity than before.
- Feel rested and better able to cope with and solve problems.
- Most report they are better able to sleep at night.

## The IBMS™ self-help without competition!

The **IBMS™ session 1** program is a self-help system completely free of any form of manipulation as the system applies your personality and character traits to realize your personal dreams, goals and instincts by giving you total control over your self-conditioning and stress reduction. The **IBMS™ session** Zone, a state developed by me, is the state you attain during your session when your body is physically totally relaxed while your brain is clear and alert, giving you total control over your session and outcome, and enabling you to holistically address the root cause of stress and stress related health problems.

*This system is the only known system that can guarantee that there is no manipulation of any kind and that all conditioning is entirely determined by you.*

## What the IBMS™ can do for you

The **IBMS™ session 1** users report the following results:
- Increased energy
- Stops slumps/dips during the day
- Improved optimism
- Improved self-esteem
- More effective management of life problems
- Improved sleep patterns; awaken rested and alert.
- Increased productivity
- Calmer nervous system
- Enhanced libido
- Increased coping skills
- Clarity
- Improved quality of life
- Reduced emotional pain and suffering

- Accelerated recovery from physical manifestations of stress
- Enhanced immune function.

## Be Yourself

I made a major discovery when I realized that human beings can only be happy, content, healthy and successful if they learn to accept and be themselves. That means that they must live according to their own unique wishes, needs, dreams, talents and skills, and work continuously toward their goals. Unfortunately, our society and environment conditions us that we shouldn't do what is in our heart.

Statements like "You shouldn't do that..." or "You should do it this way..." condition us to suppress our personalities and/or instincts and/or individual needs, replacing them with strange behavior or unfamiliar emotional states forced on us by others. Not living by your instincts, emotions and inner signals will cause restlessness and frustration, which in turn takes away your energy and causes incredible stress. The best stress reduction is to develop a stable self esteem and self confidence, use common sense and listen to your instincts, your feelings and needs. Live yourself the way you really are!

We are all created differently, and when it comes to complete health and success in life, there is no "norm" that fits every individual, making it impossible to set a standard for the "correct" or "right" wishes, needs and dreams. Every person has their own individual wishes, needs and dreams. What is right for one person could be absolutely wrong for another, which is why people have the right to live as they choose and to make mistakes, develop, mature, grow, and change their behavior in whatever way they deem best for them. At the end the only person you have to answer to – is you! You are the only one that has to live with the results created by your actions.

One of the most important requirements to be satisfied, happy, successful, healthy, and full of vitality is acknowledging that you are the person you were meant to be, and this is just fine. You must surely recognize that you are endowed with unique wonderful talents, possibilities and skills, and there is no one like you on earth. It is this uniqueness that provides you with a future full of distinctive possibilities, opportunities, challenges and successes.

It is only when you learn to accept yourself the way you are, constantly using your full potential to attain what you want, that you will enjoy a life without compromises, tension and pressure, or self-deception and duplicity. It is not until you no longer undermine yourself that you can really get on with a life that is without unnecessary stress. Only if you love yourself you can be happy and healthy. You are a special person.

You are the one and only person with whom you absolutely have the deal with for the rest of your life. You must, therefore, first learn to get along with yourself. Every human being must understand, accept, respect and love themselves first. How can you accept other people the way they are, if you have not accepted yourself the way you are? Many people live in a dream world with delusions because they are taught to believe that they do not have the right to be themselves.

**Final Observation**

Outstanding scientists are constantly proving that the impossible is possible; this is happening not just once in a while, but over and over again. Many great inventors have initially been criticized and even attacked for their inventions, but what sets them apart is their inner dream to create what they conceive in their mind.

At this point, I want you to take a moment, and in your mind create a picture of yourself and how you see your life and your future, a month, a year, five years from now and when you reach a very old age. See it completely and in its entirety, all that you have accomplished, all that you have become as a human being, and then make the decision that you are willing to do everything necessary to produce, build and achieve the future that you see for yourself. I am absolutely convinced that there isn't a goal that cannot be realized if we can both see it and really want it.

My many years of research and experience have revealed that our subconscious mind is totally aware of our unlimited possibilities, there is absolutely no doubt, and this is why I have concluded that *"Everybody, and I mean everybody, has the possibility to reach whatever goal is created in their mind."* This is possible because once the desire is planted in the mind; the brain creates the possibility for how to fulfill it. So I am absolutely convinced that every human being can achieve whatever they want if they make up their mind to do so. I must, however, reiterate that the foundation for success is the willingness to do everything that is necessary to attain the desired success. You must take action because only you can make the changes in your life that you are going to have to make to realize your dreams. The **IBMS™** can help you clarify your true goals and desires, and help you develop the motivation, perseverance and determination to act successfully!

I developed the **IBMS™** to provide you with the tools necessary to turn your life into the adventure that you dreamed it should be, full of success, satisfaction, happiness and health. It has been my goal to create a system that is easy and simple to use and reproduce. I have developed a system that helps people to attain great heights and success in all areas of life.

It needs to be repeated that you are the only person who can achieve success, health and happiness. No one but you can remove your worries, fears and sorrows - only you can resolve the conflicts in your life. Your life will only truly become yours when you fully recognize that you are the only person in the world who can have a permanent influence on your life. And that you are the only person that has to live with the consequences of your decisions, actions and apathy.

If you are willing to accept and use your individual personality, if you continue to do two or three new things every day, your life will soon become the happy adventure you want it to be.

You have a wonderful, long and healthy life ahead of you, and it can be whatever you decide it will be. Take control of your life and work with all of your possibilities, so that you can make your life into the fulfillment of your dreams.

# Section II - Chapter 1

## *Understanding Stress*

**What is stress?**

Stress is the body's reaction to a primary stimulus... danger, real or imagined. Danger is perceived by human beings as anything that threatens their mental, emotional or physical well being. Under stress, people can experience confusion, loss of control, abnormal behavior, and irrational fear. Dating from our primeval ancestors, when the body is threatened with danger, it immediately produces stress hormones. These hormones trigger fight or flight reactions, but since people cannot run or fight in normal life situations, the hormones stay in the body and alter emotional, mental and physical behavior. This can lead to abnormal actions and reactions such as binge eating, panic attacks, nervous or physical breakdowns, random aches and pain, depression, burn out; even suicidal tendencies.

**Are mental, emotional and physical stresses different?**

**YES:**

- *Mental stress* comes from **creating** or **remembering** disturbing mental images. Examples would be creating negative outcomes of future

253

events such as an irrational fear of being fired or humiliated or harmed, or recalling threatening situations, domineering parents, abusive caretakers or teachers or spouses, etc.

- *Emotional stress* comes from **experiencing** threats, severe illness, worry, hopelessness, helplessness, self-doubt, fear of failure, lack of self-esteem, or living with unfair compromise. Some examples would be suffering in a bad relationship or oppressive work environment, being physically or emotionally abused, undergoing divorce or bankruptcy or death of a family member, or being helpless to aid or comfort a loved one.

- *Physical stress* comes from exceeding normal physical capabilities that lead to physical exhaustion. Examples would be excessive drinking or eating, exhaustive physical exercise, constant extreme pain, sleep deprivation, unruly children, and working under deadlines. Also included are internal toxic and/or acidic reactions, some allergies, as well as nutritional deficiencies.

**NOTE:** All three stresses can be interdependent and interrelated.

## Is one type of stress worse than another?

Continuous, uninterrupted mental and/or emotional stress often goes unrecognized and untreated. This will sap the body's energy reserves and will eventually lead to a health breakdown and severe illness. Complete physical exhaustion (stress) will halt the body's ability to continue any activity at a specific point in time, but seldom causes a health breakdown. Physical stress can be alleviated by proper rest and nutrition and/or reducing workload.

## What are some of the symptoms of mental and emotional stress?

The **symptoms** of mental and emotional stress can be divided into two categories – physical symptoms and psychological signs.

<u>Physical Symptoms</u>:
- exhaustion, fatigue, lethargy
- headaches, migraines, vision problems
- heart palpitations, racing pulse, rapid shallow breathing
- muscle tension, aches, spasms
- dehydration
- joint and back pain
- shakiness, tremors, ticks, twitches, paralysis
- nervousness, panic attacks
- heartburn, indigestion, diarrhea, constipation, nausea, dizziness, ulcers
- dry mouth and throat
- sexual dysfunction, lowered libido
- excessive sweating, clammy hands, cold hands and/or feet, poor circulation
- rashes, hives, itching, eczema, adult acne
- nail biting, fidgeting, hair twirling or pulling
- loss of appetite, bulimia, anorexia
- obesity, overeating
- sleep difficulties, insomnia
- teeth grinding
- asthma, allergies
- increased use of alcohol and/or drugs and medication
- high blood pressure, weakened immune system.

<u>Psychological Symptoms</u>:
- irritability, impatience, anger, hostility
- anxiety, panic, worrying, denial
- agoraphobia

- moodiness, bipolar tendencies, sadness, feeling upset,
- energy swings
- emotionally exhausted, overwhelmed
- involuntarily crying, depression
- helplessness, hopelessness, lack of self-esteem
- neurotic or uncommon behavior, schizophrenia
- paranoia, claustrophobia, ADD, ADHD
- intrusive and/or racing thoughts
- memory loss, lack of concentration, indecision
- lack of motivation
- frequent absences from work, lowered productivity
- feeling overwhelmed
- loss of sense of humor.

## Why does stress affect our health?

All illness stems from a lack of energy! Emotional and/or mental stress is the greatest energy drainer affecting humans. Continuous, uninterrupted emotional and/or mental stress will inevitably lead to an energy breakdown, which in turn will be followed by a health breakdown. Therefore mental and emotional stress is the root cause of all illness and most of all of cancer.

## What else does stress cause?

Stress can cause dehydration, nutritional deficiencies, lack of oxygen and restful self-healing phases. Stress is also one of the main causes for diseases and symptoms like:

Cancer, heart disease, ADD/ADHD, Parkinson's, Alzheimer's, sexual dysfunction, bulimia, pre-aging, lowered immune function, rheumatic/arthritic/fibromyalgia, and joint and muscle pain, obesity, constipation, insomnia, memory loss, suicide , toxemia and acidosis.

**Is dealing with stress really that important?**

Untreated mental and emotional stress can shorten life expectancy and destroy quality of life. What is more important than that?

**What is the primary physiological effect of stress?**

Chronic stress leads to dehydration, one of the primary causes of physical degeneration, atrophy, and death.

**Scientifically confirmed symptoms of dehydration are:**
- DNA damage
- lowered immune functions
- inability to absorb foods, vitamins and minerals
- lack of energy supply from digestion
- reduction in efficiency of red blood cells

**Some emotional manifestations of dehydration include:**
- depression
- anxiety
- feelings of inadequacy
- irritability
- dejection
- self-consciousness
- cravings (caffeine, alcohol, drugs, etc.)
- agoraphobia

**Scientifically recognized physical signs of dehydration include:**
- fibromyalgia
- asthma
- bronchitis
- allergies
- indigestion/acid reflux
- chronic arthritic pain

- high blood pressure
- higher cholesterol
- chronic fatigue syndrome
- angina
- strokes
- ear related symptoms, dizziness, equilibrium problems
- deafness
- visual problems
- cataract
- vitreous detachment
- Uveitis
- Multiple Sclerosis

**Note:** The main cause of dehydration (other than not drinking water) is stress!

## Some facts to consider:

- Scientists at Cambridge University have evidence that the human life potential can reach 160 years.
- 112 million people take stress related medication.
- 250 million prescriptions for tranquilizers are filled annually.
- 25 million Americans suffer from high blood pressure.
- 15 million people have social anxieties.
- 14 million are alcoholics.
- 5 million people are depressed.
- 3 million people suffer from panic attacks.
- 1 million people have heart attacks each year.
- Muscles are a primary target for stress; manifesting in cramping, spasms, back and jaw pain and tremors.
- Stress can play a significant role in circulatory and heart disease, sudden cardio death and strokes.
- Stress can increase blood pressure, raise cholesterol levels and speed up blood clotting.
- Stress causes more heart disease than smoking.
- Heart disease kills more people than any other disease.

- The Harvard School for Public Health published that sixty-five percent of all cancer can be prevented by diet.
- The American Cancer Society published that at least one-third of all cancer could be prevented by diet.
- Studies have shown a sixty-six percent decrease in cancer among women with a higher oxygen level.
- Mainstream medicine agrees that your body can only heal while asleep.
- Experts worldwide agree that a positive attitude contributes to a major part of health.

## Exhilarating Health

Most heart attacks happen on Monday between eight and nine in the morning. No other day of the week, or time of day, comes even close in numbers. There are people, who at the age of forty, when they are finally able to truly enjoy their success, suffer a heart attack or a stroke, which confines them to spend the rest of their lives in wheelchairs or in bed. They no longer are able to participate in the lives of their loved ones. This is an extreme example of the negative interaction between stress and health, and it's far too common.

*Of course I know what you are thinking: "This can only happen to others – not to me."* But believe me. The people to whom it happened, they thought the same thing. If they had not thought so, surely they would have done something to stop it from happening to them.

*The results of comprehensive and extensive research show that seven percent of independent businessmen, or people in top management, suffer a medical tragedy before the age of 52. Dr. Kenneth R. Pelletier, professor of Medicine and Psychiatry at the University of California in San Francisco, writes in one of his books that there are others, the top seven percent in management that not only survive life's stresses harmlessly, but they use them to produce greater achievements and results in every area of their life. That other seven percent die from the same amount of professional stress, under the same pressure, and often in the same business!*

Therefore, you must decide whether, going forward, you will let stress have a negative influence on your career, your professional and your personal life. If so, your chances for success will be greatly diminished. You can ignore the trivialities, pain, worries, fear, cramps, tension, headaches and problems with concentration, stomach and intestinal ulcers so long that you may even risk a premature death. You can search for books, tapes and lectures, which promise a quick health fix or sell you pills to hide the symptoms, or you can take responsibility for your future, health and life by taking charge of your emotional, mental and physiological condition. If so, you should follow the instructions I am offering you. They are vital and necessary to create health and to remain in great shape.

This program has no shortcuts to cover up the symptoms that could grow into formidable life threatening problems. I will share with you the knowledge gained through research, treatment of patients, and people who succeeded in avoiding illness, or who regained their health after suffering sometimes catastrophic health problems. To enjoy health, fitness and vitality we must follow some basic rules. There are no tricks or secrets. There is only one way to holistic health. You have to use the many necessary, but simple steps that bring about the desired results. You cannot compromise your health in any field; you have to be emotionally, mentally and physically healthy! If you are not motivated enough to achieve optimum health for yourself, do it for your children, your spouse and people you love. Be a role model.

If we have not learned how to react and cope with these issues, pressures, stresses, fears and compromises, it can have a disastrous impact on our lives.

**It is not what happens in our lives, but how we react to what happens that influences our stress level.**

The AMA (American Medical Association) informs us that two out of three deaths are premature and could have been avoided. Statistics of health insurance agencies tell us that approximately one million people show up every day at their doctor's office or at hospital emergency rooms in urgent need of medical attention. The number one killer is heart disease. Two out of every four persons die of heart problems, and one out of four dies from cancer and the death rate from cancer is rising.

Several studies show that stress is the main cause of premature death and suicide. The expression: "My job is killing me." takes on an eerie reality that hits all too close to home. The consumption of tremendous amounts of Valium, Prozac, Paxil, etc., as well as other medications for depression and bipolar disease, can be often attributed to job related stress. Stress is all too often caused by financial problems, dislike of a job, a bad relationship, a difficult boss or employer, or simply a lack of career opportunities and advancement. People feel like they are "stuck in a dead-end job" and life becomes so complicated that there is literally no longer room to breathe.

Very sensitive or overwhelmed people may even see illness or death as a solution, a way out, so that they may be released from a tormenting situation. Suicide and unconscious self destruction are often the result of hopelessness and stress overload.

## It is Never Too Late to Start Over

Don't worry so much about past mistakes - instead focus and concentrate on the future. Too many people believe that after neglecting their body for years, or even decades, it is impossible to improve or dramatically change their physical condition.

This basic assumption is wrong because about ninety percent of our body cells are renewed or replaced every eleven months. Most of the cells in our body are not older than two years. Between one and seven billion liver cells are renewed every second. Every six weeks we have a new liver, all kidney cells are replaced within eight weeks, the skin is renewed in four weeks, the mucous membrane in twenty-four hours, and four thousand red blood cells are renewed every second of our life.

Remark: We are made up of atoms. Atoms are empty. This means that we are made up of pure energy; therefore, it is possible for us to continuously transform our health. Energy does not age.

## The human body is nature's masterpiece!

*If we wanted to reproduce the storage capacity of our brain, we would need to fill the Trump Tower in NY five times over with the newest microchips and computer technology. We would need all the water in the Colorado River to cool this facility and all the electricity consumed by the entire city of Philadelphia to power the installation. And all this would not be sufficient to execute a single train of thought. Our three pound brain functions with greater ease than even the most advanced computer.*

*Our heart beats about 100,000 times each day and pumps our blood through a network of blood vessels with a combined length of about 55,000 miles.*

*Our eyes can differentiate ten million shades of color and our muscles have a combined strength of twenty five tons of force if it were exerted on a single object.*
We are an unbelievable masterpiece of nature, but we take it for granted since we are born healthy, and since at first it takes no effort to be healthy, we often treat our bodies carelessly.

It is not until we get sick or have a medical problem that we fully appreciate our good health. Many people ignore their good health in the first half of their life while they are making their money, but then they spend the second half of their life spending their money trying to restore the damage they did to their health in the first part of their life. My goal is to help you avoid this experience by helping you to stop and/or avoid making many of the damaging mistakes.

*There is substantial proof that there are no incurable diseases, there are only people who refuse to do what is necessary in order to get better.*

People who refuse to recognize or believe that they are responsible for their health and maintenance have little chance of getting better.

Many people do not believe that illness is the result of personal misconduct; as such they also do not and cannot admit that they are responsible for their failing health. Anybody who believes that they cannot influence the promotion of a healthy body will not take the necessary steps to achieve a healthy body.

*Many of us find it difficult to accept that we are not perfect. We are all too often stubborn, or we hide behind ignorance and naivety and then blame other people or circumstances for our shortcomings.*

In my opinion, the term "stress" is one of the most misused words as it has become a fashionable catch phrase for a multitude of problems. We hide behind it as an excuse for not finishing a project on time, we use it as an excuse for failures and mistakes, we use it to kid ourselves when we cannot handle a situation - in other words, "stress" is frequently used as an excuse for failure.

What is damaging stress? Damaging stress (or dis-stress) is continuous pressure that results from exceeding our ability to deal with life situations. One such example would be when we have too many projects that demand our attention all at the same time, and no one job gets properly completed. Stress occurs because the brain shuts down due too much stimuli and it feels life-threatened. It does not matter whether or not the situation is really life threatening. The results are either you get regenerated or your brain will only be able use the little amount of energy remaining for its survival.

Stress arises when we inefficiently destroy our energy by focusing on what has already happened or on our problems rather than the solutions to our problems and a positive future. Typical stress symptoms grow from feelings of helplessness or from being in a situation from which we feel we cannot act effectively. Stress is the logical result of feeling out of control, of concentrating on a mountain of problems instead of the solutions. Stress triggers the fight or flight reaction that so often leads to many major problems in our life's, relationships and can lead to uncontrolled or absurd actions.

***Stress is a shortage of energy resulting from emotional and/or physiologically perceived danger or overload.***

To successfully fight or prevent stress, you must understand that you in fact create your stress; the symptoms of stress come after overworking or overloading your nervous system too much or for too long of a time without effective rest.

Pressure is not necessarily negative or dangerous because pressure is what can motivate us to grow, develop and accomplish the things that we need to do. The problem comes from ongoing pressure and strain that demands more than our nervous system can handle. And the higher your stress level is, the more you need to constantly regenerate.

Remember the example of rubbing your hand against the edge of a table, how initially your hand is fine, but if you continuously rub for an hour it will start to hurt; then if you keep rubbing it after a few hours it gets irreparably damaged. The same is true with stress. If you take regular breaks and get regenerated, your stress will not damage you.

Daily short-term stress does not cause any damage; it is ongoing stress over a long period of time that leads to serious damage. Then again using the above example of rubbing your hand over a table, if you rubbed your hand on the table and then lifted your hand and took a break for thirty seconds so that it had time to regenerate, you could then keep doing this forever without harming your hand. So is the case with stress! The most effective way to do that is to use the **IBMS™** at least once a day or whenever you feel overwhelmed.

Stress is used as a catchphrase to describe many things that cause negative reactions in people. However, some things that cause stress to one person may actually be fun to another person. The scientific division between Eu-stress and Dis-stress, positive and negative stress, does not, in my opinion, make sense because positive stress, like overwhelming joy and happiness can sometimes lead to a heart attack in the same way that sadness, fear or anger can also lead to heart attacks. If you are **mentally, emotionally and physically** strong, stress cannot harm you. Reference to negative stress or dis-stress in this work program is only to make things easier to understand.

So that we all understand clearly and in order to achieve the greatest results possible, we need to develop a new definition of the word "stress." Traditionally we have been trained to consider stress as a negative that threatens our lives, but in fact this is an artificially created concept.

**The commonly accepted scientific definitions for stress are:**
- Dis-Stress – the lack of fulfillment of vital needs which leaves us with an actual reluctance of function in our lymphatic system.
- Eu-Stress – Fulfillment of our vital needs which creates actual enjoyment in our lymphatic system.

**Assuming Control**

You need to understand that your feelings, energy and behavior altogether influence everything you do and experience in your life. Nobody but you can solve and overcome your problems. Life is not affected by all your knowledge and learning, only action and application of your knowledge and learning determine the direction of your health and life. The difference between theorizing and practical application is hard work! But it pays off in the end with good health, delayed aging and a long life. Self pity and denial can kill you.

Positive thinking is nothing more than the prerequisite for positive action. Positive thinking alone does not and will not change your life; only positive action changes your life. If you do not act, there will be others that will; if you do not make a decision, others will decide for you. If you do not give your life direction, others will take the wheel, so that they can use and abuse you.

The book and DVD " The Secret " that just became a major best seller in America, is one of the most dangerous products on the market today. It tells you about the power of expectation and that you have only to expect what you like and you will get it – and that will definitely not happen. Believe me after over

2.2 million seminar attendees, 35 000 patients and millions of readers that communicated with me, I know for a fact that only positive action will get you what you desire not positive passivity!

Our life is our life in the truest sense of the word only when we are willing to take responsibility and control and do not leave it in the hands of fate. It is our life when we do not let others decide how we are supposed to feel, how we are supposed to think or behave or let others influence our behavior and thinking in a negative way. It is our life when we stop hiding behind excuses. This is also the only way to optimum health.

We can achieve happiness, success, harmony, peace, healthy relationships and all the wonderful things we desire only when we act for ourselves and make clear, concrete decisions, develop concise strategies with goal oriented plans and work in a flexible manner to achieve our goals. We all have infinite wishes, dreams and needs within us which we all want to attain!

## A First Impression

Headaches, concentration difficulties, vision problems, stomach and intestinal ulcers, gallstones, heart and circulatory troubles, even heart attacks and strokes are just some of the typical results of stress. Problems with concentration, depression and fear, tiredness and apathy can also be symptoms of stress and are the result of a continuous overload without enough break time for recuperation. Bipolar systems, constant moodiness and feelings of anxiety or depression can also be caused by stress.

If the cause that leads to the stress is not removed, we cannot avoid the symptoms. I recommend my **IBMS™** as the appropriate way for stress reduction. Other forms of therapy, including yoga or meditation, can only temporarily suppress the symptoms like a band-aid. If you have a splinter in your finger and if you push it deeper in and cover it with a band-aid, if you leave a splinter in a wound, you cannot expect the wound to heal or to stop hurting. You need to get rid of the root cause of the problem, the splinter or in our case the mental and emotional stress.

A typical example of fighting symptoms, but not addressing the cause, would be using the splinter example. You leave the splinter in the wound, wipe away the pus, take a pill for the pain and antibiotics and cover it with a band-aid so that you do not see the problem, but you will still have stress. The cause and the stress is still the same! So to get your stress level to a normal and healthy enough level to not suffer from negative side effects, you must remove the causes of your stress. You have to remove the splinter from the wound, metaphorically from your brain, your behavior and your body because the splinter represents your intellectual and physical "failures."

In my research and therapy sessions I often witnessed the disappearance of so-called illnesses and symptoms caused by stress, such as stomach and intestinal ulcers, migraines, lack of concentration, lack of sleep, vision problems, etc., when people learned to cope with their lives. I am not saying that these people learned to deal with stress; rather they learned to organize and shape their lives so that they have control over their outcome. To simply cope and deal with stress is absurd.

If your life is out of control, you need to learn to organize, to understand your internal messages in a healthy, solution oriented way and use this information to eliminate the causes of the trouble. I need to re-emphasize that in no way should you ever think that you can cope with stress, manage your stress or accept stress as a natural part of your life. Everybody should strive for a healthy, harmonious, happy and energetic existence. You should never settle for limitations in your life. If you accept stress and stress symptoms, as a natural part of life, no matter what you will never produce lasting positive changes in your life.

*It is important to understand that you cannot live a life completely free of stress, but you can live free from damaging stress.*

To produce fast results, I must first give you an overview of my ideas, experience and modus operandi.

Remark: Modern medicine believes stomach ulcers are caused by Heliobacteria phylory, but I strongly believe that it is not true because many people have these bacteria without having an ulcer. The body actually needs to be so rundown, burned out and weak for the bacteria to do the harm. Fact is that countless people have that specific bacteria but don't have any ulcers or problems.

## If You Are Sick You Need To Act

When you are sick, feeling sorry for yourself will not get you better. Nor will complaining make you healthy, it will just make you lonely. What will help is finding the reasons why you are sick and then fixing the problem. Some people get and stay sick for the attention. They even sabotage themselves and their health. If you are seeking attention, avoid getting sick and instead be healthy, become a good coworker, spouse or neighbor to someone, and then, in a positive way from these relationships, you will get all the affirming attention that you need. More importantly, people will love you instead of pitying you or even hating you.

*Life is what you make it. Your actions in the present determine your future. You need to let go of and stop living in the past.*

I constantly hear complaints from people who blame all their problems on their childhood or their past. They claim they were abused as a child or whatever, but I believe that everyone has problems of one form or another when they are growing up. No one has had a perfect life; some people simply take responsibility and recognize that the past will not change, there is nothing they can do about what happened, but they can do something about how they take it with them. Learn your lessons and let it go! No matter what the excuses, you are the only one who suffers in the end by not letting go. Instead of looking for reasons for why you failed or why it happened to you, look for reasons for success and happiness in the future.

*Be aware that no one and nothing can fix you - you are the only one who can fix yourself, so be prepared to do it yourself!*

It is painful dealing with a negative past, but nothing can change the past. Besides what good comes from wallowing in self pity and repeating the bad times, all it does is destroy energy and your quality of life. Start afresh creating a wealth of new good memories. Complaining and self pity makes people feel badly and takes away so much energy. They need to stop concentrating on the horrible past and focus on the positive future ahead. Self- pity and whining only makes psychiatrists rich!

## The Danger of Self-Deception

Self-deception is often a problem for many people who are treating their symptoms by using techniques like yoga, self-hypnosis, breathing therapy, etc., but in reality none of these techniques really help because they do not remove the causes that lead to the symptoms of stress. The results are very short lived.

Using these techniques, the appearance of stress symptoms is addressed because we are not aware that we need to look to our emotional state and our physical behavior for the cause of the stress. In fact, unmanageable time schedules, overwhelming workloads, difficulties making decisions, poor self-esteem and more are generally the causes of these symptoms. This is why we need to address and remove these causes, not just treat the symptoms.

There are people who are diligent about practicing various methods of relaxation and regeneration, but they do so without achieving the desired results. They don't get the desired results because they are telling their subconscious mind that they are addressing their unwanted stress symptoms; ironically, at the same time it's not working, they are also trying to convince themselves that although they suffer from small setbacks, they are doing everything possible to remove the stress symptoms and so it must be working.

***The only effective way to produce lasting results is to make the decision to work both emotionally and physically to***

*address and eliminate the root cause of your stress and the stress symptoms disappear on their own.*

You can grow and build towards this goal quickly by using the **IBMS™** sessions.

## The Programs that Run your Brain

The brain can only use the programs that are installed. This means that your strongest reactions and your frequently used emotional and physical behaviors – including the bad behaviors - are programmed and conditioned into your brain with the greatest intensity. In this way, negative behavior becomes a natural part of your life, and the model for your current and future behavior. Initially when you first experience a negative reaction or behave badly, it is troublesome, it doesn't feel right, but all too soon it becomes a habit when you repeat it over time. After that, the poor behavior is no longer recognized as "poor," and therefore it is no longer addressed consciously because it feels "normal."

Feelings of dissatisfaction, inner turmoil, poor self-esteem, anxiety, and tension are all common symptoms of negative programming and behavior, and are the body's signal for help from the subconscious - we need to pay attention to them, but for most people they are largely ignored and nothing is done to correct them.

*Exercise:*

*On half a sheet of paper write down all the unwanted behaviors and failures you have experienced whether of an emotional or physical nature. You must work hard to list and identify all your unwanted feelings or behaviors. You must really be willing to explore, recognize and accept all areas of your weaknesses and inconsistencies. Then once you have addressed them, on the second half of the page write down your decisions to change, clearly developing plans and strategies to turn unwanted behaviors into new desired behaviors that will increase your energy.*

**Example:**

| Problem | Solution |
| --- | --- |
| *I get nervous, anxious and become ineffective with others when I'm late.* | *I will schedule my time to allow for delays and arrive relaxed and on time.* |

This program is designed so that you recognize, define and accept the causes and have the solutions to change them. You can start by listing the situations in your life when you behaved differently from the way you wanted, in other words, list what you did that you later regretted. For instance, you may have yelled at a spouse, a parent or children because you were overworked, or you may have been irritated with colleagues or patients in a manner that was out of character.

Now, stop reading and do this exercise! Think about situations in which you behaved differently from the way you wanted. Ask yourself what would have been the right way to act?

To improve the quality of your life, your behavior must fit your personality. If you want to be happy, but are not, you need to work on your self-confidence, self-esteem and self-respect. Never forget that stress doesn't come from the outside. It is not a virus, nor is it an illness; instead we produce our own stress as a result of bad emotional and physical behavior. In physics, the definition of stress is "pressure from the inside out."

Stress can be avoided, but it starts with taking responsibility, by confessing that: "I am not perfect, I behaved less than perfectly, but I can and will change my behavior!" In my seminars and workshops, I repeatedly see a lack of responsibility for one's own behavior as a serious obstacle standing between people and the solutions to their problems. In the end, these people cannot possibly reach their full potential, as long as they are unwilling to admit that they are not perfect. But this raises the question, who is perfect and who wants to be average? I don't have the answer, but I certainly don't want to be average, and I'm guessing that you probably don't either. Since we do not want to become robots or turn into zombies, life is more effective when we acknowledge that we are not perfect, but it is rewarding to strive for perfection!

In fact, there is great opportunity in our imperfection, as it is portrayed on this almost blank page that represents our life. It is now up to us to fill in the patterns, colors and designs that we want. The great opportunity comes from recognizing that everyone is in charge of their own life and that everyone repeatedly finds themselves in an emotional state of their own making.

*Everyone needs to recognize that life does not just happen, we are not victims of fate, instead it is just the opposite – our life mirrors our thinking and our behavior.*

### Stress the Silent Killer™

Stress is everything that the brain perceives to be a major threat - whether emotional, mental, or physical. Stress can be caused by threats to our life, financial stability, career, relationships, emotional well being, or health, real or imagined. It includes perceived threats to every part of our existence. Doubts, worries and fears are stressors that cause dramatic drains in energy. Remember, lack of energy is the only cause of illness. If your system is full of energy and has all the nutrients it needs, you cannot and will not get sick.

*Emotional and mental stress are the highest energy drains in the human body.*

The only exception is an environmental accident like a nuclear spill or any severe health problem caused by an outside force. There are many environmental problems like mercury fillings in the teeth which can cause brain tumors, and there are the side effects of some medications or medical treatments which can make you very sick or even kill you. Toxins in tap water or altered food can also make you sick. Scientists tell me that there is also the fact that it has never been proven that there is even one safe and effective vaccine and that the poisons in the vaccines could be the major cause for many diseases.

*All natural illnesses are solely based on lack of energy, usually caused by emotional, mental and physical stress.*

## Prevention is Much Better than Therapy

At the moment everybody is so concerned with managing stress that eighty-seven percent of all people chronically suffer from stress symptoms. We are in a war fighting stress or trying to live with the results of stress. When we search for the causes and then take responsibility for changing our emotional or physical behavior, we can avoid the symptoms of stress. For you to have a long healthy life, it is very important that you prepare for the responsibilities and frustrations life presents so that you can handle situations as they arise without stress.

*Avoid trying to manage stress, this approach could kill you; instead, get rid of the <u>cause</u> of the stress in your life.*

Stress and disease are not caused by a bacteria or a virus; it is the result of our own thoughts, emotions and behaviors. You may feel upset or frightened about something threatening, but this program will quickly teach you to recognize that the stress in your life is a subjective not an objective observation. Whether or not you experience dis-stress, and how you experience stress, depends on the images you allow to occupy your mind on a consistent basis.

Good health depends on the way you think about your life and how you make use of your physiology - your breathing, your posture, your movement, your muscle-tension and amazingly, your health is affected by how you speak – tone, tempo and diction. Our emotional and physical reactions are the result of our internal and external communication. If you listen to they way people speak, there is a lot more to communication than just the words.

For instance, if you talk to yourself in a monotone voice that sounds tired and weary, thinking "I cannot do this, this is unbearable, I just can't take it any longer…" as compared to saying to yourself in a confident voice, "I will take this challenge, I will work hard and I will do it as well as I can…," the result and the implications for your health will be dramatically different. Speaking to yourself in a clear, strong and goal oriented voice, monitoring tone, tempo, and diction, you will positively affect both your emotional and physical reactions.

Your train of thought significantly affects your level of stress and energy. If you focus on all your problems and difficulties at once, you will get overwhelmed and stressed out. Instead of focusing on everything you have to do, and all the things that can go wrong, focus only on what you can control at that moment - the difference will be enormous. By focusing on what you can control this moment, you are directing your thought process, not the other way around.

If you focus your attention on solving your immediate problems and not wasting time on obstacles, problems and demands, you will find that your life will be filled with more energy, progress and successes. You will enjoy looking forward to the future instead of always being afraid of the past. Having successes are very important in the building of self-esteem and self-confidence, fostering energy, strength and vitality. The more successes, the more strength you have to produce even better, quicker and more effective results.

In contrast, if you focus on problems, problems will determine your life, take over your thinking and run your behavior. If you focus on solutions, solutions and progress will fill your life. Thus, you must learn to control the images, sounds and feelings that come from your thoughts by constantly communicating with yourself in a positive manner. I understand this is not easy to achieve and this is why I offer this program.

## Health and a Stress Free Life Begin in the Mind

Our core values and beliefs are one of the most basic elements of health, but they are often overlooked because we are inclined to focus only on the symptoms of illness and refuse to look at the causes responsible for the disease and illness in the first place. The causes come from stress.

Some of the causes of poor behavior are from negative thinking which comes from a poor belief or value system. Remember, what you think about determines your life. If you value health, and believe you will be and are healthy, you will be healthy; if you focus on illness, and believe you are going to be sick, you will certainly become sick. If you only focus on problems and obstacles instead of solutions, you will suffer from the symptoms of stress. You could argue that poor physiological behavior, bad nutrition, faulty breathing and lack of exercise cause illness, and it would be true in so far as faulty breathing, bad nutrition and lack of exercise are the results of a poor mental state. This means you need to cultivate a positive belief system about yourself by focusing on success and good health.

If you let fear control your life, you will suffer from anxiety and physical tension. This will result in poor circulation, a shortage of oxygen and medical complications. If you focus on problems instead of solutions, you will experience a shortage of energy resulting in your not having enough energy for your emotional and physical needs - this will cause stress. These and many other basic elements of poor emotional behavior lead to the causes of illness and the deterioration of your health.

We need to start by separating out the causes from the symptoms of an illness. We need to fight the symptoms by removing the cause. There are many sensible and natural ways to regain health and avoid stress discussed in this book. You can begin by taking responsibility for your health. The more we try to avoid this responsibility, the more obvious the symptoms become, forcing us to do something or suffer even greater consequences later on.

It was from all my practical experience that I recognized help cannot come from outside. The only true help is self-help. If you are sick, you made yourself sick and as such only you can make yourself well. This is because you are the only person who can reduce your stress level; no one else can do it for you.

*"No doctor, treatment or medication can heal a sick person. Only the person's own self healing system can heal them!"*

Of course, practicing basic good health principles play an important role, but you must personally take responsibility for your health and your quality of life. To enjoy the best health possible, you need to do everything necessary for good health. In fact, this is what led to the development of my **IBMS™**. This system gives every person some guidelines to activate and stimulate their own personal self-healing ability so that they feel regenerated and ready to enjoy health for the rest of their life. The results will speak for themselves!

I believe there are solutions for every problem, and answers for every question. However, it starts with being aware and accepting our challenges by doing everything necessary to realize the results we want to achieve. The power of the mind is limitless. Start by believing in yourself, so that you can activate and use the strength of your subconscious mind.

*You have the power within you to turn your life into the wonderful experience it deserves to be.*

## The Hidden Causes of Stress Symptoms

Stress emanates from the most unlikely areas and often where we least suspect it. Usually stress is associated with heavy burdens, a life crisis, or difficult dilemmas in our every day life. We tend to overlook the everyday activities that generate stress symptoms resulting in loss of energy. We might actually be in a stressful situation or we might be simply worried that everything might go wrong when it isn't, or we may dwell on being scared by focusing on bad things, but **nothing happens in our life that we don't control/influence whether it is our thinking, feeling and/or behavior!**

*In reality, we are only influenced by our own emotional and physiological reactions to what happens to us and we have a choice about how we react.*

Whether we feel that we are vulnerable or whether we feel totally capable of getting the result we desire, our feelings about ourselves will have a direct influence on our emotional condition and, therefore, this will directly affect our energy level and our ability to function in a positive manner. In a crisis, we tend to give in more willingly and not look for solutions as we stare at the obstacles and the problems before us. Knowing this, now concentrate your energy solely on the task before you in a positive way looking for a solution and an effective way to act.

The images we create in our mind determine our feelings and our behaviors. The same is true for the mental pictures we have of another person or a specific situation. In the same way our mental images and what we say to ourselves about those images, and the way we say it, determines our feelings and, therefore, our behaviors. Your behavior is radically different when you picture a person as a formidable and undefeatable opponent like Goliath, radiating strength and towering over you, versus your behavior when addressing a person who is intellectually equal, that you look straight in the eye, and you speak to confidently on whatever topic you choose.

The pictures in your head dictate your behavior because it is in this way that you program your brain and nervous system to react - exactly as you have already experienced it in your mind. This means that a person can program a pattern of fear and failure into their nervous system that they will experience over and over again. If a person sees themselves easily and effectively handling a situation, then they will experience a more positive result over and over again. In other words, if you see yourself doing it well, you will do it well. If you see yourself feeling and behaving badly then the result will mimic your image.

In this regard, it is possible to program changes in the nervous system using the basis of the techniques in the **IBMS™** . The subconscious mind cannot differentiate between an *actual* experience and an *imagined* experience created in the mind. The illustration of telling a friend about a wonderful happy experience that happened to you long ago, when you notice that as you talk about the experience, you simultaneously feel the same emotions that you felt at the time of the original experience is a perfect example. Your subconscious mind experiences the event as if it was happening right now for the first time, triggering all the reactions in your mind and body that were a part of the original event. Naturally the same is true for a negative, sad, frustrating or depressing memory; you experience all the frustration, anger, and depression that you felt at the time of the event.

In the case of a negative experience, you re-create all the stress and loss of energy that you originally felt. By constantly repeating this event in your mind, you needlessly suffer from becoming sad, frustrated and/or depressed, over and over again, when in fact the event was long ago in the past. Many people suffer from the energy drain this causes simply because they do not let go, and they are never able to stop repeating these situations in their mind, but the **IBMS™** teaches how to change this habit.

I want to clarify that there is a big difference between seeing things in an associated or disassociated manner. In other words, if you see and hear the events as pictures in your mind and it is as if you and the people around you are like actors acting in a movie, and if you observe the events and pictures as if you were in the audience watching a movie in a theater, that means you are *dissociated,* you are at a distance from the event. In contrast, the **IBMS™** of conditioning is one of personal contemplation; that means you experience and feel in your mind the event as it would really happen. You are in the picture, experiencing and feeling what is going on directly including all the sights, sounds, smells, sensations, and meanings of your experience.

In order to better understand the full extent of the applications of my system, I want to give you an overview of the **IBMS™** model. Basically, the **IBMS™** originated from working to consciously activate the bioelectric and neuro-chemical processes in the body. I began working with self-help and self-healing techniques after studying every form of therapy, self-help, hypnosis, personal development and success training. I took the best and most effective aspects of all the therapies and combined them into an easy to understand and easy to use system. Effective, long-lasting conditioning only occurs when dendrites (brain cell connections) are created.

I have designed the **IBMS™** to activate the body's self-healing and regenerative ability as quickly and as easily as possible. This works by stimulating the nervous system to create neuro-chemical and bioelectrical processes that enable the body to heal faster. The program is both easy to understand and easy to use.

Once I integrated my research with practical experience, I was asked to lead a research program that addressed prevention and preventative therapy for health problems in mental and physiological situations. This experience afforded me the opportunity of learning even more so that I could further refine my newly developed therapy. All this research and experience led me to conclude that it is not possible to achieve a lasting successful result by using outside therapy or intervention.

As a result of my findings, I developed a scientific and philosophical system of therapy based on the concept of "help to self-help," in other words, helping patients to heal themselves. This system is a work-program for personal achievement, perfect health and lifelong success in all areas of life which I called NAPS®-Therapy and Self-help system. The **IBMS**™ is a part of the original NAPS®-Therapy and Self-help System.

*I concluded that every human being has the ability, the opportunity and the possibility to deal with all of life's challenges and emerge as a winner.*

## The Realization and Acceptance of Facts

You will not be able to reduce and eliminate the stress in your life as long as you do not recognize and accept what that stress is. It is no different than the situation of an alcoholic who cannot overcome his drinking problem until he admits to himself that he is an alcoholic.

Often arrogant and irresponsible behavior stands in our way when dealing with conflicts because we do not want to admit that our emotional and/or physical behavior is not only hurting ourselves, but might also simultaneously hurt others. It is often so difficult to admit that our life is not how we would like it to be.

Human weaknesses and failures are a natural part of human existence; be prepared to acknowledge and accept these weaknesses and failures, and instead focus and work on your mission in life. Your greatest challenge in life is the willingness to admit, address and define your errors as without recognizing these factors, you cannot control your life and determine your fate.

Deception and manipulation of others and dishonesty, deception and denial with oneself, along with repression, cause a tremendous amount of stress, and therefore are a massive energy drain. It is important that you now think of all the situations that you can remember in which you did not behave as you wished and all the times you can remember when you behaved in a way that would have not been the proper way to behave. If you haven't already, start a journal for "optimum health" in which you write useful ideas, techniques, remedies or experiences you have had, also list what you did or didn't do for your health and stress reduction.

## Fear – Murderer of Dreams and Health

Everybody lives with fears of some sort or another. Components of fear are the doubts and worries that bring with them feelings of helplessness and hopelessness. Knowing that there is no way to absolutely guarantee the safety, happiness and success of our future, we can be consumed with worry. To avoid these feelings, you need simply to believe in yourself, trust your instincts and rely upon your abilities.

One of the biggest stressors in people's lives is constantly worrying about things that they cannot control. These people need to work on the problems that they can control by making action plans and setting clear goals for what is achievable. Because once you do everything possible to attain your goals, you relax and the stress goes away on its own. You cannot control the weather, not even if you plan a pool party, but you can be prepared by having a tent ready in case of bad weather with the result being - less worry, less stress!

If you find you are worried about something that you can address and act on, do not procrastinate, take care of it immediately otherwise you will get more and more stressed out the longer you wait. A general rule of thumb is to start by asking yourself if it is possible for you to help yourself, weigh your options and be prepared for the worst possible outcome. Then focus on what you can change and take the first step then next step until you've reached your goal. Be sure to take time to have fun and regenerate along the way, make time for yourself. Learn to take life events the way they come and to deal with it the best possible way when they arise.

In my opinion, everybody needs about twenty minutes twice a day relaxing by themselves in order to regenerate from daily tasks and stresses. These breaks provide the energy to address whatever challenges appear. You will feel recharged and ready to meet those challenges head on. Otherwise the ongoing and/or accumulated stress will eventually harm you. Sometimes spending quality time with family or friends can be energizing; plan time to get together, organize events that you can look forward to attending. The **IBMS™** twenty-minute sessions are the best and fastest way to get regenerated and to take charge of your life.

Your immune system functions on a reward based system. It needs a reason to stay healthy; if you don't give it a reason then it will not keep you healthy. If you cultivated reasons to feel good, your immune system simultaneously will work better. If you harm your immune system by constant partying and overeating or eating bad food, your immune system will eventually fail.

Nothing in life functions in extremes, in fact, life is based on a perfect balance, which is why people should not live in extremes because it throws off the natural balance in their body. In nature, everything is balanced, and if it is not in balance, it does not last long. Nature always gets rid of extremes; there are always consequences to imbalance.

Many people's health actually suffers from extreme dieting when they go on all protein diets, fasting diets, or rapid weight loss programs; they think by losing weight they are getting healthier, but they're not. For one thing, their body's get so far out of balance that the weight comes right back on. In my opinion, if you are a healthy person and you want to stay healthy, you can eat unhealthy food thirty percent of the time, as long as seventy percent of the time you eat a balanced diet of healthy food. But if you are sick then you need to do everything right 100 percent of the time until you are completely recovered.

Health needs to be conditioned into the nervous system, and it takes approximately three to six weeks to make a noticeable change. Any faster and you create imbalances and possible negative consequences.

Remark: Nature doesn't do anything in extremes that survives. Everything is an accumulation of many different things. Every extreme is wrong! Extremism is a mental illness.

*Humor and laughter are great stress reducers that stimulate your immune functions.*

**Fear as a Stress Factor**

**The Emotion of "Fear," and How to Overcome Fear that Causes a Great Deal of Stress.**

Ironically, there are some fears which we ignore or even dismiss as absurd like the "fear of success," or "fear of happiness." These particular fears, in fact, prevent many people from moving ahead, keeping them from ever making the attempt to become successful or even trying to reach their full potential. The person suffering from fear of success subliminally connects negative side effects to their idea of success, like having to work long hours, the pressure of increasingly greater expectations, more people making demands on their time, and having to give up their family time, all these things keep them from allowing themselves to be successful.

Additionally, people worry that their success may result in the loss of personal relationships because with success comes a growth which sometimes exceeds the growth of those near to you. Since the fear of success can be caused by many different things, in order for you to discover what might be causing this, you must first define all the drawbacks and negatives you associate with success.

*Exercise:*

*Write down everything negative that you think could happen to yourself or to others when you become really successful and achieve your goals and realize your dreams.*

*Now write down why it would be worthwhile by making a list of all the good things that will happen to yourself and others when you achieve your success and realize your dreams.*

*Then write down how the "negative" aspects could be turned around into positive results as you achieve your success. Make an action plan for how you would deal with these situations or circumstances every step of the way on the path to your success.*

The fear of negative developments far outweighs the fear of positive results. The fear of not being able to handle success is usually a subliminal fear, which we are hardly aware of as it is happening to us, but all forms of fear stem from our internal communications and are a result of learned behavior patterns. Basically, it all comes down to lack of self esteem, which is why I developed the powerful individual **IBMS™ sessions.** See **www.instinctbasedmedicine.com**

Fears come from being afraid of losing someone or something we already have, but most of the time if we truly address our fears we discover that rarely do our fears turn into reality. All automatic processes like fear of success or fear of true happiness have been installed in our minds through repetition. This is why we need to get rid of the bad programming and replace it with new desirable programs. The **IBMS™** programs can be very helpful with letting go of your fears. Look at the sessions: trauma erase and take charge of your life!

If you want to benefit from this system and you want your energy, vitality and ability to work for you in a manner that is

285

no longer adversely affected by unknown causes, you must use what is in this book to define your personal conflict areas.

The **IBMS™** was developed so that you can personalize the system to suit your needs. Permanent and positive improvements in one's life must come from within that person. No outsider or external situation can have a permanent impact on the life of another. For instance, if you do not learn to get along with yourself, you will never learn to produce a permanent positive result, and you will not come close to realizing your potential in life. You can start by installing a new pattern of behavior by working on the exercises in this book to the best of your ability. This way you will ensure that your life improves in a positive way.

*Exercise:*

*Write a list of all the things you worry about, all of the fears you experience in the next five days, including small fears, big fears - any fears you experience once or repeatedly. Write them all down and keep track. Notice how often each fear repeats in your min; write down each and every time you experience it.*

*At the end of five days, go over your notes and list the worries, anxieties and fears you lived through that turned out to be nothing more than "figments of your imagination."*

You probably already know the answer, but do it anyway. This should show you that the fear in your head has little or nothing to do with what is really happening, nor does fear or worry have any positive consequence if it does happen. However, you may notice that if you play negative pictures repeatedly in your mind, they may become a self-fulfilling prophecy.

All human behavior is based on either conscious or subconscious conditioning. If the focus is always on negative developments or bad endings, i.e., worries and fears, then the nervous system gets programmed for exactly that! It expects and creates what you fear, in other words, your brain responds to and creates an experience of what you precondition in your mind. But most of all, it creates and enormous amount of stress and therefore energy loss.

*It is important that you only concentrate on real problems and events, not on hypothetical or imaginary fears. Do not spend any time focusing on solutions to fabricated mental fears that may never come true in the first place.*

From the exercise, you know the difference. It does not include difficult real life situations or crises for which you need to be prepared to develop solution oriented behavior and goal driven thinking. You need to change the negative behavior patterns in your nervous system and respond appropriately only when real dangers or a crisis arise. By focusing on solutions, you *minimize* the fear because the solutions empower you, providing self-esteem and self-confidence, while avoiding the negativity associated with fear. This works every time because your brain, your subconscious accepts that you are in control, and therefore you will find you behave effectively in crisis situations.

**The Basics**

The only way to minimize stress and handle your actions in a way that will not lead to negative stress symptoms, is by identifying the situations that lead to negative stress. How and why do we experience dis-stress situations? The answers to this question will provide the information for you to develop a personalized anti-stress program.

First learn to see problems as challenges, as opportunities for growth as this will dramatically lower your dis-stress level. See yourself as part of the solution in your mental world; see yourself as able to make solid good decisions. The manner in which you see yourself determines whether you experience negative stress or not. The way you view your situation determines whether you can turn dis-stress situations into eu-stress situations for both yourself and others.

You are the only person with the ability to turn the most difficult of life challenges into motivating eu-stress situations. You can do it by using the right self-communication. In other words, whether a stressful situation makes you unhealthy or sick, versus driven, motivated or confident, depends entirely on your personal and individual approach to that stress situation.

Since you are aware that stressful situations and ongoing stress can lead to a loss of energy and a health breakdown, you should realize that all stress reduction, avoiding stressful experiences whenever possible and overcoming stressful situations when they occur, is very important. In fact, you don't avoid the life situation, only your negative stress producing reaction. Once you learn to identify and confront obvious stressful situations with new mental and physiological self-programming and conditioning, you will avoid getting energy drained and you will not be constantly risking a health breakdown.

There may be a slight misconception that people's jobs cause stress. Generally speaking, only people who dislike their work, who are disorganized or not in control end up being literally destroyed by their job. If you see your work as your life's work, more like a calling with a higher purpose, and you give it your best shot, then it will not cause stress, and it will give you feelings of fulfillment. Don't make compromises against yourself. If you can not stand a job or relationship get out of it!

Of course there are many different factors that contribute to our stress level, such as the demands and duties of our private, business and social life, financial demands, family problems, etc., but how they affect you totally depends on you! The question is, how do you confront the problems that lead to stress with problem solving solutions and strategies? Or do you feel sorry for yourself, whine, and stay overwhelmed doing nothing? If you only think in terms of the "what if..." or the "if only I had..." your problems will intensify, but if you focus on accepting the facts and on finding solutions and acting on those solutions, the problems will diminish and your quality of life will steadily get better. It is all about your values and the attitude you have in confronting the issues.

Work takes up the majority of people's lives and that perhaps explains the reasoning that most stress is considered to be work related, but as you have learned, stress is the result of lots of negative mental communication, resulting in an overload causing the symptoms of stress. This can happen when a person feels overwhelmed and suffocated by their work as these feelings make the subconscious feel like it is a prisoner. This feeling of being a prisoner, unable to escape, feelings of being restricted or limited, trapped in some way, has such an enormous deleterious impact on both the self-confidence and self-esteem of that person that they are unable to find any solution to their problems. This will inevitably lead to a nervous breakdown because instead of addressing their challenges, they flee emotionally and mentally, only focused on surviving.

**It is constant hard work to take control of one's life, but the price is worth the effort** as there is such a feeling of satisfaction to be gained from knowing that you will have a healthy and successful life, going forward from this day on towards greater levels of success and good health. Freedom means to be in control of your life!

## Finances and Relationships as Causes of Stress

Practical experience has taught me that our relationships with our partners, spouse, children and family can cause major stress in our lives. Other people's peculiarities and habits can drive us up the wall, as can our feelings of being hemmed in by private commitments, duties and pressures, but if this happens to you, inform them about what is annoying you, realizing that everyone has their own peculiarities - even you! Learn to accept that everybody has the right to live their life the way they think is right for them, in the same way you would want others to respect and accept you the way you are.

But remember: If you are in a relationship that kills you in the whole meaning of the word you need to get out of it.

Remember that you are the only person who can impose limits and pressures on yourself because at some point **you decide** whether you will do something, not do something or do it differently. Use common sense and follow your instinct.

Financial worries are a basic fear that often leads to loss of energy and strength, which can also make us sick or paralyze our ability to function. Differentiate between whether the financial fear is rational, a real problem, or simply a possibility in the future. Fabricated fears about future possibilities can only be overcome with good preparation. You must realize that you cannot solve future problems in the present; you can only do something in a solution oriented way if and when the problem actually arises.

Hypothetical problems that only exist in your mind cannot be solved simply because they do not exist in reality – however, they can cause a tremendous amount of dis-stress.

It is important to learn to react to stressful and crisis oriented situations only when they happen or when you are certain that they will become a reality. Avoid focusing on past problems because it is not possible to change the past, and since you can't predict the future, there is no need to worry about what might happen - it will most likely be very different than anything you now envision anyway.

I am sure you have experienced worrying about a bad situation which ended up being easier to resolve than you had imagined. In the case of financial problems, the only possible solutions are to find new or better sources of income, and/or get a grip on your financial situation with a budget that you follow. Worrying, whining or complaining about the problem and not finding a solution leads to massive stress and a possible health breakdown. If you are afraid creditors will call you because you haven't paid the bill, worrying will not change the fact that they will call you.

If you have problems with being in social situations, you need learn to not be afraid by focusing on solutions - or suffer endless stress and an enormous waste of energy. If you have an overwhelming fear of public speaking, but you have to speak, you must train yourself by giving your speech in your mind several times a day pretending that you are in front of a real audience. This will condition a calm, deliberate and confident behavior in your subconscious mind so that when you deliver the speech, you behave accordingly.

Please note that you should not dwell on the negative judgment of other people as it can cause serious dis-stress. If you feel regularly stressed by the comments of some of the people in your circle of friends, confront them with what is causing you the stress, ask for a positive response and you will alleviate some of the problem. However, if this does not work, avoid these types of "friends" altogether.

We all know that anxiety, nervousness, irritability, insomnia, muscle cramps, headaches, and dizziness can be symptoms of stress. We also know that these stress reactions can have a deleterious impact on the quality of our life, our health, and our ability to function. It is, therefore, very important to learn what triggers our stress, what risks are involved and how to prevent them. In other words, how can we deal with the problems that cause those symptoms?

## Positive Stress is Eu-stress.

Although "stress" usually denotes a negative connotation, there is in fact positive stress which promotes our well-being and can drive us to achieve; this stress is called eu-stress. This positive stress can be generated after or in anticipation of a wonderful experience.

Holding onto negative stress without taking a break will inevitably lead to a breakdown, like an engine that keeps running in the red zone. You must learn to catch your dis-stress before it damages your nervous system. The more you keep pushing yourself without taking time to regenerate, the harder it becomes to find your way back to normal behavior.

We can teach ourselves to experience as many eu-stress reactions as possible. An example of how to achieve this would be to start by acknowledging with pride your good work. If you <u>turn even small successes into great accomplishments</u> – eu-stress, your energy level will increase exponentially.

Eu-stress is healthy, stimulating and essential in our life as it determines the degree of our happiness and the quality of our life. Be sure you set aside enough time for recreation, and ensure that you get enough oxygen, nutrition and exercise. And most importantly, remember that you work to live and not that you live to work.

Only solution focused, goal oriented thinking produces eu-stress, ensures positive results, and creates positive expectations preventing negative stress reactions. The more a person focuses on problems instead of solutions, the weaker and more helpless they become. The longer they stay focused on the problem, the greater the risk that they will remain feeling inadequate and weak, thus causing a dis-stress cycle.

Without regeneration, excessive and ongoing dis-stress could lead to feelings of impotence, as well as stomach and intestinal ulcers, cramps, digestive and concentration problems. Although you should always seek the advice of a medical practitioner, it is also helpful to pay attention to your own physiological and emotional reactions to stressful situations.

By planning to stop working after a certain amount of time, allowing yourself time for some freedom and recreation, you will spare yourself from experiencing dangerous dis-stress and find more enjoyment in your life and your work.

## What Stress Really Is

### Physical Stress

The normal stress we all experience, apart from physical pain, is similar to the feeling we have when being forced to listen to loud machinery running constantly. It disturbs our concentration and keeps us from accomplishing anything. Another example would be when you are on the telephone and your child interrupts you begging and nagging for something, or when you are overloaded with things to do and there's not enough time to do them all. This kind of daily stress uses up physical energy, but generally a good night's sleep will take care of the regeneration. However, ongoing or damaging stress without relief is emotional and mental stress, which causes long lasting damaging effects and will lead to a health breakdown.

It is possible that physical stress can eventually lead to emotional stress, but as long as it does not turn into emotional stress it can be alleviated by taking breaks, a walk, deep breathing, a good night's sleep, a fun time with friends, a great movie, a relaxing time, laughing with fun people to list a few ideas.

Physical stress has never been much of a problem, but many people think that they can overcome all their emotional stress with meditation, yoga or other relaxation techniques. **In my experience,** as I have previously mentioned, these techniques are actually a waste of time and money, and at their worst, they can be dangerous because they do not deal with the underlying problem that's causing the stress.

Every kind of technique that manipulates you in some way can harm your personality and your sense of self. They will never help you to develop and grow as a human being, but they can make you addicted, helpless, or schizophrenic. Also beware of passive techniques, which can be dangerous because they give a person a false sense of doing something about their problems while actually doing nothing.

Meditation may be good for the people who need to impress others, but when used as a stress reducer it is nothing more than a waste of time **because it does not address the real causes of stress and will not have long term effects on stress related symptoms.** Real benefits and development only come from actual stress reduction and health prevention.

I am avidly against any kind of positive thinking without positive action as it is a waste of time and not a long-term solution. For instance to constantly repeat "I am going to be rich!" without doing what is necessary to become rich, will not make you rich, it will only cause more stress. The same is true with praying! If a parent only prays that their child will stop doing drugs, drinking, committing crimes, getting tattooed and/or pierced or getting bad grades and does nothing about the behavior, the child will undoubtedly continue with everything it's been doing. Parents need to be active in raising the child in a healthy positive way!

## Mental and Emotional Stress, the Cause of all Trouble

The only way that people get sick is by having a breakdown of energy, which leads to an internal breakdown of body functions and mutations in the cells and organs. An energy breakdown takes away both the ability to think clearly and the means for the brain to think on its own at an optimum level.

Some examples of severe emotional stress come from when someone close to you dies, if you lose your job or you get divorced. The only way to address this stress is to go to the root cause of the problem, deal with it, end it, and regenerate afterwards. This is possible with the **IBMS™**

With the **IBMS™** you will be able to identify and eliminate the stress from these kinds of problems in your life. The **IBMS™** stress reduction vitalization self help sessions on the CDs, along with the included handbook, are the end result of thirty years of experience, research and unmatched success. I have helped countless people to cure themselves from every kind of illness and most significantly, from cancer and other auto-immune diseases.

Before I developed my system, I had already cured many people from so-called incurable diseases. What I realized was that it's not that I am a healer, I simply figured out what buttons to push to achieve the right response and provide the correct information to the patients so that they could cure themselves. My system was basically developed organically, which is why I have no competition and my success is unmatched. **I discovered that if you get rid of the root cause of an illness, the body heals itself. I help people to find the root cause and solve their problems themselves. I had cancer patients that got instantly better when they decided to get out of a bad marriage that was the root cause of their illness. I even saw spontaneous healing when the root cause of the illness was resolved. I could help a patient that was 5 days before a breast cancer surgery to be tumor free at the last test before the surgery. ( her Name is Gerda G. )**

**How Stress Affects Your Immune System**

It takes a long time for energy to actually breakdown; in fact, you have to be worried and unhappy almost all the time to restrict your optimum health. Sleeplessness is ninety percent of the time caused by stress, but if you cannot sleep, you cannot regenerate or repair your body, which is why it is important to find out what stress is keeping you from sleeping, and fix the problem.

When you get really stressed your muscles constrict, thereby impeding your blood flow and your breathing. Your entire body is oxygen deprived, including the air bubbles in your lower lungs.

As mentioned, studies at many universities, including U.C. Berkley and Irvine in California, proved that a lack of oxygen leads to the mutation and death of cells. If you are constantly stressed, your oxygen level is constantly down and you are constantly dis-stressing your cells. Stress can cause nutritional

## Dr. Leonard Coldwell

deficiencies and dehydration and therefore all kinds of degenerative diseases and autoimmune diseases.

Otto Warburg and Max Plank each got the nobelprise in medicine by proving that a body that is filled with oxygen cannot develop cancer.

***If the situation is not corrected the result could be mutated cells turning into cancer.***

So-called free radicals (prospective cancer cells) are produced by toxemia and acidosis, but most of all from the lack of oxygen and energy. Several Nobel Prize winners have received their awards by proving this fact one way or the other. Stress is one major cause for acidosis.

When you have emotional stress, do not concern yourself with the physical stress, you need to eliminate the emotional stress first because this is what causes the shallow breathing and internal breakdown. If you do not feel good, you often do not make the right choices and may try to suppress these feelings with drugs, alcohol, medications, or food by overeating.

For instance, there is no illness called "depression," it is only a state of mind and physiology of the body. You cannot be depressed if you are happy, energized, have exciting goals and are actively working on achieving them. Often depression is an excuse for laziness, cowardice, self pity or an excuse to fail, or justification for failure. It begins with the "loser" attitude and behavior, followed by the biochemical changes in the body. The behavior causes the depression, not the other way around. Only very few people with depression truly have a physiological reason for being depressed. You need to feel hopeless, helpless and focus on the negative to fell depressed.

It is important to uncover the causes of your emotional stress because in order to learn to deal with your emotions you must know why they are there in the first place. The **IBMS™** will help you to learn the necessary techniques to produce fast effective results.

Physical stress can be caused by a lack of nutrients in the body. When the body feels threatened, in this instance from the lack of nutrients, it needs to survive so it produces stress hormones which cause flight or fight reactions. These hormones bring on feelings of being fatigued, excessively nervous, hectic, and panicky. The stress hormone cortisol is also responsible for obesity.

The moment your body gets the signal of danger, it produces stress hormones, which invariably cause your body to become weaker, ultimately causing a health breakdown if the situation is not corrected. A blocked or pinched nerve in your spine can cause back pain and headaches. The blockage can actually be caused by stress. Basically, pain can be the physical symptom of stress. Fibromyalgia and Migraine head agues are often caused by stress.

## Immune System Dysfunction

The immune system is so sensitively intertwined with the visceral organs, glands and cells that any immune dysfunction or immune suppression can have a deleterious effect on the entire health and homeostasis of the body. The thymus gland and T-cell functions play a pivotal and important role in generating and regulating immune response. A deficiency or imbalance in their function will cause immune system dysfunction and immune suppression to occur, leading to a certain health breakdown.

There are some sixty-five million Americans suffering from immune system dysfunction. That number is growing at a rapid rate primarily due to the aggressive and invasive approach of medical treatments that often focus on symptoms instead of restoring and maintaining the proper function of the immune system.

Immune disorders manifest in autoimmune disorders, these occur when the cells of the immune system confuse normal body cells with foreign antigens, and attack them. In immunodeficiency disorders, which typically refer to a weakened immune system, the response is often associated with chronic infections and inflammation.

Typical autoimmune disorders are rheumatoid arthritis, asthma, allergies, lupus, diabetes and multiple sclerosis. Typical immunodeficiency disorders include Epstein-Barr, AIDS, viral infections, otitis media, and even cancer; all of which may result from immune suppression.

We need to ask ourselves: if my body worked fine from the day I was born, why did the body stop doing its work? The reason is lack of energy. Lack of energy is usually caused by mental and emotional stress.

*The exact cause of autoimmune and immunodeficiency disease has yet to be completely understood, but there are obviously many factors involved in its origin. Some researchers, including a Nobel Prize winner in medicine - Dr. Gunter Blobel, have been studying the cell-to-cell communication of the immune and nervous system believing, that this may be a leading contributor of immune system dysfunction. Every cell communication in the body needs electricity (energy), so if we have a deficiency in energy, there can be non communication or misleading communication between the cells and the nervous system.*

**Immune Dysfunction and Stress**

Substantial research has clearly demonstrated that a wide range of stress can deplete immune system resources and adversely affect neurological and biological communication. A lack of communication between your nervous system and your immune system can result in abnormal levels of B and T cells, and fewer IGA antibodies secreted in the saliva, all of which are vital to good immune system function.

Stress can be defined as "a state of disharmony or threatened homeostasis provoked by psychological, environmental and physiological stressors." Stress is also invoked as an important part of the normal response to stimuli and should not be thought of as an abnormal reaction since it involves the "fight or flight" mechanism necessary for survival. Much of this response is mediated through the hypothalamus which monitors and controls certain functions such as the sympathetic nervous system and endocrine system.

Although stress is generally associated with negative connotations, it is a double-edged phenomenon. In times of real physical danger, the body would not be able to survive without the acute stress response, as it prepares the body for short, emergency responses to potentially life threatening situations. However, a lingering stress response to non-emergency situations is bad and can lead to chronic health conditions.

*Stress becomes a hazard to the body when the communications systems of the body are interrupted or overwhelmed by a variety of physical, chemical or emotional stressors.*

# Section II - Chapter 2

## The IBMS™ in Action

### The Way to Conquer Stress

Stress is often the result of trying to do too much without enough time or resources. Do not try to think and work on several jobs at the same time; instead focus your attention on the solution of the work at hand. The brain is not able to focus on two things at the same time, and you will inevitably cause unnecessary stress as a result of failures.

Another source of stress can be found in relationships. For instance, if the behavior of your colleagues bothers you, tell them. If coworkers give you constructive criticism, accept it. Get your finances in order so that you avoid financial trouble, the number one cause of stress in relationships. If you are already in financial trouble, develop solutions and strategies to get out of trouble.

If someone disturbs your peace or concentration, address the issue and develop a two-pronged approach to help and support each other, ending one-sided demands. We all make mistakes, but we must learn to accept constructive criticism. It is not a personal affront to listen to and cogitate over the information, proposals or opinions of others.

To be better understood and avoid unnecessary conflicts and/or stressful reactions, you should address and communicate your feelings to the relevant person. This will steer you from many unnecessary conflicts. If people do not appreciate your successes, don't be upset or stressed because you must learn to do things for yourself, for your own sake and for the enrichment and quality of your own life. Do not seek approval from others as this will only produce stress!

We often self-impose time pressures on ourselves that cause a tremendous amount of stress, which is why it is so important to learn to simply say "No" to people or work when you are overloaded. You need to learn how to manage your time and delegate.

Other situations that can lead to stress are problems that come from dealing with people in general, superiors, colleagues, family members and/or friends. Because of this, it is so important to learn communication skills to avoid major conflicts. This skill alone alleviates being exposed to the stress caused from lack of communication induced problems.

If you try to get along with everybody, you will eventually lose control of both yourself and your life. Learn to find people in your life that fit with you and your true personality, with whom you can be yourself so that you do not have to pretend. Keeping up fake idealistic pretenses contributes to one of the most dangerous stress factors of all. By behaving differently from your true self whether to please others or otherwise will almost always lead to your losing your own identity. That leads to insecurity, fear and ultimately stress.

No matter what, all you can do is the best that you can do! Knowing this, if you feel overwhelmed, remember that you are responsible for this feeling. You are the only person who can ask more of themselves than you can accomplish.

A good way to reduce the amount of stress in your life is to set realistic goals and have an action plan. It is important to write down your thoughts, plans and goals, because by putting them on paper, you provide your subconscious with the information and control over what will happen, which in turn makes your feelings of helplessness and dis-stress disappear.

Examine your work, behavior and successes to determine what gets you closer or sabotages you from achieving your goals, this way you will identify how fast or slowly you will realize your goals, dreams and wishes.

Do not chase pies in the sky and always be prepared for difficult situations! Remember to spend ten percent of your time and energy on dealing with the conflict, but spend ninety percent on finding the solution

Prepare yourself mentally to accept and react to new and unknown situations calmly. Even if something odd, strange or new happens unexpectedly, be flexible, thorough and composed when reacting.

It is also important to give yourself the time and opportunity for personal fun time so that you can work on your hobbies and the realization of your desires and dreams. It is just as important to enjoy free time as it is to work so that you can produce eu-stress situations, having fun, so don't use your free time to worry or try to solve conflicts or problems.

If you have muscle tension, it is a sign of lack of movement or poor breathing, nutritional deficiency, dehydration or not enough relaxation breaks. If this is the case, it is important to develop, perhaps with the help of experts, a program that provides a balance between regeneration, relaxation and good breathing and a good diet.

It is essential that people not swallow their frustration, anger, hatred or hostility, but it can be useful to air your feelings, in the truest sense of the word, by simply going into the woods or some vacant area and yell at the top of your voice. It is my belief that women grow considerably older than men (twice as many men die from stress reactions than women) because women have learned to communicate their stress.

Women are much better at airing their feelings thus releasing the pressure. Men, on the other hand, have been trained/conditioned to behave like "men," meaning they are not allowed to cry or show their feelings; they must swallow and hold in their negative energy and are literally killed in the process.

Never walk away from a conflict because it will follow you and become a burden at the same time. Once a conflict is resolved, it is no longer a burden.

If you are asked to perform too many things at the same time, instead of reacting in an aggravated manner, learn to manage the situation by communicating how long it will take you to perform all the tasks. Nobody can ask you to do more than you can do!

Some of the best eu-stress responses are gained from stimulating activities, experiences of personal development that lead to the enjoyment of personal success - these activities are imperative for your future.

Generally speaking, people are never really helpless, yet many people suffer from feeling helpless. In studying the philosophy of success, there are many examples of how people found a way even when the situation seemed hopeless by changing their lives in a positive and profitable way.

In reality, a person must convince themselves that they are helpless to be helpless. The fact that people are perpetually capable of finding new solutions or starting over is what separates humans from animals. Don't tie up your thinking with this negative thinking or you will suffer from emotional and physical symptoms.

If you feel that you are either physically or emotionally not up to par, look for the reason and eliminate the cause permanently. Medication and over-stimulation must not be used to cover the symptoms, you need to focus on the solutions.

We need to realize that we can never be better than everyone else! Do not try to be the best all the time; in fact, we can only do our best at any given time. Do not pressure yourself by always trying to be better than everyone else, just be the best that you can be.

If somebody does not like you, don't take it personally, simply recognize that not everybody will like you nor will you like everybody. We all have the right to like or dislike each other.

It is important to learn to say "No" if you want to avoid stress. Doing something repeatedly that you do not like just to please others will double your stress level because first, you are annoyed doing something you do not want to do, and secondly, you are angry that you are doing it at all.

Seeing a positive future reduces and prevents stress because it produces eu-stress. The more opportunities you create for your future, the happier and healthier you will be.

Learn to regulate your energy with regular periods of regeneration, breathing exercises and good nutrition, so that you will not overwork and become overly stressed. To avoid being exhausted at the end of the day, give yourself a boost with a **IBMS™** session.

The feelings of guilt people suffer when they take a day off often leads to an incredible buildup of dis-stress. If you feel the need to do absolutely nothing, your subconscious is giving you a signal and you need to listen to it! Your body may need to relax, regenerate and restore, or maybe it needs all the energy available to boost its self-healing system to fight off an illness or virus that you are unaware exists, or perhaps your brain may need a break in work to transfer information from short-term memory.

For people looking to retire it is imperative to make plans and set goals for the future, if not, the subconscious will be programmed to turn off all the energy which is one of the major reasons why people die shortly after they retire.

I cannot end this segment without clearly stating that you should stay away from sleeping pills, tranquilizers and pep pills make the decision now that you are much too important to unnecessarily destroy your body. Medication can and will not help you to resolve your life's challenges. Be aware of the true value of your body, life, personality, abilities and capacity for work, and know yourself as a loving, intelligent human being. Make the decision to pay more attention to the signals and messages of your body and mind by listening to your intuition and responding in a natural way.

## There always is a Solution

There is an answer to every question and a solution to every problem. However, having said that, it must also be said that to find the answers and solutions, we must be willing to do the necessary work and have the determination to persevere until we have achieved and realized our goal.

The "fear of failure" plagues approximately eighty-seven percent of all people and is one the worst stress factors. In the psychology of success, there is no such thing as failure; there are only results, you either get what you wanted or you don't. You will have much less stress in your life if, when you don't produce the result you wanted, you learn from your result, so that you modify your approach and start over working until you reach your desired goal.

If you follow this solution oriented rule your life will be free of failure because failure comes from giving up, not trying and/or not finishing.

In life, it is important not to focus on the negative, those things that may go wrong or not work out, or situations that are out of our control. Concentrate exclusively on what you want to achieve, finding solutions and strategies, learn from your mistakes, so that in the end you can reach your goal. Be sure to picture successes and personal triumphs in your mind when you look to the future.

To react negatively to criticism is usually a sign of poor self-esteem because people who respect themselves and recognize their value and ability enjoy constructive criticism; they delight in the opportunity to improve themselves. On the other hand, they also can reject the criticism without taking it personally because they know when the criticism is wrong for them and that it has more to do about the other person.

Only people who have lost their self-esteem and self-confidence feel personally insulted, assaulted or hurt, and then respond with anger, hostility or fighting back. Cooperative, solution oriented action, so that everyone gets the best results, often includes constructive criticism. Develop your self confidence and self esteem with the specific **IBMS™** session. See: www.instinctbasedmedicine.com

In life, you will encounter people who are envious and even resentful of you, but to react negatively gives them exactly what they want and this is exactly what you should not do. You have to earn envy; pity on the other hand is dished out for free. In this regard, it is important for you not to allow yourself to be envious because as soon as you begrudge someone something, you send your subconscious the message that success, possessions and accomplishments are all negative. Your subconscious, in turn, fights to keep these so-called negative traits (success, accomplishments, etc.) from happening to you so that you will never achieve, be, or possess what you envy in others.

Daily overload and the unlikelihood of finishing all the jobs and tasks on the schedule is one of the real stress factors from which we all suffer, but starting today, change how you manage your scheduling by asking yourself the question, "Can I get this done today?" If it is not realistic, explain your dilemma. In this way, you manage the expectations of the people around you so that they do not have false hopes because disappointment often leads to anger, aggression, hostility, and a lot of stress.

If you practice goal setting and develop action plans, you will discover that you actually take charge of your future which in turn translates into a life where you determine and shape your fate. A person in charge of their fate controls their life and does not need to fear the future.

Because the **IBMS™** provides the technology and opportunity to learn new ways to deal with your life, you no longer need fear physical or emotional lows - you now determine your emotional state. Use the goal setting **IBMS™** session to find out what you really want.

**Fears lead to Inappropriate Behavior and Bad Results**.

This happens because you preprogram your mind with the fear so that it becomes a self-fulfilling prophecy. Instead concentrate on only what you want, focus on your desires and achieving the best results.

Poor concentration also leads to an accumulation of stress. Regular breaks to regenerate, along with breathing exercises and good nutrition, will quickly get rid of concentration problems, unless they are the result of a medical problem.

Another huge stress factor is the "fear of loss!" This fear is often the result of focusing on the negative and becomes something you attract into your life by visualization. To understand and eliminate these fears, ask yourself:

- Is this fear real?
- Is this fear justified?
- What is the worst thing that can happen?
- What could I do and what are my options if the worst happened?

*Being prepared is the best stress reduction!*

If you suffer from stress because you are overworked, the problem can easily be solved by being more organized, managing your workload better and keeping your work under control. You owe it to yourself to learn to say "no!"
Take your CD player with you to work and use the **IBMS™** sessions.

You must pay attention to your spinal column, as the mobility of your fingers, your eyesight and your ability to concentrate all depend on your spine being flexible and unobstructed. By exercising, breathing deeply and fully, and taking regular breaks, your ability to work will greatly benefit as will your health, energy and vitality. Use the specific **IBMS™** session.

Fear of infection or disease, in and of itself, increases the risk of infection as every fear measurably weakens the immune system. It is important to protect oneself, but it is also important not to get caught up in unnecessary fears or imagined negative situations. Infections or an outbreak of herpes for example usually happens only when you are stressed. You will never see an excited energized positive action person getting the flue or the cold. You need to be run down first to get sick.

Sometimes bad habits are learned behaviors that have been passed on from generation to generation. Others are simply developed as bad habits. Never having enough time is one bad habit that can be addressed and resolved easily with some organization and delegation of work and responsibility.

By simply experiencing **IBMS™** sessions every day, you in fact save a lot of time because the sessions provide the regeneration and relaxation you need to be more effective and efficient. In fact, if you try going to bed just twenty minutes earlier at night, and getting up twenty minutes later in the morning, you will start your day full of energy and strength to take on the world! If you add a healthy breakfast, preferably with fruit and fruit juice, the sky is the limit!

One of the results of not having any relaxation and down time is a poor quality of life and eventual suicide. Without the enjoyment of success, without stages of recreation and regeneration, if your subconscious cannot make some sense out of your work and pursuit it will not make the huge efforts required to keep you healthy or even alive. We need to feel rewarded for our actions or we could feel unworthy and depressed.

Allow enough time for hobbies, friends, family and personal interests, and if your free time is unexpectedly disrupted, do not worry or get angered, instead focus on fast solutions to overcome the disruptions and obstacles, and you will not be afraid or stressed. Reward yourself regularly.

### The Danger of Compromise

Every compromise leads to emotional and physical stress, which manifest in anxiety, poor self-esteem, lack of energy and eventually to illness. A compromise is when for one reason or another you feel pressured to make a decision that you would really prefer not to make. Compromises are the decisions you made when you accepted a result other than the one you wanted. In other words, you agreed to a less than satisfactory solution instead of the one you really wanted. A compromise against yourself, who you are, what you really stand for can kill you.

In a compromise you settle for restrictions and limitations, which gives a signal to the subconscious that you don't have to shoot for the stars, give a hundred percent. A compromise is something you do not really want to do, but you do it anyway. It is not a compromise if you knowingly accept and are willing to do something even though it does not really meet your needs. For instance, if a doctor decides to keep treating a patient that does not pay after already treating the patient for say twenty hours without pay, but the doctor wants to keep going because the patient is important to them, then this is a compromise, but not in a negative, illness-causing way. Basically, it is not a negative compromise if you make a clear decision to do something you want to do, but that you could refuse, if you were so inclined.

The manifestations you produce when you compromise show up in low self-esteem, a poor self image, self-confidence and energy. In addition, compromise produces tension and negative feelings which lead to massive stress. If compromises are made over and over again eventually it will result in a medical tragedy and can be seen as one of the main causes for cancer and other chronic illnesses. For example a woman, who compromises by staying in a marriage for the sake of her children when her husband abuses her constantly, emotionally and/or physically, generally ends up getting a chronic illness.

*Exercise:*

*Identify the areas in your life in which you repeatedly make negative compromises because you feel pressured or need to*

Dr. Leonard Coldwell

*accept the compromise to avoid conflict. This does not include conscious decisions made after serious thought for a good reason. If you constantly make concessions for the sake of peace, or to avoid tension, and they are in conflict with your goals and desires, then these are compromises that impede your energy and endanger your health.*

After you have identified the compromises in your life, make the decision right now to avoid them from this time forward. Be willing to accept the fight, the energy drain, and the necessary behavior changes you will undoubtedly have to make, and develop plans and strategies to avoid any situation that compromises you as a person.

**I suggest following my code in life:**
- *Never allow yourself to be blackmailed.*
- *Never sell yourself out.*
- *Never make a compromise against yourself.*

**How to Define the Symptoms and Eliminate the Causes of Stress**

Stress is the greatest energy drainer in our lives! And energy is the foundation of health and success. It is imperative that everybody learn to control their stress so that they will have the energy to realize all dreams.

Dis-stress and Eu-stress can loosely be defined as stress in the negative sense and stress in the positive sense respectively. Having said this, stress and stress symptoms in this book are not discussed or approached in the traditional or conventional way. Instead you must understand the causes that are responsible for the stress that you might either experience or suffer.

A stress factor can be any stimulation that you recognize, directly or indirectly, as a threat. For example, criticism from a respected close friend or family member can cause lots of

310

stress, but here there are no objective stress factors, only subjective stress factors since many people experience criticism as constructive and helpful.

The release of stress hormones depends entirely on your internal acceptance of a situation or whether or not you receive and accept the information as stress or not. It is, therefore, very important to recognize that stress is typically not generated by actual physiological damage. At least eighty percent of our dis-stressful experiences are self-induced, that is, they are created in our minds by our emotions.

*In the science of "stress psychology" we claim: "It is not what happens that determines our stress level, but it is how we react to what happens that creates stress."*

And that is exactly how it works. The way you react to stressful situations, will determine whether or not the stress hormones cause chaos. The fight or flight reaction is a natural response to the release of stress hormones. Our early ancestors needed the ability to react in seconds and command immediate bursts of physical energy to escape from or engage in combat with the daily dangers in their immediate environment.

Do not look for massively stressful situations in your life; there are, in my opinion, very few actual circumstances of real danger. There are far more little things, things that accumulate over time that cause real damage to your health.

Today, physical danger plays a lesser role in our lives than many centuries ago, but mental danger has taken over and has become an increasingly greater threat. Because our subconscious cannot distinguish between real experiences and emotional fears, whenever we think of a frightening image, our subconscious sees it as a real threat and releases stress hormones even if we are only thinking about insignificant fears of future events.

Because we cannot simply physically fight everybody or run every time we are threatened, the released stress hormones are absorbed by our body and instead of being broken down, they become a poisonous threat.

## Dealing with Stress

Each person is totally responsible for allowing the images produced in their mind to become dark, gloomy and threatening pictures, instead of seeing bright, positive and cheerful pictures. In other words, you control whether you see a situation as a problem that creates trauma and stress, and you control whether you see it as an opportunity to grow and learn. The choice is yours.

The manner in which you handle a situation in your mind will dictate whether or not you produce stress hormones. In other words, if you allow your thoughts and attitude to be negative, dwelling on the problem not on the solution, then you will produce damaging stress hormones. Behavioral therapy and preventive medicine have proven that negative statements and thoughts can become self-fulfilling prophecies like "My job is killing me!" In this regard, if we remember that we do not live to work, but work to live, immediately our attitude changes and the pressure is relieved as the stress hormones are diminished.

We only have "X" number of years of life, and since our life expectancy depends on the amount of energy we have at any given time, it is extremely important to ensure that our energy level is not weakened in order to be healthy and enjoy our lives.

The **IBMS™** focuses on improving the quality of life for everybody because ultimately, quality of life means the ability to enjoy your life and to enjoy success with others. However, most of us spend about two-thirds of our day on the problem solving, running errands, meeting challenges, etc. and only a third or less on regeneration, recreation and positive stimulation. In fact, our energy could simply be refueled by a kind word to or from a friend, a family member, or a partner, which would provide the strength to tackle our obstacles yet again.

Unfortunately, most of us function under the absurd conviction that in order to be successful we must work ourselves to the bone at the expense of our private lives. Then when we become sick or suffer a breakdown of some sort or another, all of a sudden our priorities change, but by then we often have already caused so much damage with our bad behavior that it is hard to restore our good health. Not working harder, working smarter makes you successful.

One of the worst kinds of deleterious stress is caused by bad relationships. Some of the best ways to protect yourself from this stress are to learn to be a team player, creating a team, and ultimately having some flexibility in the world around you. If you are lonely, it is hard to be happy, healthy and content. And success is meaningless if you have no one to share it with, nor can you be successful if you are alone. People don't just need their spouse, children and families; they also need friends to fill their lives. Of course, stress is also caused when your relationship with your spouse or business partnership is an ongoing battle instead of an enriching asset to your life.

The fear of failure and loss are serious stress factors, but spending time simply worrying about finances, health, friends and family members can consume a tremendous amount of energy, needlessly causing serious damage from the resulting stress. In order to control your stress level, it is important to analyze each worry to determine whether or not you have any influence or control over the situation, if you have control then you must take action and leave the worry, and if your analysis is that you have no control then you can stop worrying because there is nothing you can do about what will happen. For instance, remember the garden party example, if there is a forecast of rain and you fear that your party will be ruined, then you can take action by renting a tent, or making arrangements to move the party indoors if the rain comes, instead of simply worrying about it! If you give in to the fear of a rainy day and feel powerless, you will produce harmful stress hormones.

By repeatedly thinking about our worries and fears in our mind, we tend to make them bigger and more important than they should be. How often have you told yourself after something happened that it was not as bad as you thought, in fact, now that it is over, it was not bad at all.

In dealing with stress of paramount importance is our ability to control our thoughts and the questions we ask ourselves. For instance, if you keep asking yourself what could go wrong or what terrible thing might happen, you will live in constant fear. Whereas if you ask yourself what is the best way to deal with a situation, and you take action, fear and desperation will disappear.

The **IBMS™** session can help you with that.

It needs to be understood that fear is not a method of prevention for anything. In fact just the opposite is true; fear attracts the negative because by our focusing on what we do not want, that is what we attract. It is like what inevitably happens to the driver on a slippery country road who keeps staring at the tree they want to avoid all the while heading straight for it until they crash into to the one thing they wanted to avoid. Haven't you ever wondered how a driver, out in the middle of nowhere, hits the only tree or pole for miles around? Your life goes where you are looking for it to go. Because of this fact, it is important to screen fears. You must determine whether or not they make sense or whether or not you even have control of the situation. By preparing yourself to expect the worst, and once you have a possible solution, then you can let go of fear because there is nothing more that you can do.

Everything we build up in our mind imagined or real, has a basis in reality as far as our brain is concerned because what you think of in your mind transmits a direct message to your nervous system. The primary problem with fearing something that might or might not happen in the future comes from actually experiencing in your mind, over and over, a negative outcome because it drains from the subconscious the same amount of energy it would use if the event really happened! Worse yet, you do it on an ongoing basis every time you repeat the fear in your mind. The way you form pictures in your mind, light or dark, close up or far away, threatening or pleasant, is completely controlled by you. If a negative image pops into your head, you can immediately change it into a pleasant image by creating an image of the best possible solution or outcome in that situation. Take charge. Get in control of your thoughts.

If you see yourself as a loser in any given situation, you will behave like a loser when the situation occurs because you will have conditioned it to happen! If, on the other hand, you prepare yourself mentally for desired results, you will feel that you are in control, and your self-confidence will grow and simultaneously your stress level will be lowered or avoided altogether.

It is, of course, important to recognize, define, and change the actual physiological dangers that cause stress, like the dangers from overworking, undernourishment, lack of oxygen, not enough rest and regeneration, environmental toxins, etc.

In conclusion, be warned against the dangers associated with ignoring and suppressing stress signals in your body. A signal must be stopped, corrected and worked through, so that any damaging effects can be avoided. Never repress stress signals because that only leads to more accumulated stress and ultimately this can have catastrophic health consequences. It is like boiling water and closing the vent so that the steam cannot get out, in time it will explode.

*Mental images that you create in your mind are neurological stimulations that create a blue print for future and present actions!*

## It is the Many "Little Things"

It is amazing how many seemingly little things in our every day life contribute to the increase or decrease of our stress level. Instead of looking at stress in the traditional way, by searching out the causes of stress, you can eliminate the damaging effects that stress causes.

Optimal stress reduction can only take place when you become aware that stress is a learned and conditioned behavior as it is completely dependent on how you personally evaluate a situation, your inner representational system and your mental communication. Remember that stress is only a survival mechanism that is put into action when we feel danger. Stress produces fight or flight reactions that stimulate the body to act in a fight or flight manner. It is the little things that regularly keep piling up that damage our ability to achieve and maintain the highest quality of life and health.

**Self Analysis of Dis-Stressing Situations**

It is important to analyze crisis situations that occur frequently in your life. In this you can be prepared because if you are well prepared, you will have positive solutions in mind and you will produce fewer stress causing situations in your life.

*Exercise:*

*Write down any situation where you repeatedly experience the fight or flight response, any situation that makes you feel like there is a threat to your life as a person, either mentally, financially, emotionally or even physically.*

*Then add what you will change in your behavior so that this situation will no longer cause dis-stress in your future. (For instance, "If someone swerves into my lane on the freeway, I will slow down to make room for them, take a deep breath, and let it go.")*

## Looking at What Stress Means to You

Everyone has a completely different definition and understanding of the term "stress" and of a typical "stress situation" because something that causes anxiety or even panic to one person may not bother another person at all. The basis for these different reactions lies in the "how" we represent the situation to ourselves and the resulting internal communication concerning the situation. Therefore, we need to first define what stress and a stressful situation means for each person.

*Exercise:*

*Using a journal or notebook with plenty of blank pages for writing, answer the following to the best of your knowledge:*

*1. What does stress mean to you personally?*

*2. List some typical situations that cause you stress?*

*3. How do you usually react in these situations?*

*4. How could you change your reactions in the future?*

*5. List the reaction that you would like to change in each of the following categories?*

*Professionally -*

*Privately -*

*Physically -*

*Financially –*

*To set clear goals and develop effective strategies, you must first know who you are and what you really want. In order to*

317

*discover the answers to these questions, please answer the following:*

1. *How would you describe yourself - your personality, your skills/abilities, your positive and negative attributes?*

2. *How would you be described by others? (How would somebody describe your personality, your skills/abilities, your positive and negative attributes, and your accomplishments and achievements?)*

3. *What changes do you need to make, but have not yet made? Write down everything that comes in your mind!*

4. *List the changes you should make and how to do so.*

5. *Next write down two things you can do today or no later than tomorrow to make these changes. Repeat this task every day, until you reach your goal!*

6. *Examine the demands you place on yourself ensuring that they are realistic and do not cause more unnecessary stress. Do not demand the impossible. Now write down all the demands and expectations you have of yourself.*

7. *Then realistically list the demands you make of yourself professionally and privately.*

8. *Now write down what you can delegate from your professional life, how, who, when and where.*

9. *Now write down what you have been doing to regenerate, for your self-esteem, your personal development and your personal success.*

10. *List what you want in the future for your personal development, your quality of life, regeneration, health and vitality.*

**Please answer the following:**

1. *What are the personality traits you would like to acquire or improve?*

2. *In what areas do you not use your full potential?*

3. *Why not?*

4. *What can you do to change that in the future?*

5. *List all the obstacles that are standing between you and reaching your life goals:*

6. *How could you best prepare to reach those goals?*

### The Principle of Self-motivation

You can only be healthy if you have enough self-confidence, energy, vitality, self-esteem and enthusiasm to deal with yourself, your life and your future. Success is not simply about reaching a goal; working daily towards reaching it, is a goal in itself.

Keep reminding yourself of the importance of being healthy. Do not wait to appreciate your health until you have lost it; do not sacrifice your family for your job, the one cannot survive and thrive without the other. Remember that success is always dependent on team play, both professionally and privately. Use the motivational **IBMS™** CDs.

## The Personal Characteristics of Successful, Healthy People

The following is a summary of some of the basic characteristics of successful and healthy people:

- Individuals who see problems as challenges and opportunities that will help them to grow to be even more successful.
- Individuals, who take responsibility for their work, are not lazy and persevere no matter what.
- Individuals, who take charge and act, have a strong value system and are responsible.
- They turn negative stress into positive and productive energy.
- Because they have clear values, they know exactly why they act in a certain way and for what reason.
- They have a good sense of humor and can laugh at themselves and the ironies of life.
- They know how important good relationships and team play are for their health and success.
- They are aware of the value of their health, their energy and their appearance.
- They are physically active, knowing that they need to exercise and breathe for their health and energy.
- They make sure that they get enough sleep, so that they can recover and restore themselves during the night.
- They take calculated risks; they believe in themselves; they live without fear with a positive attitude.
- They make time for recreation and regenerating, knowing that they will work harder, better and more efficiently once regenerated.

## Believe in Yourself

The importance of positive self-esteem cannot be over emphasized. Your self-image is imprinted in your mind according to the messages you give yourself. If for example, you communicate with yourself saying things like "I could never do that!" versus "Of course I can do that!" you can immediately imagine what the effect is on your brain. In fact, you develop healthy self-confidence by picturing/seeing your strengths and possibilities in a positive light in your mind.

If you do not believe in yourself, and you tell yourself that you cannot do something, you will not be able to do it. It is only when you stand fully behind your decisions and actions that you will behave in such a manner that your peers, family, friends, clients, etc. will have faith and confidence in you. Why should anybody believe in you if you do not believe in yourself to start with? Your self-esteem determines which tasks you will tackle and/or how enthusiastic and confident you will be in finding the solution to a problem. Basically, concentrate on everything you can do, and how you could do it even better.

*Exercise: Developing a Deeper Belief in Yourself and Your Abilities*

*The key is believing in yourself and having confidence in your ability to deal with challenges and problems.*

*Start by looking at your past - focus on your successes and achievements. See yourself as a doer, as someone who has goals and standards. Picture yourself as a person who makes decisions, reaches their goals with perseverance and flexibility. Now think of something that is important to you, but that you have been putting off for one reason or another. Take a moment and make the decision to take action - now picture yourself setting goals and making an action plan to accomplish your goal.*

321

*Make a mental picture, seeing yourself in action taking the first step, then moving forward to successfully completing your goal. Say something like, "Yes, I can do this!" Notice how good you feel about yourself when you do this. The fact is if you can see yourself doing something, no matter how difficult, you can do it!*

Whenever you think of yourself, you must see yourself as a problem solver, a doer and a winner. This mental programming is eighty percent responsible for how you see yourself and contributes to your feelings of self-esteem and self-confidence. Finally, your self-image determines everything you accomplish in life. Remember that the brain can only program the input that you give it, consciously or unconsciously.

## Family and Friends - the Foundation of Health and Success

A solid strong support system gives us energy, security, strength, vitality and success. Loneliness and isolation often lead to feelings of helplessness, which then leads to illness. It is extremely important to remember your family, friends and supporters that helped you along the way to your success. To be lonely and successful is a contradiction in terms.

In my therapeutic work, I met many patients who at first appearance seemed successful, happy and content; in fact, I thought they had it all! However, I soon discovered that the higher they climbed on the professional ladder, the lonelier they became even though they had material wealth and professional success. The problem was that they had lost their support system along the way. Their family, friends and children all left them along the way and they ended up alone, unhappy, dissatisfied and sick.

Loneliness generally leads to bitterness, which in turn leads to a lowered immune system. Bitterness arises as we become aware that we have not lived up to our potential as a human being and that the things that are really important in life have eluded us. Without family and close friends there is an emptiness to life no matter what the level of success. This feeling leads to self-pity and a negative attitude which depletes our energy thus lowering our immune system with the result that we suffer a health breakdown.

I can honestly say that the people that I met that were the truly exceptional and successful people, in every case, were as attentive to their personal team (family, friends, etc.), as they were to their professional team. In addition, they were filled with energy and vitality, and their immune system was very healthy, thanks to the emotional support they received. Having a team and being a member of a good team are the best therapy against depression and frustration. Playing on a "team" enhances our desire to work and has a positive influence on our energy and health.

Yale University concluded in a research study that each person in their life influences at least 250 people who in turn influence another 250 people. Even if we reduce their number to 200, it still means that every person directly and indirectly touches 40,000 people (200 times 200). With this in mind, we should remember to behave as if we are influencing 40,000 people and that it is extremely important to our own success to treat everyone as if they were the most important person in your life.

If you have a personal and professional social network, it will catch you if you fall financially, emotionally or physically. Having people to help, bounce ideas off or work with saves strength, effort, and energy. In fact, comparable studies performed at several universities derived the following similar conclusion - only eight percent of the things that cause our fears and worries can be consciously influenced by our own thoughts and actions. As a result, since we cannot control ninety-two percent of our anxieties and fears, it is futile and a waste of time and energy to worry about the things you have no control over like the economy, world politics, the weather, etc.

Instead, concentrate on the eighty percent that you can do something about and forget the rest.

Your relationship with your spouse or your life partner affects approximately eighty percent of your health and success. If you are very successful professionally, but your personal life is a disaster, your energy will be adversely affected and eventually your professional life will suffer as you feel more and more burdened with failures and setbacks in your personal life. The result is that you continue living feeling apathetic, indifferent, lethargic, and frustrated, all of which manifest into corresponding medical problems.

Studies performed at both Harvard and Yale Universities show that the most successful salesmen, managers and self-employed individuals have a healthy and happy personal life. They make time for their personal life including family and friends, and they incorporate equal consideration between both lives. It is extremely important to be attentive to your spouse's or partner's needs so that you can build and enjoy a future together. Team play in your private and professional life is one major factor for stress reduction.

In conclusion, success depends on team play. It is much easier to eliminate feelings of loneliness and helplessness with someone we love and who loves us. It is easier to cope with feelings of frustration, indifference and anger if you can share them with somebody! To experience lasting success and health, it is crucial to have a well-balanced and contented personal life, which is why your personal life should always be the highest priority when you set your goals.

To create great relationships you need to be yourself. Don't play a role just to satisfy others. Show the world who you really are. Then you have only people in your life that like, love and accept you the way you really are and you don't have to constantly produce stress by denying yourself to be the true you.

# Section II - Chapter 3

### The Healing Process and the IBMS™

"The body can only heal and repair while in a restful state, which means that if we do not rest, there is no way for the body to find the strength and energy to repair and regenerate itself."

If you are sick with the flu or a cold and do not rest, you will run your system into the ground until you eventually drop. It is no different than running your car in the red zone, but instead of slowing down and letting the car cool off, you keep on going and block out the red light so that you cannot see it. The result is that it is only a matter of time until the car dies and needs major repairs. The same is true if when you are sick; you deny your body the rest it needs and ignore the symptoms. It is only in a restful state and with deep sleep that the body can repair and heal what is wrong. It is for this very reason that the **IBMS™** was developed because the **IBMS™** sessions can provide the equivalent restorative benefit of hours of deep restful sleep during the twenty-minute session.

The **IBMS™** system is unique as no other system known to exist can boast achieving the results that are constantly repeated over and over again by this system. What separates the **IBMS™** system from everything else is that during a session, as the body relaxes, the brain becomes more and more alert. This basically means that the brain has the ability to function more effectively, which allows for clearer, more alert and efficient thinking than you have ever before realized.

325

In a state of total physical relaxation and total mental clarity, you are in absolute control of your thinking process and all of your decisions. As such, you are capable of taking responsibility and control of your entire life! Your nervous system is stimulated so that it gets regenerated in the most effective way possible. The results from a **IBMS™** session are actually measurable on brain scans or with blood tests which clearly show the positive chemical and bioelectrical changes. This is, in addition, to the obvious improvements in self-esteem and the self-confidence levels.

The only way to help a person is to help them to help themselves! If you feed a hungry person, they will still be hungry the next day, but if you teach them how to find work and make money to buy food, you will have taught them something really valuable because now they know how to get food for the rest of their life. The **IBMS™** is a total self-help education, training and coaching system that enhances your individual talents and enables you to take control over your life. There is no magic pill, trick, system or person that can get your life in order for you. You need to do it yourself and the faster you do it, the faster you can enjoy you life on the highest possible level.

Since in my opinion, the only reason we have for living, is personal growth and development, it is damaging and dangerous to our personality and self-esteem to let someone else fix our problems. I believe that anyone who tries to take the responsibility from your hands is damaging you. If anyone tells you that they will take care of you, solve all the problems in your life, or they will fix you, you should run as fast as you can. Only you can fix yourself!

I believe it is a crime against humanity to manipulate people from the outside even if you think you have their best interest in mind. No one has the right to manipulate another person, which is why I am so avidly against hypnotism or NLP techniques as I have already made clear. Even if we are not consciously aware of this, our subconscious mind knows that we cause our own problems, and we need to fix them.

Acting on your instincts is the safest way to heal yourself since your body knows what is best for it. If you do not follow your instinct, you will be unsuccessful in whatever you do, but if you follow your instincts then you can achieve whatever you want. Simultaneously, if you give other people the power over "fixing" your life then you will inevitably get hurt because this takes away the means to grow on your own, stunts personal growth and development and leads to many problems. Nobody knows what is best for you except you! If something does not feel right to you, then it is not right.

The **IBMS™** sessions help you reconnect with yourself and get back to your instincts so that your instincts become finely honed. If you live the way that you instinctively feel is right, you will automatically stay healthy. People generally get sick because they do all the wrong things, and the only way they can get healthy again is by doing only all the right things!

Artificial or drug induced relaxation has no long term benefit nor does it have any effect on stopping or preventing the causes for your stress related problems. As previously explained, hypnotism and massage induce relaxation, but if you are in a state of relaxation for more than seven minutes, your body produces sleep hormones making you feel tired for the rest of the day. In contrast, a **IBMS™** session provides only five and one-half minutes of total relaxation within the twenty-minute session so that your body never produces sleep hormones. After a session you feel extremely energized and after a few sessions, the quality of your life improves dramatically because quality of life is based upon your energy levels.

If you want to be pampered and want to be touched for comfort, massage is wonderful and helpful. But it does nothing for your mental and emotional stress level.

## The Speed of Healing

I have such a problem understanding how people can think that a problem with their health that took thirty years to develop could or should somehow be fixed with a pill in a couple of days. If it took that long to develop, it certainly will take some time and doing a hundred percent the right thing to get rid of it! In fact, using the **IBMS™** sessions gives you almost immediate results, but you still need to continue to use it daily for the much needed breaks and to get motivated to do the right things.

Don't try to "hang in" when you know that you need a break because you make more mistakes when you are tired. It only takes twenty minutes to regenerate, when it could take you all day to fix something you messed up when you were tired and not thinking clearly. Instead take a break and get regenerated in twenty minutes with the **IBMS™** sessions.

We have **IBMS™** sessions for many of life's challenges and we are always adding new sessions, but we are also able to create specific personal sessions to suit individual needs. In addition, we are in the preliminary stages of planning the **IBMS™** Coaching Centers like I have it set up in Europe, and providing it in one on one workshop settings; if you are interested, please let us know by writing to the address at the end of this book.

**Program Your Health**

Please recognize that we all use pictures when we think because the only language of the brain is a symbol, that means a picture. Therefore scientific visualization is the only way to use your brain. Christians should be aware of this fact because it is the only way for the brain to function. It has nothing to do with new age or other religious techniques. Use your free will and take charge over every part of your life by self conditioning. ( specific faith-based **IBMS™** sessions on CD are available: www.instinctbasedmedicine.com )

It is important to immediately start programming your health, despite whatever emotional or physiological shape you find yourself in at present. You should begin picturing in your mind exactly how and who you want to be, not what you fear or might get or have. If a person who is sick does not believe that they can get 100 percent healthy and strong again, they will not put in the effort to regain their health, strength and vitality. But if they believe in a healthy and vigorous future, they can start to fight and will persevere in reaching their goal. In the modern psychology of success, it is said, "If you believe you can do something, you can, and if you believe you cannot, you will not!" This is because no matter what you are always right! Our belief system triggers the matching part in the brain to activate or immobilize specific regions. So if you believe that you can do something, the corresponding areas in the brain and throughout the rest of your body are stimulated, enabling you to realize your goal. In reverse, if you believe that you cannot do something, you automatically shut off the area of the brain that is responsible for the realization of the action. This is why what we believe becomes a self-fulfilling prophecy.

Everybody knows people who are always saying: "I knew it would not work." And the end result was that, it did not work! Well, it did not work because they did not believe it would work and sent the message to fail to the brain so it failed!

To change your belief system, you need to find evidence and confirmation that you can accomplish what you want so that you can reach your goal. A belief system is nothing more than a gut feeling that something is right for you. Belief has nothing to do with truth or falsehoods; it is only instinct that something is okay.

If you need affirmation all is possible, educate yourself by reading stories of people who have achieved the "impossible." By filling up your mind with these positive results oriented stories, your brain will start to accept that everything as possible. Once you condition your subconscious to believe that you will succeed based on sound knowledge, you have already taken the first step on your way to success.

*A study was performed on the behavior system of conditioned fleas. At the outset, fleas were put in a glass covered with a lid and then studied. At first, the fleas jumped seemingly endlessly up against the lid, but after a while they stopped jumping so high, in fact they jumped lower an lower indicating that they had learned escape was impossible so they jumped less high. Because they were newly conditioned not to jump so high when the lid was removed none of the fleas even tried to jump high.*

This same conditioning is also possible in a negative way and often happens from being around negative people. Without realizing it, we are influenced by their negative remarks or we actually believe them. On the other hand, we condition ourselves to believe that since we were unsuccessful in a previous situation, there is no reason to aspire to try again or for another. However, simply because you did not previously succeed or because somebody else failed, does not in any way indicate that you won't succeed this time!

I was impressed by the story of an eleven-year-old girl, who was the only survivor of a shipwreck thirteen miles off the coast of Miami. When found, a newspaper reporter asked her, how she, not an experienced swimmer, had managed to swim to shore. The girl answered, "With every stroke I told myself: One more time, I can do it one more time." This is the way to get to your goal! Remember to keep repeating to yourself: "One more time, I will try one more time, I can make it!" Get closer to reaching your goal, one step at the time.

The world has been working on convincing the public that there is no cure for cancer, even though this is absurd and not remotely true as can be seen by the many people who have been cured without surgery, radiation or chemotherapy. In fact, there are even cured AIDS patients who literally changed from being HIV positive to HIV negative although how is still unknown, but the point is that even AIDS is not incurable. Peter Duesberg did, however, prove that HIV positive does not lead to AIDS (refer to his book *Why we will never win the war on AIDS*).

When you have a mountain to climb, think about all the people that have gone before you and succeeded because if you do not convince yourself that you can overcome the situation or crisis, you won't. Remember John D. Rockefeller, the richest man in the world in his time? Well when he started he was a starving bookkeeper who slept at his desk because he could not afford to rent a place or a bed.

*Everything is possible! In fact, we are born to be healthy! We are born to be successful and healthy! This is the way nature intended it to be.*

If you are suffering from a medical crisis, or you have been told that you have a chronic illness, and you find it difficult to believe that you will ever be completely healthy again, think and focus on the many people who have totally recovered. You may think that with surgery or therapy, the best you can expect is a semblance of health, but in fact, if you take charge and decide to win the battle then you will.

Over the last thirty years, I have had the opportunity to assist in the healing of many patients suffering from cancer, rheumatism, muscular dystrophy, multiple sclerosis, high and low blood pressure, gout, asthma, neurological problems, insomnia, weak concentration and memory problems, sexual dysfunction, depression, anxiety, nervous disorders and diverse emotional, neurological and mental problems. I used the **IBMS™** to achieve an above ninety percent success rate. It is when the patient develops the belief system that they can win that they take back control of their body and start the fight back to health.

Even if you cannot entirely believe that you can get better, it is important to start telling yourself, "It is possible, I may be able to do it, I can possibly do this." This will start opening the door and reconditioning you to a new belief system, a healthy and successful future.

Once you accept the possibility that you may overcome your health crisis, start by improving your health with good nutrition, breathing and exercise. You can influence your future health with many small improvements, which will reassure you that you can do it. The little improvements will show progress, which in turn, will give you confidence and thus begins the new computer program in your mind that tells you: "I can do it." You need to have a clear goal outlined in your mind before installing this new program.

## Energy Drainers

The people who surround your daily life have a tremendous impact on your health. Are you surrounded by people with a negative and critical attitude? If you are, you are at risk of absorbing their negativity, which can ultimately affect your belief system negatively. Even if you have a strong personality and a positive attitude, you will eventually be ground down by these types of people. I call them energy drainers! Nothing is worse for your health than the company of negative, unhappy, critical, envious or vicious people.

Here is an example of what I constantly experienced in my practice. I sent home completely cured patients that originally came to me seriously ill. These patients were sent home having been taught to help and regenerate themselves by applying our methods, but when they come home, looking radiant and healthy, claiming that they felt great and had no more pain, etc., they would be confronted with quizzical questions like, "Are you sure, you're okay? Is this really going to last? Don't you think that you are just imagining this? Are you sure that you have no pain? You must have some pain? How can you be cured so quickly and without all the normal conventional treatments?" Hearing this over and over again has a wearing effect that erodes their belief system and all the newly programmed positive input eventually disappears. These doubting comments are often said in ignorance, but nevertheless the end result is the same, the development of a negative belief system and images implanted in the mind.

What is the point, if improvement is visible in a very ill patient, of obstructing, eliminating and preventing them from any "hope" of getting healthy again?

## Remove the Energy Drainers from your Life

Everybody experiences difficulties in life, but over time, it is not so much what happens to us as how we cope with what happens to us that is important! Some people whine and complain all the time, while others are always searching for solutions. It is much easier to whine, complain and blame others for your misery, but it does not help you in any way and only creates losers because it is always easier to complain than it is to look for and work on the solutions.

If you are approached by somebody seeking advice with a problem, listen, help, and try to find a solution, but if the person whines and is looking for you to solve their problem so they don't have to, then run, don't stop, get away from them because they will suck you dry! You have neither the time nor the energy and strength to waste on losers. You need to use all of your energy on improving your own life and helping those who will appreciate and really need your help. Realize your dreams and goals, work for health and success, and enjoy hobbies, fun and all other things that are important to you and your family.

*Life is simply too short to waste on negative people.*

Whiners should know that statistically eighty-five percent of the people to whom you are whining are not interested in your complaint, while fourteen percent of your listeners are delighted that the problem is yours and not theirs.

It is vital that you not focus on how much you were hurt in life, how badly you were treated, how rotten your childhood was, etc., nobody is interested nor do they care, but more importantly nor should you. What you want to accomplish and do is what matters, not what happened to you.

People need to let go and remove all negative people, energy drainers that are in their life. Unfortunately, we often have family members that are energy drainers, although perhaps well meaning energy drainers, nevertheless they need to be told:

> "I love you and you are very important to me. But, from now on, if you undermine my actions in any way, I will have no choice, but to distance myself from you. Either we can avoid any questionable subject, or we can discuss everything in a positive manner. Either you support and help me find solutions, or we go our separate ways!"

*Exercise:*

*Write a list of all the people who have had a negative influence or impact on your thought process, actions and/or feelings. Include the people who leave you feeling badly after you have talked to them! Anybody who undermines your talents, future, ideas, behavior, achievements, goals, etc. fits this profile. Then tell these people that you will no longer accept their negative influence on your life or simply remove them from your life!*

Get rid of the spoilsports, energy drainers and party poopers who are only out to spoil everybody's happiness. Get rid of the people, who are responsible for the misery in their own life because of their negative attitude, otherwise they will keep you from realizing your goals. We are all directly affected by our environment and poor associations are all too often responsible for people not reaching their potential.

**Perseverance is the Key to Health and Success**

You must believe in yourself! You will keep reading this because it cannot be over emphasized! You must keep on telling yourself that "you can do it, and you will do it." Having said that, just saying it does not make it happen, you have to take control and make it happen. No matter what, in every process of life there will always be ups and downs, smooth sailing and setbacks, but with the desire, the belief system and the inner programming you need to rely on when life puts you down, you will bounce back. This is possible because you will have programmed yourself to expect difficulties, yet to act, which will get you to move in the right direction. Ups and downs are a part of life, only the degrees change!

Another important insight that you need to understand is that you should not focus on whether life treats you fairly or unfairly. When a hurricane hits Florida and destroys hundreds of homes, there will always be the people who whine and complain and do nothing, while the industrious people are busy rebuilding.

Whenever life deals you a blow, shake it off, get up and move on. This is ultimately the true secret of success.

## A Program for Self-Image

To condition yourself for desired success, first decide that you will dedicate the time for daily regeneration and follow the exercise. For best results, regenerate two or three times a day with **IBMS™** sessions.

*Exercise:*

*Begin by seeing yourself in the place where you want to be with everything you want to accomplish then write everything down on an index card. Be sure to write everything in the present because the brain does not understand the past and can only be conditioned in the present. So, for instance, write: I am a healthy, successful person, full of determination and vitality, I have this or that car, work at a nice desk in my office, I have this kind of loving family, etc. Even if you do not feel that you are very healthy and fit at the moment, for conditioning sake, you must speak in the present tense - I am healthy and full of vitality. Simultaneously, picture the corresponding images in your mind, seeing yourself in an imaginary mirror looking healthy, radiant, successful, full of confidence, etc.*

Remember that it is very important to **contemplate, that means** to always see yourself playing yourself not as though you were watching a movie; you need to be actively playing in your images. In other words you must experience the mental programming as though it were real, seeing, hearing, tasting, feeling and smelling everything with your own eyes. Conditioning is not possible if you disassociate or see yourself as an outside observer. Regular and continuous repetition of your mental pictures will eventually change and improve your self-esteem and behavior in the manner that you have programmed.

*Exercise:*

*What does success means to you? How do you see your life with your success in five, ten or thirty years, and what does a totally successful life mean to you? Now picture these images in your mind and take mental possession of everything you would like to experience and have in your life. This is how you mentally permanently program your desires.*

# Section II - Chapter 4

## The Commitment to Health

If you want to be successful with your health, you must be committed to do everything necessary to achieve your goal. You can begin by setting clear goals, deciding how to reach them and not allowing for the possibility of failure or giving up to enter your mind. Being committed to success means that you are willing to do everything that is necessary to achieve success.

If you don't have a mission or dreams and desires in life, you will most likely be unhealthy or sick. Have you ever accepted or tolerated obstacles in your life without doing anything about them, but then suddenly you decided that "Enough is enough." After that you took control and acted stopping the humiliation, insults or limitations from going further. This comes from commitment, determination and perseverance. If you live your life according to your own values and rules, you will enjoy and be prepared for all of life's demands. You will not be a victim and suffer from all the negative stress in spite of challenges, because you will be realizing your dreams.

Dr. Leonard Coldwell

**The Paths to a Good Attitude**

There are some conditions that need to be met in order to achieve excellent physical, emotional and mental health and the resulting abundance of energy. These conditions are as follows:

A. You have to accept responsibility for your life, including control over future developments.

*Losers refuse to take responsibility for their actions or for negative developments. Losers also always blame other people, other circumstances and other situations for their demise. Their failures are always the result of how life has unfairly treated them. Their failures are never the logical result of their behavior. These are the people that always say: "I should" or "I ought to," never "I have decided" or "I will do that."*

B. You have to set meaningful goals.

*You will develop a greater sense of self-awareness and self-understanding when you realize your goals while developing a new sense of self-worth and self-confidence. By improving your self-image, your confidence and behavior grows respectively.*

Goals give you direction and they program your future. Goals help you to take responsibility and control of your life so that you determine your own future and give you motivation to act and to persevere. Winners take responsibility, learn from their mistakes and move on until they have reached their goal. Losers, on the other hand, avoid making mistakes by doing nothing, which is of course the ultimate mistake. There are only two ways to lose, either by doing nothing at all or by stopping doing something. Having few or no goals makes you feel lost without direction and hope resulting in feelings of depression, irritation and failure all of which create stress.

**Losers prefer to live by the rules, value systems, directions and goals of others, so that when they fail or lose, they can blame all of the foregoing for their failure or loss.**

**Winners prefer to make their own mistakes, learn and move on.**

**Losers are forever looking for excuses not to act, so that they can avoid failure.**

**Winners look for answers and solutions.**

You start by first considering what is important to you then set your goals accordingly. Remember to ask yourself, "Why do I want to achieve this and what will be the end result?" Then develop an action plan, having first analyzed whether or not you are willing to pay the price necessary to reach this goal. You must be honest, realistic and clear about the sacrifices you will be forced to make then you need to decide if these are worth it! Some goals may not be worth the sacrifice like for instance sacrificing your family for career!

Then develop the determination and commitment to reach your goals by always speaking to yourself in the "I want and I will," not "Perhaps, I could" form about everything. As an example of commitment and determination, let's say that your child swallowed some poison, but the telephone is broken and your car will not start. Now are you going to wait and hope for the best (perhaps, maybe if…), or do you grab your child, run into the street, stop a car and persuade or demand that the driver rush your child to the hospital? This is the difference!

*Focus your energy on creating valuable and important actions, not on wasting time and energy. Follow the Pareto Principle, which states that twenty percent of our efforts produce eighty percent of our results so concentrate on expending twenty percent towards your goal so that it will produce eighty percent of your success.*

C. Break down the bigger goals into smaller more manageable parts so that you can handle them in the most effective way. Have a positive attitude because it is only when you believe in your possibilities that you will you act accordingly and be successful.

D. Find work that you enjoy because successful people always look for what they enjoy and then turn it into a profession, so that you can earn money doing what you enjoy.

*If you are in a job or a relationship or anything that you do not like for a very long time, it will eventually make you sick. If you are doing something that you have decided to do even if you do not like it, your health will not be in danger. If you are happy in your job or whatever else, you can enjoy health. Consider problems as challenges to expand your creativity and grow.*

E. Be a team player because all the success in the world is worth nothing if you end up lonely and alone.

*You are a failure if you end up alone so do not lose your team and your dreams on the way to the top as they are the foundation for your future, your career and your success. Without a team, there is no balance in life and a loner always becomes discouraged, distrustful and much stressed.*

F. Be attentive to all the problems that could and do arise.

*Denial of problems always results in catastrophes, therefore, recognize, accept and eliminate problems before or as they happen, do not ignore and think they will go away. Losers ignore signs that should alert them that there is something that needs attention whereas winners immediately address them.*

In life, face challenges, enjoy finding solutions and delight in the battle so that you will emerge a winner. Have the right attitude and tell yourself "I will do it myself, and I will succeed." Take responsibility and take charge of your life because you only have one life to live so live it well!

## Taking Charge

One of the most basic elements of good health and self-esteem is the knowledge that you are in charge of your life. People, who feel that they are being manipulated, become tense and suffer from stress related problems. People get a sense of freedom from feeling that they are in charge of their life. It is crucial for everyone to act, make their own decisions and be in charge of their own life.

Medical research has repeatedly shown that people who are or feel that they are trapped or manipulated, are more frequently ill than people who do not feel that way. Life expectancy is also dramatically reduced for people who feel trapped or manipulated.

If you can influence your life and health in a negative way, then you obviously can also influence your life and health in positive way. If negative emotional or physical behavior can bring about negative reactions, positive behavior can, of course, lead to positive neurological processes.

If we consciously take charge and accept responsibility for our actions, simultaneously, feelings of helplessness diminish and the corresponding distress is reduced.

A feeling of helplessness, of being at the mercy of others, is an important stress factor, which has a significantly negative influence on our health.

If instead of talking you act, the action automatically generates a feeling of being in charge and provides the insight that you have influenced the outcome.

A feeling of helplessness creates, among other things, a negative self-image because your feelings of self-assurance and self-confidence gradually diminish, leaving you unable, after a while, to perform on a high level.

By breaking down your goals into manageable sections, you can reward yourself along the way continuously strengthening your self-esteem and self-image.

Celebrate your successes in direct proportion to its importance while increasing your possibilities for improvement.

The more opportunities you have, the greater your sense of freedom and security. When crisis situations or opportunities present themselves, you will be able to control their outcome.

The more options you have to resolve obstacles and hurdles, the less stress you will suffer, which will enable you to look with greater confidence and less stress at your future.

Many people have actually died when they discovered, realized or felt that they had lost control over their life and their future. Suicide is often the result of people realizing that they cannot defend themselves nor do anything to change this feeling or circumstance.

Visualize tomorrow as a new birth, imagine the person you always wanted to be and in reality already are within yourself.

Never forget that you can start over every day of your life to live up to be the person you have always wanted to be. After all, every day is a new beginning, if you are willing to leave the past behind and live in the present.

***Remark: Self destruction or suicide is usually the result of depression caused by stress.***

## Use the Principles of Control

To take charge and be in control of your destiny and to live in accordance with your own value-system, you must answer the following questions:

    1. Why do I feel helpless?

2.  How can I change this situation for the better?
3.  In which situations do I feel confident, and what can I do to feel that way now?
4.  Where and how do I start?
5.  Who do I know that can help me?
6.  What information do I need and where can I find help?

*Exercise:*

*List the areas in your life where you want more control so that you can reach your full potential. Broad and loose descriptions are not acceptable so you must clearly identify and specify what areas need change and improvement. Define all the areas in your life that need improvement.*

Start by identifying the areas in which you want to take control that are most important to you. For example, prioritize listing the situations in which you have previously felt completely helpless because they are influenced by negative neuro- associations.

Instead of asking yourself "Can I take charge?" tell yourself "How can I positively change this situation?" Do not worry or concentrate on things that you cannot change, rather concentrate on your desired result, not on errors and failures. Prepare yourself for the possibility of contingencies then move on.

Recognize and give yourself credit for the fact that you have already overcome many small and large problems in the past so you can tell yourself "I have succeeded before, so I can do it again." or "If others can do it, so can I!" or as the **IBMS™** teaches "Nobody has done this before, so I will be the first!"

Never attempt to solve everything at once, nobody can, but worst the failure could discourage you so that you may feel too helpless and overwhelmed to continue at all. Remember that a one percent change every day translates into a 100 percent change in 100 days. Think about what that means over a 365 day period? If you focus on dividing up all the obstacles prioritizing the most important as your immediate target, you will consistently progress towards your ultimate goal and with each success you will be better prepared and ready to deal with the next obstacle

Do not set your individual goals too unrealistically high as you will sabotage your success and instead you will feel like a failure. Be sure to give yourself a realistic deadline so that you will be successful. For instance, if you decided to quit drinking coffee, but you drink half the amount of cups the following day, you should consider that a success. In other words, give yourself credit for your achievement even if it is not the end result – it is progress!

Find people who recognize and support your skills, talents and potential to help you. Like all world-class athletes, you too want to find a coach or a trainer who is able to advise, push and help you to consistently grow to reach your full potential.

In fact, I see my role with this book and the **IBMS™** as your coach and friend, who educates, works and trains with you developing concepts for your individual success. Our goal is help to self-help, by using the newest and most effective information, training methods and knowledge available today. This information is flexible as it can be adapted to help everybody to produce unlimited success in every area of their life by helping themselves. Never be afraid to seek help, especially from the people that can help you to make the most of your life.

Please understand that all manipulative techniques are dangerous and can destroy your life and health. Instead, seek out education and training programs that enhance your development. Stay away from any kind of program that tries to change your personality or tells you what to do and when to do it.

Every person in the universe is absolutely unique, which is why you have the possibility of producing unique and unusual success. Do not walk in somebody else's foot steps, do not follow a leader, instead look for leaders and guides to assist you to develop your original concept of success. You have only yourself for the rest of your life so work with your emotional and physical self!

Learn, above all, to feel good about yourself by always doing the things with which you are most comfortable. You can learn from the success stories of others, but do not try to copy them instead take what you can use for yourself to apply towards achieving whatever you want and is good for you. You must feel good about your actions! Be wary of manipulating techniques that try to influence your thinking, feelings and behavior as they will have a deleterious effect on your life and health. As such you must carefully choose who if anybody you allow to have influence on your feelings, thoughts and behavior. My advice is not to completely trust anyone; only trust yourself when it comes to your health! Help to self-help is, in my opinion, the only way to achieve a strong, positive self-image and self-esteem, and it is the foundation for happiness, health and success.

You cannot learn how to lose weight and stay slim from an overweight person. A heavy smoker cannot tell you how to quit. A loser cannot teach you how to become successful. To fashion a long life with health, energy, strength and vitality, you must find your way by searching, trying and making your own mistakes then growing as a result of those mistakes. Mistakes allow you to learn and grow, as they provide the foundation for future successes.

Use your knowledge and experience to lay a strong and stable foundation for your future. A skyscraper is only secure if the foundation is sound which is why two thirds of the concrete is in the foundation.

Never build your future and success on the backs of other people or luck! Build on yourself because you can only create a successful future if you enjoy a good feeling of self-confidence and a strong positive self-image.

Work on problem solving so that you will better handle problems as they arise. This experience will provide invaluable life lessons, more energy and better health.

Stress is often the determining factor of a heart attack, a stroke or suicide. Stress affects your health, and it makes you feel miserable and dejected. Do not avoid, ignore or deny stress, rather turn it into healthy energy.

Stress can be your emotional and physiological reaction to change. All things are completely neutral, until we give it our personal positive or negative meaning that causes our emotional, mental and/or physiological behavior.

Enjoy change because change means growth and growth provides the wisdom of life.

By expecting and preparing for change, you control your life.

## Deadly Compromises

Everybody strives deep down for independence and freedom; in fact, in the Western World freedom is considered one of the mankind's most valuable possessions, which is why the moment you compromise, or act in a way other than what you consider the right thing, you get yourself into trouble.

If you compromise, but the decision is made of your own free will, it will not harm your health. For instance, let's say you decide to work an hour longer every day, so that you will get a four or five day weekend at the end of the month. This will not affect your health. However, a compromise is deadly if you constantly are forced to repress your negative feelings and ideas in order to get along with another person. It is also deadly, if you have to force yourself to behave in specific ways and make decisions that you do not agree with because you are being controlled by an individual. The reason these are deadly compromises is because they can affect your energy level, your health and the longevity of your life if it continues over time.

Compromises destroy self-esteem, self-confidence and eventually people's health. A deadly compromise is a decision that you not only consider to be wrong, but you also know it is bad as it is an action that contradicts your ethical and moral values.

*Exercise:*

*Clearly define and outline the areas in your life, in which you feel very uncomfortable. Why are you uncomfortable and what are you doing in these situations? How would you like to behave in these situations to feel comfortable in the future? Everybody should be happy with their behavior; therefore, it is important to live by our own rules and values because only we know what we can and cannot accept about ourselves.*

What is right for one person may be totally wrong for another, and what someone else thinks is wrong or even impossible may actually be right for you. If you continuously suppress your moral and ethical values to please others, you will never be happy or satisfied, nor will you stay healthy or successful. You can only be successful if your goals correspond with your personality.

People cannot change their true personality and character, although they can change their attitude and behavior, but the core of a person is inborn and unchangeable. Certain characteristics will never change, but this does not mean that behavior cannot change and improve.

## The Physiology of Strength

Have you ever noticed that when you are in a stressful situation your muscle tense up, your breath is shortened and your movements are rigid? This is because your nervous system is signaling danger and sending stress hormones with negative messages to the body so that you lose some control over your behavior and sensations.

When dealing with a stressful situation, it is important to hold yourself up high to stimulate your brain in a positive way.

Take deep slow breaths and focus on your goal looking straight ahead not down at the floor. If you do this, you will simultaneously feel stronger, more confident and behave accordingly.

In fact, you will behave as you feel and not the other way around. In the past, everybody thought that it was the other way around, but now we know that it is a cybernetic loop as we respond physiologically to our emotional awareness, meaning that our behavior comes from our feelings of frustration, depression and fear, or from our enthusiasm, determination, strength and energy. This is why you will discover that when you are in a positive situation and have achieved success, you act and speak enthusiastically because you feel it.

Another example would be if you find yourself on a difficult stressful telephone call, which requires your full attention, either stand up straight and walk around while talking/listening, or sit up straight, erect, under no circumstances slouch. Proceed with confidence, inhaling deeply and exhaling slowly incorporating your whole body; this alone has an immediate calming effect. Whether you are sitting or standing, maintain a position of being ready to jump into action with your head held high. On a side note, it is hard to feel down if you hold your head up high, simultaneously, it is almost impossible to feel depressed or down if you smile.

You can positively influence your health, energy and emotions in many ways if you are willing to exercise all your possibilities. Remember you feel as you act so carry yourself with confidence, strength, energy and vitality, and you will feel that way! By looking forward to your success and focusing on succeeding, your expectation will influence fifty percent of the remaining work, and more importantly you will have taken emotional and physical charge of your venture in a positive way.

It is important to note that you must never leave anything up to coincidence, luck or hope instead you must take charge and work towards your goal. You need to program the future according to your personal image and then go for it! If you look forward with passion and enthusiasm to the challenges of tomorrow, you will not only feel good when you succeed, but you will also feel good along the way. This is a great form of stress reduction. This is why you need to enjoy the present and cherish every accomplishment, every challenge that is overcome, every goal that is achieved, every step forward, in fact all the things that bring you closer to your ultimate goal. Find pleasure in your work, your actions and your solutions to your problems. Meet each day with enthusiasm and confidence believing in yourself and your abilities. Make a resolute decision that you are willing to do everything that needs to be done in order to achieve the desired result. Plan to always go the extra mile while being prepared to get up one more time, each time life throws you down, and remember to keep the motto "failure is not an option" as your number one resolution. The more you feel in control of your life, the lower your stress level will be.

Once you have decided that your goal is to have a long, healthy and successful future, the next question is how can you realize this result as quickly as possible? You need to set some minor goals that lead you in the direction of your main goal. You give your life direction by setting goals. When you have clearly defined goals, your fear of the future disappears along with any feelings of helplessness or worry of being manipulated by others. You provide meaning and direction to your life by setting your personal goals. In fact, by having personal goals, you keep yourself from expending unnecessary energy.

When you set a specific goal for yourself, like what you want to achieve in a meeting with a customer, be sure to incorporate how you will feel and behave, as well as the result you want to achieve. The developing and following action plans applies for all aspects of your life, as this is how you make your life your own.

***Never take an unnecessary risk, but always take necessary risks.***

## Back to Nature

Regeneration is extremely important so be sure to seek our activities that you enjoy that give you a feeling of well-being. Whatever you like to do be sure to find the time to do it whether horseback riding, walking your dog, seeing a movie, hiking, lying in the sun or whatever it is you like to do alone or with somebody you care about. Also listen to enjoyable music that makes you feel good because it is the good feelings that help you regenerate and increase your energy. If you can, watch comedies as laughter is the greatest way to generate good feelings! Nothing is a better stress reliever than doing things that you love with the people that you love.

*Exercise:*

*List the activities that make you feel especially good, and the places where you can relax and get regenerated.*

**Note**:   It is not the length of the regeneration time that makes a difference; it is the intensity and regularity of the occurrence. (**IBMS™** sessions offer in twenty minutes the most effective regeneration available!)

I developed systems for many corporations that address reconditioning overworked managers by teaching them to take effective breaks with specific exercises for regeneration several times a day. We do this by teaching the participants to withdraw into their ideal recreation place in the mind, so that they can regenerate themselves within minutes. Today many doctors, psychologists and dentists offices use my program.

## Exercises for Regeneration

It cannot be overstressed how important it is to learn to relax because otherwise you will wear down your energy;

therefore, I propose some of the following as some relaxation exercises that I feel have been the most effective:

*Exercise:*

*Lie down on your back and slowly start focusing on relaxing your feet, wiggle your toes and gently move your feet from right to left, now consciously relax your legs, first your calves then your knees and your thighs. Once that is done relax your lower body, your spine and your upper body, move your neck gently back and forth while relaxing your head, your face, your forehead, eyes and jaw. Move to relax your arms, starting with your fingers, your wrists, your lower arms, your elbows and the upper arms. Let your body go so that it feels heavy...., warm... Let the heat spread from your solar plexus (stomach) through your whole body.*

*Now breathe in 5 times concentrating on the left side of your lungs then breathe again 5 times this time feeling the air in your left shoulder, then again down into the left side of your abdomen. Repeat the same 10 breaths, this time incorporating for the first 5 breaths your left arm including the fingers of your left hand and the next 5 breaths incorporate your left leg, foot and toes. This entire exercise is for the left side only of your body.*

*Once the left side is completed, start the entire process over again this time doing the exact thing with the right side of your body. Once that process is finished, breathe deeply 6 times normally, then repeat the process from the beginning again this time concentrating on both sides of your body, including your abdomen, legs and fully expanded chest sending the air up to both shoulders, head, arms and fingers. Now exhale, imagining that you are exhaling from every area of your body.*

*After exhaling, now imagine inhaling a golden bright shiny light that fills your abdomen and spreads throughout your whole body. Imagine inhaling vitality, strength and energy. Let the golden bright shiny light be the symbol of all things that are good for you. Then exhale a dark grey cloud that symbolizes all your fears, worries, doubts and tension. You will notice that you feel lighter and freer every time you inhale the golden bright shiny light and exhale the dark grey cloud.*

*After this exercise, you will feel renewed! As another addendum, you can incorporate taking a mental vacation to your special place wherever you choose to go and then repeat the golden bright shiny light and dark grey cloud experience. The golden bright shiny light can also be a beam of light from the sky, showering you with energy and vitality while all the negativity in your life is washed away.*

*These exercises are very powerful because as you supply your mind with the symbols of relaxation, strength, health and vitality, your brain assists by stimulating the corresponding organs to revitalize your whole internal physical system.*

The **IBMS™** sessions take you through this exercise and more accompanied by special music for the best regeneration possible in twenty minutes.

Note:   For people who are very tense and/or suffer from cramps, these exercises are of great help because of the warmth that is sent and felt in the troubled areas.

**Dealing Effectively with Stress**

- Do you suffer from tense muscles in your back or neck?
- Do you have pain in your shoulders, stomach or intestines?
- Do you feel sick or nauseous at times?
- Do you lack concentration?
- Do you sometimes feel dizzy, weak or tense?

- Do you have difficulty breathing?
- Do you feel nervous, restless, aggressive, frustrated, depressed?
- Do you have clammy hands?
- Do you have sleep problems or sexual difficulties?

Many of us live with these symptoms compensating and hardly noticing them over time acting as though they are normal. This is not normal and can be remedied with stress reduction that targets the cause of the stress. The Wilkening Institute conducted a research study of 387 employees who were suffering from chronic stress symptoms to find the causes and solutions of their stress. The results were as follows:

They responded that their professional stress was caused by:
- ✓ *Time pressures*
- ✓ *Pressure to perform*
- ✓ *Professional conflicts*
- ✓ *Team pressures*

And their personal stress was caused by:
- ✓ *Unpaid bills*
- ✓ *The paper-boy did not deliver the paper*
- ✓ *One of their children refused to eat*
- ✓ *The cat ruined the sofa, etc.*

As you can see, it is often the accumulation of many little annoying things that cause stress.

Other causes that lead to chronic stress are:
- Fear of the future
- Fear of losing a job
- Overwork
- Too much responsibility or the responsibility in itself
- Competition
- Working with people you do not like

- Common insecurities

*Exercise:*

*List all the things that caused you stress over the last thirty days.*

Since most stress is caused by many little things, the way out of stress is also through little things. People often think that they do not have the time for working out or playing a sport, but in fact without knowing it the message they send their brain is that they do not have enough time for themselves. This is bad as it simultaneously sends the message that they are out of control. Spend time on finding solutions as this is the best way to avoid stress and preserve your feelings of being in control which will also provide you with the ability to make important necessary decisions.

**Stress and the Dangers of Stress**

When we experience positive stress, like the joy of reaching a goal, mastering a skill, getting a promotion, closing a deal, increasing our performance, etc., it contributes to the pleasure and enjoyment of our life, and simultaneously strengthens our immune system.

Distress always leads to feelings of fight or flight and results in our reacting somewhat beyond our control because these feelings originate in the part of our brain that takes over in life threatening situations with the sole purpose of surviving. When after a stressful situation we do not remember something that happened, it is because the brain was in the survival mode. In the past, if you found yourself in a similar situation, you probably could do nothing to change your reaction, but now recognizing what happens physiologically, if you experience a sudden feeling like you want to run away or to fight, look for the cause and get out of the way!

Once your body produces stress hormones, it is important to get rid of them so that they do not poison the body. It is, therefore, important to find an emotional and physical outlet. Some helpful physical outlets are sports, climbing stairs and deep breathing exercises. Emotionally, it is even more important that you either see the situation or the people who have angered you differently, in a comical way, so that they lose the negative power they have over you.

With regards to an individual who has caused you tremendous stress, it is important to be able to forgive. Although you do not have to become their friend, you must not allow negative or destructive feelings to control you as it will wear you down and ultimately zap you of energy. Some suggestions would be to write a letter about how you feel then burn it, don't send it, or you could talk to the person and tell them how you feel then forgive them. While you are at it, forgive yourself for all the thoughtless and harmful things you have done to others, so that you are free of guilt.

Psychologically speaking confession and forgiveness, as practiced in the community of the Catholic Church, provides tremendous release and, therefore, is a positive influence on stress release, but you can also achieve similar results by talking to friends, relatives or anybody you trust.

It is a statistical fact that women live longer than men! One reason is because women have a much easier time discussing their feelings and problems while men repress their feelings and problems - probably in line with the motto "Men don't cry or show their feelings." I personally feel that it is more "macho" to show your feelings than to slowly die every day by living by a credo that invariably results in being terminal.

It is also possible to be stressed by outside influences like heat and cold, or a poorly ventilated room lacking oxygen. Feelings of oppression, claustrophobia, combined with headaches and lack of concentration, tension and muscle spasms can be the result of being cooped up too long in a confined area, needless to say all of these have a deleterious effect on your health. In order to stress out their business associates, some negotiators would hold their meetings in confined, overheated and oxygen deprived rooms in order to speed up the closing of the negotiation in their favor.

**Observing the Symptoms**

Weakness, fatigue, exhaustion, lack of concentration, feeling frustrated and annoyed, and fight or flight responses are all symptoms of distress that could jeopardize your health. Anger, aggression and irritation are often the result of the fight reaction. The flight reaction manifests itself with a desire to avoid, isolation, avoiding having to make decisions, etc.

Basically healthy stress is as productive in our life as distress is destructive, so it is important to learn to intelligently and sensibly manage stressful situations. One thing to remember is that every situation in life is in fact neutral until we personally evaluate the matter, and consciously or unconsciously give it a positive or negative score.

Stress reactions produce stress hormones called cortisol, adrenaline and other accompanying components, which are the body's way of responding to a crisis situation by providing extra energy and capabilities. All the energy and strength produced is for sheer survival, as in the case of an auto accident. In fact, the survival part of the brain exclusively takes over to control our actions in crisis situations. Once the crisis is over without damage to our physical health, our body and mind usually return to their normal state - this is considered Type-A-Stress.

Type-B-Stress is the result of continuous, undefined anxiety, fear, worry, doubt, poor self-esteem and self-confidence, feelings of being at the mercy of others, of being helpless, manipulated or restricted. These emotions have no precise or identified cause so they cannot be avoided and are always present. This continuous invasion of distress destroys our health, because the factors that cause this stress are not restricted by time and cannot be overcome in one period of regeneration.

Over the course of my life, I have seen dramatic positive changes happen with people who were suffering terribly from ongoing stress and work "burnout" which was affecting their health. In one case, I forced a group of burnt-out managers to cut off their work, private life, in fact everything, by taking them to a remote and isolated rural place where they were forced to leave their phones and computers behind. I had them go horseback riding, fishing, and participate in barbecuing, playing team sports, enjoying nature and the companionship with friends. By forcing these stressed-out managers to switch off their worries, doubts and fears and live only in the present, after the first three days of regeneration, most of them did not want to go back to their regular lives. The first three days were extremely and often unbearably difficult as they fought every inch of letting go of their regular life. So that these managers did not simply return to their jobs repeating the same bad behavior, they were taught technical and social skills so that they would be better able to cope in their private and professional relationships. Dis-stress no longer threatens their health.

For a typical business manager who already suffers from serious stress and illness, the idea of relaxation, turning off the brain or regeneration is almost unrealistic or at the very least hard to imagine, particularly as they usually think that they have absolutely no time for themselves. However, in the same way that the health damage caused by stress is the result of an accumulation of many small negative things, so is the benefit of many small positive experiences as these will lead eventually to health.

The moral of these stories is that if you do not take the time for regeneration, relaxation and for some kind of balance in your life, the stress will eventually cause your body to use the little energy available to strictly survive, putting you in danger of possibly experiencing a heart attack, a stroke, stomach or intestinal ulcers, etc., but it does not need to happen! You have a choice; do not let your stress get so far that a physical collapse is not only imminent, but also unavoidable. The best way to avoid illness is preventive health, so follow all the suggestions, do the exercises and experience the **IBMS™** sessions.

## The Ability to Act Sensibly

In order to change the way you deal with stress, you must learn to identify and define "a stressful situation."

*Exercise:*

*Refer to your list of stressful situations in the past thirty days and identify the situation in which you remember getting a headache, tummy problems, cramps, or when you felt any physical manifestation whatsoever. These are the situations that clearly can be defined as the ones that lead to your stress, but now you can learn to deal with them more effectively.*

*Now write down how you could react in a better more sensible manner to these situations in the future.*

## Self-doubt as a Stress-factor

If you do not believe in yourself, your abilities and your future potential, it has a lasting deleterious effect and can be disastrous to your health. As a result, you must recognize and acknowledge that you are a terrific person, and then concentrate on using your unlimited potential.

If you find yourself believing that you will fail in a given endeavor, you might physically experience tension, poor circulation or breathing difficulties all resulting in a lack of energy. It is for this reason that you need to be aware that there is no such thing as failure, defeat or error. Everybody behaves at every stage in their life according to their knowledge, experience and potential, otherwise, they would do nothing at all. If you always try or do give your best, you can never blame yourself for the result as nobody can do or give more than give their very best.

If you produce a certain result, it is not a success or a failure, it is simply the result, whether you wanted that specific outcome or not. It is your personal evaluation that turns the situation or result into a positive or a negative. If things did not go the way you wanted them to go, do not consider them failures, mistakes or defeats, but see them instead as positive lessons enabling you to further develop. Experience is the foundation for success and for moving forward in every area of our life. If you do something that does not work, you have produced a result that teaches you how it does not work, and the result is that you have moved forward and become wiser. Now you know one more thing that you should not do to reach your desired result.

*Back to Edison who said after failing 10,000 times in his search to develop a light bulb, "I will succeed very soon." And when he was asked "Why?" he answered "I am running out of possibilities for failure." If you run out of possibilities for failure and keep on trying, you will without question inevitably produce success. Edison was also asked if he considered himself a failure after 10,000 attempts, but he replied "Why a failure, I now know 10,000 ways how not to make a light bulb." Experience leads to success, so see every outcome as a lesson, as a step on the ladder of success, so you can build your life according to your desires.*

**Exercise:**

*To develop unique self-esteem and self-confidence, you must first create a picture in your mind of the person you want to be including the corresponding intellectual conditioning.*

*One way to accomplish this is picture yourself on your ninetieth birthday. There are lots of people around you giving speeches in your honor, praising you for your life achievements, for who you were, who you have become, for what you did, what you have and the people who are your friends! Now write the speech you would like to hear when you are ninety years old, including all your credentials and qualifications. This is an easy way to quickly see and determine your true goals and who you want to be at the end of your life! This way you can set your goals in stages so that you can arrange to produce the desired results.*

## Needless Stress

Underlying chronic stresses are failed ambitions that were either too ambitious or lacking commitment, or mistaken following of rules made by other people which resulted in failures and disappointments. They cause the aforementioned catastrophic health problems. You should have big dreams, visions and goals, as big as possible, but your capabilities, abilities, performance and your time available, mean that the setting of goals should be realistic and feasible. Otherwise you will produce failures, keeping you from observing your schedule, thereby damaging your self-esteem. Setting a half hour to force a deal with a difficult customer, who usually needs three days to feel comfortable with a decision, can lead to unneeded pressure and stress. Remain realistic, but set your mind on the highest achievable goals.

## Stress as Healer and Stress as Destroyer

We recognize that there are two types of stress. Type A stress is the stress we experience in a crisis. It releases hormones and gives us the energy to cope with life threatening problems. Stress type B results from undefined or less palpable predicaments, like vague apprehension, worry, doubt, fear of the future, a feeling of overwork and helplessness, anger and hatred. This type of chronic stress cannot be removed while the causes and solutions are unknown. Therefore, it does long term harm. Be aware that a single cause can usually be overcome, but the coming together of many single factors causes exhaustion.

A panic reaction is a clear sign of excessive demands and strain that has exhausted a person's energy, so that he can no longer react positively to a stressful situation. This "explosion of release" can lead to total confusion and lack of control, even to undesired reactions.

Long-term stress factors could become a cause of illness. Stress leads to an accumulation and therefore, an elevated level of adrenaline, cortisol and other hormones.

Extreme levels of the above mentioned hormones lead to several illnesses and reactions, if they are present over an extended period.

Tears may appear in the arteries when the blood pressure is too high. This can lead to an elevated level of cortisone and a diminished blood flow, with the possibility of a stroke or a heart attack.

Adrenaline and noradrenaline take care of fat removal, which could deposit itself in the arteries. This, again, is an onslaught on the body caused by stress.

Changes in hormone levels, resulting from stress, can diminish the body's immune capacity, which can lead to other illnesses, even to cancer. We could say, the longer a stress situation lasts, the more dangerous it becomes.

**Don't just react**

The reduction of stress or the attempt to change negative stress into positive energy simply means that we have a positive response to demands, crisis and obligations as opposed to just a reaction. In therapy when we speak in the positive sense, we say that a patient "responds" to medicine. If we say that a patient "reacts" to medicine, it is usually meant in a negative way; the patient suffers from complications, i.e., an allergic reaction.

Do not just react to life, but respond. Accept what happens and make the most of it. Change your outlook, do not look at problems as difficulties, but as challenges and opportunities so that you can change, grow, learn and show your hidden talents. The way we look at things determines how we see something as a challenge. Do we see a catastrophe and react in panic, or can we see a challenge as an opportunity to grow and develop?

Focusing on success and a wonderful future gives us strength and energy. If we focus on failure, possible problems and defeat, stress makes us weak and incompetent. When it is dark behind and in front of you, look inward, look at your possibilities and hidden resources, and use them to lighten your future path. If you demand of yourself to look for answers and solutions and try to find them within, you will quickly decide that you have far more resources than you believed. See a crisis as an opportunity that offers many possibilities, which you should not hesitate to exploit.

Women usually live longer than men, while men learn from role-play and their upbringing to bottle things up. They have a tendency to swallow their worry, doubt, anger and fear. This leads often to the same type of explosion as a water kettle with a valve that is too tight. Women talk easier about their problems, their anger, about things that happened and get rid of their pent-up energy. Political prisoners and soldiers, who were able to talk about their horrible experiences, recovered faster from physical and emotional calamities than those who could not. The ones who talked lived longer and healthier lives.

Team play is for this reason an important foundation for health and success. Develop a social network, so that you always have enough friends, acquaintances, coworkers and family members to catch you when the bottom threatens to fall out from under you. Friends with whom you can laugh and friends with whom you can cry will have a beneficial influence on your health. Therefore, be a team player, be part of a team for balance and release.

I am not talking about whining and self-pity, or about psychoanalyzing your life to death. Just talk openly about what is bothering you and look together for solutions and ways to deal with what is wrong, and then let it go! This will offer release and help you.

The ability to ask others for help is an important facet of health and success. Nobody can climb the ladder of success by himself. "upwards together" should be your motto. There are no "self-made millionaires" because many people were on the team and contributed to this man's accomplishment. People who are afraid to offer or ask others for help will never become successful and reach their full potential.

You are not afraid to consult a physician and ask his help if you break your arm or have acute appendicitis. But people who suffer from an emotional or mental breakdown, have a crisis or other problems, are often unwilling to ask for help. But it should be just as natural to ask for emotional aid as it is to ask for physical help.

Get together with your team and use the wisdom, skills and talents of all the members by brainstorming their ideas; in this way, you can exploit everyone's talents in the best interest of all concerned.

## You Are Not Indispensable – You **Can** Take a Vacation!

During my work I have concluded while dealing with top managers from all over the world that every one of them considered himself indispensable to his company. Many of them oversaw the most absurd details themselves like the ordering of paper and office supplies. Never allow yourself to say, "If I can hang on just one more week," or "In three months then I will take my vacation." Some people even bring their work along with them on 'vacation.' These people consider themselves indispensable. They actually believe that in their absence everything will fall apart.

Avoid the thought that you are irreplaceable. Even if you can't leave completely, find time for regeneration, relaxation, hobbies and time to spend with your family. Please, believe me! Listen to your body, because illness is always a cry for help. If you refuse to pay attention, your body will assert itself more intensively. Remember, there is no illness without a cause, no symptoms without a shortage of energy. Keep this saying in your mind.

Please consider objectively how dangerous it is to keep pushing yourself while your body is crying out, and you yourself are suffering from overwork and discontent. Suddenly and unexpectedly, without being able to prepare, you could be torn from your work by an acute illness, stomach or intestinal ulcers, inflammation of the nerves, or even a heart attack or a stroke. If that happens, there will be no time for preparations, no time to train new people and no time to get the necessary items out of the way. You will be torn away from your work with many things left undone. You would determine neither the time nor the duration of your collapse, but this could really cause the failure of your business or your career. And this could happen because you were not willing to take the time, when needed, for regeneration, relaxation, compensation, hobbies, family, friends and the enjoyment of life. If you had acted wisely, you could have picked the time and duration yourself.

You can be certain that the body will take a rest when needed, whether you are willing to give it the rest it needs or not. So it is smarter to plan time for vacation and regeneration and really use them. Listen when your body cries for help; don't ignore the signals, but instead react intelligently.

We have the genetic potential to live a healthy, fit and vital life for 160 years. If you want to live this long, you must be conscious of your health and take measures to achieve and maintain good health, right now, not when it is too late and you are forced by ill health, disability and bodily limitations.
It depends on you; the fate of every area of your life lies in your own hands. This includes the very most important sector, your health. As each year goes by, you lose some of the potential to live 160 years because of poor breathing, poor

nutrition, poor exercise or lack of it and also by a poor emotional state or negative mental attitude. It is not too late to start over.

## The Danger of One-sidedness

Life is characterized by diversity. To achieve and sustain optimum results, we need comparable diversity in our life. We can create this by bringing balance into our life. You cannot just live for your job, nor for your private life, nor for your children, or even recklessly for yourself. You must strike a balance between hobby, family, work, recreation, regeneration and pleasure which helps to give your life an integrated, successful, and fulfilled quality. A one-sided burden brings imbalance to life, no matter in what area of your life, and always leads to wear and tear, stress, tension, deterioration, monotony, apathy, frustration and depression.

For instance, make sure that you do not just take care of your own retirement, but also of the retirement of your employees. Take care that there are challenges and interesting possibilities for all. In this way, you and your fellow workers will remain flexible, active and curious; you will all enjoy your work much more when there are new challenges, progress towards your goals and good results. Mental and physical exercises are a requirement for vitality and contentment in life.

## Needless Worries and Fear Take Your Energy

You have no influence at all on the development of the world economy, or on the collapse of large companies or banks and even less on tomorrow's weather. It is therefore completely absurd to fear, stew, or worry over things you can't do a thing about.

Do not waste your energy on fear. Concentrate on the best way to improve your personal and professional situation. Do not concentrate on what others are doing or on those who may be your competition, or are in the same line of business.

Remember that you are unique in the universe and can therefore produce unique results. Focus only on your results and performance, while keeping your goals clearly in front of your eyes.

Life is characterized by diversity! To conceive the ability and achieve and sustain optimum results, we need comparable diversity in our life which can be created through balance. In other words, you cannot just live for your job, your private life, your children, not even recklessly for yourself. You must strike a balance between fun, family, work, regeneration and happiness to give your life an integrated, successful quality. Too much of one thing, no matter in what area of your life, always leads to wear and tear, stress, tension, deterioration, monotony, apathy, frustration and/or depression.

## Burnout Can Happen In Work or Relationships

Constant strain from doubt in yourself and your abilities leads to the so-called burnout syndrome. Burnout leads to a feeling of being burned up, empty, weak and helpless. Burnout often results when people with low self-esteem, low self-confidence and a negative image of themselves try to overcome what they perceive as deficit, weaknesses or shortcomings. Those people spend more time at work because they believe that they can overcome quality with quantity. This is, of course, never the case.

Another cause for burnout is that they do not have sufficient self-esteem, self-confidence and discipline, and therefore do not live according to their own values, rules and principles but follow the views of others. They try to realize unfamiliar goals, which are not their own and which do not give them a feeling of accomplishment, even if they realize them. These people do not receive any feedback, have no sense of contentment, but are left with a feeling of emptiness and burnout. They often are missing the strength to say "no."

Only when you set your own goals and work on the realization of your own dreams will you have a feeling of accomplishment. A feeling of accomplishment will give you strength and increase your self-confidence and self-esteem as a generous return for the work and effort you put in.

However, doing work that makes no sense either because it has nothing to do with your goals, or is against your ethical and moral values, can leave you feeling empty and completely exhausted, even when you complete it successfully. No one who leads a life full of compromise can be healthy or even stay healthy if he does things or is forced to do things that are against his moral and ethical values.

It is the same with people who feel forced to stay in a catastrophic marriage. They stay because they fear other people's gossip, because there are children involved or because they are in business together. Those people are destroyed by compromise. Whenever you do something you absolutely do not want to do, you risk your health. Long-term demanding compromises kill people in the truest sense of the word. They are in my opinion, the main causes of serious illness, even cancer.

Our body speaks in a symbolic language. In my observation: women who suffer over a long period from relationship problems are inclined to suffer from illnesses of the reproductive organs. Women who have many problems with their offspring or who cannot give birth often get breast cancer when the conflicts last a long time. People who are in situations they can literally not digest suffer frequently from stomach and intestinal problems.

You cause your own tension and stress because it is not what happens in your life that causes the stress, but your reaction to what happens. It is therefore important that you program your behavior. Only then can you be sure of not becoming overwhelmed by difficult situations. Prepare yourself so that you are ready to act correctly when you are facing a dispute or attack. Picture the desired outcome and the best behavior in your mind.

## How to Create a Strong Immune System

You can resist illness and stress successfully only when you are in top shape, and you are working efficiently on the realization of your dreams. Your body is the foundation for the fulfillment of your goals and it presupposes a mentally, emotionally and physiologically healthy mind.

Today we have unambiguous scientific proof of the necessary steps, which can be summarized in the four following requirements:

- Regular and sensible exercise
- Good nutrition
- Restful sleep and relaxation breaks
- Independence and freedom from addictions

Real health is based on constant improvement. Health and vitality cannot be achieved with a quick fix, like "You can be slim in seven days," "Lose ten pounds on the ten-day super diet," or similar and often dangerous nonsense. Our attitude, our philosophy of life, is the blueprint for our health. We have to decide on a path that enables us to realize our dreams.

The foundation for success is accepting our weaknesses and doing what we think is right. Too many people ignore the signals their body sends. They get more and more accustomed to the limitations and restrictions they accept as part of life. Examples include regular use of alcohol, over eating, irregular sleep, nicotine, too much coffee, as well as pain and lack of energy.

I am no advocate for a hundred percent vegetarian diet or any other one-sided approach to life. I know very well as a researcher in health issues that a healthy person can drink a cup of coffee each day or a bottle of wine now and then. But when somebody consistently eats unhealthful foods, or frequently overeats, the wine and coffee do have a significant effect.

I would like to point out that every form of extremism is fundamentally wrong. Extremists are hysterical people, who suffer from a mental problem. Extremism is not a natural phenomenon; it is abnormal and undesirable behavior. Life and quality of life is made up of many combined but separate factors. Life is not black or white, it is not even gray, rather it consists of as many as ten million different shades of color that we can use to shape more colorful and beautiful lives.

## Regular Sensible Exercise

Please remember that our body starts breaking down, in the true sense of the word, by the age of twenty-eight. We can do nothing to stop or slow down this process without putting in more effort than before. One-third of our population suffers a heart attack that could have easily been avoided simply by being active in sports before the age of sixty. Problems with joints or the spinal column can also be avoided when they are caused by lack of movement or are due to geriatric problems.

If you are in poor condition you have to struggle and work harder. The circulation, detoxification, energy and oxygen supply will become insufficient, and you will lack energy. Muscles shrivel when they are not used. This diminishes the blood circulation and they will waste even more energy through lack of oxygen. You have less chance to heal when you are hurt or ill and the time needed for restoration becomes considerably longer. You become more susceptible to infections, feel weak and start acting listlessly. Degenerative illnesses will certainly follow.

Physical activity is the most effective way to reduce anger, strain and stress. Several years ago we introduced a 'Go-program' with regular light activity, four times a day, for top-managers and other leaders to help them to reduce tension and conserve energy.

If you have not been physically active for a long time, start small and build up slowly. Regularity leads to success, it won't happen in one peak all-out performance. Do your exercises in a natural manner. Twenty minutes of exercise a day is sufficient, thirty minutes a day is good and sixty minutes is excellent.

**The Basics of Good Nutrition**

Another essential point is nutrition - a delicate subject that we must discuss intensively. I would like to provide a general summary of the essential basic ideas:

*Your nutrition represents the building blocks essential for the renewal of your cells. Ninety-eight percent of our cells are totally and completely renewed within the short time-span of eleven months. Our body forms those cells with building materials found in what we eat during that time. If you offer your body inferior material (nutrition) for the building of the cells then your body can only make inferior cells and the health of your cells determines the health of your complete body.*

Please learn to eat when you are hungry. That means you only eat when you are truly hungry and not out of habit or emotional need. Do not eat uncontrollably, especially, do not eat when your body does not give signs of hunger. Don't eat everything on your plate just to be polite. Always eat when you are hungry, but eat healthful "living" food, such as fruit, vegetables, and salad and then only as long as you are hungry. Do not eat at prescribed times because your body will find its own rhythm, independent of the hunger of others, or times set by convention. Hunger is a very dangerous and tension producing need. Absolutely do not starve yourself, no matter what 'they' are telling you today. Hunger emits stress hormones, cramps and discomfort. Long-term diets that leave you hungry all the time can lead to chronic stress with catastrophic results.

Hunger and diets can lead to a deficiency of iron, stress, a deficiency of vitamin C and calcium and of many other electrolytes. Hunger is responsible for iron deficiency. But eating too much or bad food is just as bad. Tension and hunger, alcohol and coffee can lead to arterioscleroses, problems with circulation, increased production of insulin, and a serious deficiency of *calcium*. Nicotine destroys oxygen and diminishes the content of oxygen in the bloodstream. Oxygen is of course necessary to supply the energy for all forms of life in our body.

Take care you supply your body with a balanced amount of vitamins and minerals with fruit juices, fruit and vegetables. Drink, when possible, water or natural fruit drinks because nothing is better for your health or against thirst. Avoid mineral water because the minerals cannot be absorbed or digested by the body and tax your energy supply. Carbonated drinks have, moreover, a corroding effect on the kidneys.

## The Importance of Restful Sleep

Sleep is important for restoration, relaxation, health and the ability to work. Certain elements our body needs to live and survive are only produced during sleep; one of them is serotonin, a substance of the utmost importance for our existence.

During sleep it is important that every ninety minutes your body is in the REM-phase, because only in this phase can we receive optimal regeneration. Only when we follow this normal cycle is restoration possible. Alcohol, for instance, disrupts the brain's regularity and therefore the rhythm of sleep, which is absolutely necessary for our health. Sleeping tablets lose their efficiency after about two weeks, and then we usually sleep worse than before. If you suffer from poor sleep you should change your way of life and improve your diet so that you can sleep well without sleeping pills.

Sleep reduces tension. If we do not sleep well because of stress we increase our stress. Try to break up this deadly cycle by accepting and solving your problems. Enjoyable music, sounds of nature, beautiful forest scenery, the sound of a rushing stream, mental training and our **IBMS™** programs can help you in the conditioning of a healthy sleep.

Even when you cannot sleep well you should stay in bed with your eyes closed so that your body can at least have the opportunity to relax and restore.

Dr. Leonard Coldwell

Remark: The body can only heal itself during sleep or very deep relaxation.

**Freedom of Addiction**

The freedom from addiction is not just important for our health, but also for our self-esteem and self-image. Even reducing one simple addiction, like the addiction to coffee, restores our ability to deal better with stress. Coffee destroys several minerals, calcium among them. Besides leaching the calcium from the bone, caffeine dehydrates our body of water. For each cup of coffee, it takes two 8 oz. glasses of water to restore hydration. Coffee gives us a quick shot of energy then we plunge deeper than before. Try herbal teas or hot lemonade.

Use of alcohol, nicotine and pills to solve our problems can be deadly in the truest sense of the word. Denial of addiction is the addict's main problem that makes a solution of the problem impossible. If you do not believe that you have a problem you can't and won't work on solving the problem.

Smokers insist all too often that they could easily quit, but just don't want to. Alcoholics often assert that they do not drink regularly or all that much, just now and then, or not at all.

*Exercise:*

*Keep track of your drinking or smoking, note how much alcohol or how many cigarettes you use every day or week, and how much coffee you drink. Write everything down for at least a week and add it all up so it will really grab your attention.*

You can only get rid of an addiction by changing your self-image. This means that you can no longer see yourself as somebody who smokes, is overweight, drinks alcohol or swallows pills. You have to see yourself as a free, healthy and vital person. There are several ways to achieve this. It is possible by consciously changing your self-image, by using principles of pain and joy or with the **IBMS**™ of conscious mental programming and conditioning.

Ask yourself whether the way you live reflects the image of the way your life could be, or should be. Do not get into extremes; strike a balance instead. If you, for instance, came home late from a party last night where you ate and drank too much, give your body at least fourteen days to restore itself before you indulge in a similar bash.

Good living means striking a balance. If a party adds to your "quality of life," do go and enjoy it. But remember what the eating and drinking does to you and your body and give your body sufficient time to recover.

If you practice the four following aspects together in a balanced manner, you should be healthy. Do not overdo any one aspect, rather live with balanced regularity. It makes all the difference.

**Remember:**
- Regular, sensible exercise
- Good nutritional habits
- Wholesome sleep and stress reduction sessions
- Independence and freedom from addictions

**Start Tomorrow in a New Way
and Give it One Hundred Percent**

When you get up tomorrow, clap your hands and shout, "Yes!" Stretch and reach up high. Pace to the bathroom, look yourself in the eyes and say: "This is my day and I will use it well." You will find that in this way you give yourself more time for working and solving problems. You give yourself not thirty or forty, but 100 percent of your capacity for work because you do not need two hours just for waking up and getting started.

Start your day healthfully, with fresh pressed orange juice and a fruit salad. Give your body the necessary energy to get started. Support your body mentally, emotionally and physically by building self-esteem and self-confidence regularly with positive, goal directed self-communication. Say to yourself before you tackle a problem, "I can do it! I can fix that." When others try to dissuade you with negative opinions: "That is not possible! You cannot do that!" Respond with the **IBMS™** formula: Everything is possible! And use the appropriate **IBMS™** session, **www.instinctbasedmedicine. com**

Nothing has happened, no invention, not one great change for mankind, from which people did not say that it could not be done. It was so with the airplane, electric lighting, batteries, the gramophone, the rocket to the moon and many other inventions. If it has to be done, and no one has yet achieved it or succeeded in doing it, then you are the person to do it.

**A special tip: I recommend starting the morning with fresh pressed carrot-celery juice on your empty stomach! It may not taste all that good, but it is excellent to detoxify your body and it will give you lots of energy.**

*The best way to avoid stress is to develop the knowledge that you are in control of your body.*

### Humor versus Stress

Someone who relishes being alive and enjoys his work stimulates his mind positively and reaches an anabolic state. Stress, on the other hand, produces a catabolic state; it produces destructive, immune suppressing hormones.

A good example of the effectiveness of humor is a story of the recuperation of Norman Cousins. In his book *Anatomy of an Illness*, the then very ill actor, who suffered from cancer, writes how he literally laughed himself healthy by using comedy videos and tapes.

Laughter has an even greater influence on the immune system if you can combine it with physical activities. Use humor for your own benefit and that of others. It will strengthen your own immune system and theirs. A friendly smile generates warmth, openness and confers energy. Negative humor (irony or sarcasm) destroys team play and effectiveness. It leads to disharmony, competition and isolation. A feeling of helplessness, an inability to work and illness are often the result.

But humor should never be at the cost of others. It is important that you can laugh about yourself and make yourself the butt of a joke. Humor reduces stress for all concerned, especially in tense situations. Don't take life too seriously otherwise it is like becoming blind from staring through a tube at the picture at the end.

*Communication combined with laughter helps us to relax and solve problems. A nine-year old girl in a psychiatric hospital in New York, who had not actively participated in anything for one-and-a half years, started to participate within twelve minutes with the help of a professional clown. She called out his name and her behavior was, after only two hours, completely as that of a normal child. In the same hospital a depressed seventy-two-year old man threatened to kill himself by refusing to eat. Thanks to the help of the same clown the man was discharged and pronounced healthy in two weeks.*

Think about people who make you feel good, because they make you laugh. Those people can see the irony in problems and in life itself, and they can certainly laugh at themselves. Consider how you can bring more joy in your life. Surround yourself with witty, positive people. Ask yourself what you can change in your life and how you can add some humor. Learn to look at life with more joy and optimism and try to live that way.

**We should know the following:**
- If you have to eat meat, eat it in combination with salads and vegetables, not with potatoes, pasta or rice.

- If you eat potatoes, pasta or rice, eat those also with vegetables and salad.
- Fruit should really only be eaten in the morning on an empty stomach because fruit begins to ferment immediately if it is consumed in combination with other food. Poisonous gasses emerge causing flatulence, discomfort, cramps and tiredness.
- Fruit eaten as dessert burdens the digestion. Start the morning with fruit, so that the body, which has fasted during the night, can process the fruit that is rich in fruit sugar, vitamins and liquids, all great for energy.
- When possible drink freshly juiced fruit and/or vegetable juices and lots of non carbonated water, because the gas can affect the function of the kidneys. The minerals in mineral water cannot be absorbed by the body.
- Research in nutrition has proven years ago that milk products (all dairy) are not suitable for human consumption. If a child suffers regularly from mucus and has difficulty breathing, or already in the morning frequently suffers from a stomachache, feels bloated, has a headache or diarrhea, or allergies, I would dare say that this child had milk with breakfast.

Milk in the acid environment of the stomach coagulates and curdles just like the milk in tea to which you have added some lemon. This glutinous, clotted mass is hard to digest; it moreover contains casein, an enzyme that the body cannot process. Casein clogs the capillaries which are needed for the transport of nutrition and oxygen. Milk may also carry minute leftovers of bacteria and antibiotics which were given to the cows. And we are all, no doubt, familiar with the consequences resulting from regular administration of antibiotics. See www.notmilk.com

- Because our body consist mostly of water, it is very important for our organs that we drink plenty of water and that our food is rich in liquids. The liquids absorb the toxins and remove them. This is only possible from drinking lots of water and with nutrition (juicing) that is rich in vitamins, minerals and enzymes. If you change to a diet rich in liquid, you should have, after fourteen days, a younger skin, a more beautiful complexion and an abundance of energy.
- Please be aware that one-sided diets are dangerous for your health. If you have already tried several "weight loss" diets, you have probably found that shortly afterwards you were even heavier than before. The body reacts to the diet by storing the food for your protection/survival, in preparation of your next fast. You lose, moreover, mostly water in quick weight loss diets, thereby damaging the heart and muscles. You can only become and stay slim with plenty of movement, healthy nutrition, correct breathing and by making this a part of a basic lifestyle. Every fantastic diet that promises miracles is no long-term panacea.
- Counting calories does not work either. Take for snacks only some nuts, seeds; eat fruit only until noon. You can eat as much and any fruit you like without gaining weight. Fruit leaves the stomach in twenty minutes, only bananas take about thirty-five. After that you can eat anything without the risk of causing heartburn. If you want to experiment and find out how easily this happens, just eat one or two apples after a normal lunch. During the rest of the day, you will enjoy the miseries of flatulence and gas.
- Make your coffee or tea, if possible, with well or spring water and avoid tap water that contains chlorine and other dangerous chemicals. *Fluori*de

*is a cancer causing radical.* Fluoride is a waste product in the production of aluminum; it is poisonous and was once used as rat killer. When I was living in California, there was at on time a warning on TV announcing, "Please do not use tap water for your aquarium in the next three days as it could kill your fish."

***You have the right to be happy healthy and successful!***

**Living Without Guilt**

You came in this world with a strong and incredible need for further development, for growth and for the use and expansion of your human skills and talents. Therefore, you not only have the right, but also the duty to shape your life the way you see fit so that it agrees with your own needs, wishes and dreams. Don't let anybody take it away from you!

However, many people do not believe that they have the right to do everything necessary to be happy, content, healthy and successful in every area of their life. This was already drummed into them in their earliest childhood. Ignorant religious teaching often causes a lot of misunderstanding. The waiting rooms of psychoanalysts and psychiatrists are filled with people who suffer from guilt feelings caused by the preaching of others.

It makes absolutely no sense to live in humility with guilt feelings; such an existence is not natural. Rather every human being has the right to be happy, successful, healthy and content. Everyone has the right to regularly do those things that give him joy and allow him to be joyful.

**Internal Signals**

You know of course that pain and small irritations in our body indicate that something is not quite right. They are warning signals of our subconscious to let us know that we are doing something wrong. There are of course several ways to deal with a conflict situation. You can look for a quick fix and swallow a few pills. You can fool yourself and look for reasons why it cannot be serious. Or you can get a book that offers quick and easy answers, like a vitamin cure or some other program.

Many so-called health programs are responsible for the complete destruction of many people's health, because they promote a one-sided approach or element to take care of our health. Important information is neglected, relevant signals overlooked or put aside and the necessary steps are never taken.

We will not become healthy simply by spending a lot of time doing a certain sport or by regularly exercising too much. This will necessarily lead to negative stress and the body will react when it feels threatened. The body can be, for instance, overloaded by jogging that is too intensive because with overloading we produce too many stress hormones. By hiding behind a fitness program and overlooking the necessity of putting the same effort in our emotional fitness, and by not paying attention to stages of regeneration, we often bring about a catastrophe.

The assumption that good nutrition can prevent illness is also basically wrong, because no single discipline can keep us healthy. Several factors play an integral part in our effort to become and stay healthy. Remember lack of energy is the only cause for illness.

Someone who pushes aside his needs and feelings unavoidably ruins his health. We all know that we cannot keep our automobile engine in third gear, and that we must regularly replace the spark plugs and oil to keep our car on the road. So, why do we not do the same for our bodies?

If we want to stay healthy, a necessary requirement for achieving success and attaining a good quality of life, we must pay attention to the signals in our subconscious, to stomach aches or headaches and intestinal troubles. We must explore the causes that made us sick and change our behavior.

Dr. Leonard Coldwell

## Egotism

Egotism is good. Because egotism is nothing but a component of self-preservation, without it humanity would have died out long ago. But I want to make it clear that I do not mean inconsiderate behavior, rather I mean that everybody must realize that the most important person in his life is he. He must either suffer the pain he brings to himself or is caused by others, or he can enjoy every victory he has won. The enjoyment will bring happiness and the suffering must be overcome. Egotism does not mean recklessness, ignorance or aggression against the feeling of others.

People who do not concern themselves with a good quality of life do not deserve your attention or assistance. You will be happy, content and healthy only when you live in accordance with your own personality with your needs and desires, as only then can you achieve success in every area of your life. To realize the success you are dreaming about, you must pay attention to your own intuition, listen to your feelings and needs. Do not chase the directions others give you, because you will run the risk that, although successful, you may become unhappy, lonely or ill because you did not realize your own goals, but those of someone else.

A father, for example, can force his son to realize the dreams he did not realize himself although the interests, talents and skills of the son point into a totally different direction. In this way, we breed failures and losers because we rob people of their own personality, their wishes and dreams and we replace those with alien pursuits. These people live alienated from their own personality and will be in emotional or physical stress.

But egotism plays another important role. You must be aware that you are the center of our own life because only then will you build up enough energy and strength to play positive roles in the life of others. If you exhaust yourself, become weak and ill, you will not be able to help and improve the life of others. You cannot pull somebody from a swamp by jumping in; rather you need to stand on a solid foundation to pull him out of a morass. Become a self-sufficient person with good self-esteem and self-confidence; be financially and emotionally independent. If you are emotionally and physically robust, you can start to help other people, those who are important to you and have the same dreams. The only true help is self-help, helping others to take responsibility, helping them to help themselves.

If you really want to help your spouse, your daughter or son to change their lives by helping them to improve it, then it is absolutely necessary that you are strong, self-confident, healthy, and successful.

Learn to take yourself seriously and grow into a mature strong person so that you can have confidence in yourself and will be able to define and work on the realization of your feelings, needs, and dreams.

*And never forget, you are born to be successful!*

**Pay Attention to What you Let Enter into your Mind.**

Once you acknowledge that it is you who determines how you feel and how you act and that you are responsible for long term success in your life, a great new world with adventures and escapades will be open to you. You will recognize that you can turn your life into a masterpiece, an answer to your dreams, and that you can reach unbelievable heights. Remember that all people who made great inventions for improvement in the world were originally ridiculed. Not until after their breakthrough were they applauded.

Even though many people are afraid of change and therefore fight innovators, inventors, and people who rock the boat, do not let them change your mind. Many people are even unwilling to accept positive changes if they are tied to large emotional of physical expenditures. Therefore, do not be concerned what others consider right or wrong for you, because you are the only one who knows what makes you happy, content, healthy and successful. Conditions such as happiness, satisfaction, peace and love are emotional conditions, they are feelings, and how you reach those feelings nobody knows but you. So you have to create those feelings in accordance with your own rules and values.

I want to warn you against a serious danger that is standing between you and success. They are the energy robbers. Those people who with a negative attitude and by continuously questioning your success, ideas or possibilities, try to divert you from action and drain you of your strength and energy. Just as you must be aware of the thoughts that engage you and of the thoughts that enter your mind, you must pay attention to the people that surround you and the influences that touch you.

**An Overall View of Basic Elements**

Your behavior is determined by your self-esteem and the way you see yourself. Therefore, you must let go of negative experiences in your life because they will otherwise influence your self-esteem and as a result your future negatively. Thanks to experience, knowledge and development, you are a new person every day. You are no longer the person you were fifteen years ago when you made your past mistakes and experienced certain failures. You can therefore let go of those situations and people with ease.

Too many people give up because they keep looking at the past and cannot see that life is different. But it should not be that way. Problems and challenges can help you to a higher level in life. See problems as an opportunity to grow and tackle old problems in a different way. Walking away or denying problems increases the tension and can lead to chronic stress. Consider yourself the actor and producer of the film "That is my life," not just as the actor. Write the script, be the director and don't be a marionette at the mercy of someone else's wishes. Don't dance to somebody else's tunes.

Let go of the past and do not fear the future, for you can only live for today. You must, of course, determine your own future, goals and behavior.

Sensible time management is an essential fundamental element of stress reduction or prevention.

Pursue active stress reduction with regular regeneration sessions (preferably IBMS™) to reduce stress, exercise and engage in positively changing your mental dialogue.

Focus on solutions, not on problems. Many people see life as an obstacle course and are their own greatest obstacles.

Do not let others stand in your way of success; you are the only one who can stop them. Not until you say, "It is over," is it indeed over.

Always remain flexible and creative, and always live in the present. Avoid chronic stress by avoiding living in the past and the future.

Only three percent of our fears become reality, an even smaller percentage is catastrophic.

Avoid people who drain your energy, and search for people with whom you can build up effective team play.

A smile is worth a thousand words! Shatter loneliness with friendliness with a smile. Be interested, encouraging and caring in your relations with others; communicate and motivate yourself and others by saying, "You can do it if you want."

Health is an integrated factor, which cannot be isolated. The freedom of dependence or compromise is just as important as it is to live by your own values and goals.

Taking risks offers you the opportunity to use your talents more effectively than before. The premises in which you find yourself can also lead to stress, for instance you might be too warm, too cold, too loud or lacking in oxygen. Find out what causes you stress, then change it.

Avoid being pressed for time; instead plan your time realistically. Also don't let others put you under time pressures that you cannot handle. This can have catastrophic consequences leading to stress and it can affect your behavior.

# Dr. Leonard Coldwell

You alone can turn you into the healthy, successful and dynamic leader you are meant to be. Do not rely on others, on fate or luck, but take full responsibility and control of your health and future yourself.

# Section II - Chapter 5

## A Long Life in Excellent Physical and Mental Health

### Health Starts in your Mind

Almost every physiological illness originates in our behavior, based on a poor value system or on emotional situations we can't control. Many sick people know that this is so, but instead of concentrating on the cause of the illness and planning some changes in behavior, they fight the symptoms with all means and measures and are surprised that this does not work very well in the long run. We can of course raise the objection here that wrong physiological behavior, poor nutrition, and incorrect breathing can also lead to illness. That is relative, because incorrect breathing and bad nutrition result from bad emotional behavior. And those who protest that viruses or bacteria cause illnesses are also partially right because people who have a high energy level are immune against infections.

A person who, instead of working on solutions, focuses his attention completely on the problems in his life, will soon find himself short of energy. This will remind him that he needs more energy, so that he may have enough energy for good emotional and physical health. If we do not make the effort and examine the causes that ruin our health, and if we furthermore try to cover the symptoms with medication, as we frequently were taught, we behave like someone who pushes the splinter deeper in his finger and covers it with a band-aid and takes a pill against the pain. This does not solve the problem, but just the opposite; things will get worse, until the situation becomes unbearable.

If we want to banish a problem forever, we must tackle it by taking it by the root. This includes the recognition that ultimately we are the ones who are responsible for our health. We have the responsibility, whether we like it or not. The more we withdraw from this responsibility and control of our health, the more obvious the symptoms become. They will force us ultimately to act, if we don't, they will destroy us!

As I keep repeating, practical experience taught me not to count on help from outside. The only real help is self-help. The only one, who can truly help a sick person, is the patient. Advice for the very best nutrition, correct breathing, and other essential components of a long healthy life are of course very important, but if a person is not willing to take responsibility and do everything necessary to take charge of his health and the quality of his life, then he will not enjoy excellent health.

I am convinced that there is a solution for every problem and an answer to every question. We must just be willing to accept all challenges consciously and do everything necessary to realize the desired result. This includes, above everything, our health. The power of the mind is limitless. We must start to believe in ourselves, so that we activate and use the limitless strength of our subconscious. In that way, we can reach everything we want.

I want to point out that a trusted and experienced physician should be regularly consulted if you are ill; he should offer guidance and help you along the way.

**The Neuro-physiology of Health
– Conclusive Action Summary**

**What is the use of all your success,
if you are ill or die early?**

We all know examples of people who go through life as if they were chased by an unseen force; they run anxiously through life, from one job to the next. They have no time for themselves, their family, their friends or hobbies. By the age of 35 and up, they enjoy great recognition, they are highly respected, have accumulated great wealth and enjoy social and professional recognition, but at age forty or forty-five they suffer a heart attack or stroke and end up in a wheelchair, or suffer from some other limitations.

If we observe those negative examples, we realize that it is completely nonsense that we try and overcome every job with force, perseverance and self-discipline, thereby completely neglecting our needs and ourselves. Many people work without ever enjoying the results of their labor. Scientific research shows that twenty percent of all people suffer serious health problems resulting from work, because they could not deal with professional stress; seven percent died of the illness.

The same research showed that another seven percent did just the opposite. They are successful, healthy, vital and fit; they enjoy excellent relationships, their family functions very well, they have good friends, pleasant hobbies and enjoy a wonderful quality of life. Those seven percent belong in the same category as the seven percent who were destroyed by their work. I keep asking myself what the difference could be between the positive seven percent and the negative seven percent. The results point, in my opinion, to the attitude of each person, whether they see life as problems or as challenges.

**Create your own Success**

To model, therefore to mold our pattern of behavior, our belief system and thought patterns, is a natural way of learning to live. We are trained by imitating emotional and physiological behavior. People acquire a belief system, a value system, and inner convictions from their parents, grandparents, teachers, ministers and friends. This includes their gestures, mimicry, physiological and emotional behavior as well as their approach to health. They either teach us to satisfy our needs and enjoy times for regeneration or they may teach us to live our lives with old wife tales and ignorance. All this behavior is taught, they are acquired patterns of behavior.

*If a parent smokes, for instance, the chance that a child will smoke is about sixty-five to seventy percent. If one of the parents is an alcoholic, there is a fifty percent chance that a child will become an alcoholic, if both parents are alcoholics, the probability becomes seventy-five percent. Seventy percent of all children live a life as fit, or unfit, as their parents. They either take regular care of their health, or they completely neglect the care for their physical needs. We must absolutely eliminate poor behavior patterns and learn to live with the changes.*

I have become successful in my work by studying and modeling my life after that of healthy, vital, successful people, people who have succeeded in creating solid relationships and maintained these over a long period of time, people who were very successful in every area of life and who were brimming with health and vitality. You must, just so, learn to understand the patterns of behavior, belief systems and thought patterns of your colleagues, friends and others around you and pattern your own life accordingly. You will save yourself many disappointments, time and strength because you can learn from the successful concepts of others. From the way they deal with stress and take care of their health, you will find it easier to reach your goals.

## Basic Elements for a Wonderful Quality of Life

Self-confidence is an essential aspect of health, because the more you accept yourself, the more gratified you are, the better you will like yourself and the readier you will be to do something for your body, your health and vitality. You will gladly make the effort. We must learn to recognize and view problems as challenges. We must use them as opportunities, so that we can grow and develop and not run the risk that we push them aside. We must force ourselves to persevere, to make our own decisions and set our own goals. To persevere so that we can fulfill our dreams is one of the most important decisions we can make in our lives. If we are willing to pay the price of success and are not willing to succumb, we will succeed in reaching our goal, no matter what happens.

*Even F.D.R., who was chained to a wheelchair, realized his dream to become president of the United States.*

Therefore, we must take charge of our lives by setting ourselves long and short-term goals. We must accept that life will hand us many challenges and that we will have to face a lot of interference on our way to a wonderful life. We must learn to see ourselves as the ocean waves, the waves of life, not the victims of waves.

## The Danger of Emotional Conflicts

To repeat one more time, neuro-chemical changes will take place in our body if we are exposed to real danger, for instance, an automobile accident. These chemical changes protect us by putting more energy at our disposal; they may also prepare the body for the possible loss of blood, etc. All this energy is focused on overcoming the momentary crisis physiologically. When the crisis has passed, all our bodily functions will return to normal.

It is nevertheless very dangerous to dwell on fears and conflicts that are not yet real. We weaken our body, mind and energy capacity without being able to change our emotional outlook. Our bodies will keep running overtime in a dis-stress situation and suffer damage. If this artificial dis-stress situation is repeated, we introduce permanent negative physiological changes. If the crisis does not end, the body will never return to its normal condition and migraines, backaches and even a heart attack can be the result.

The seven percent of the people who are in excellent health do not suffer less stress than you or I; rather, they have learned to cope with stress. They know how to deal with the stressful situations in their life. An unhealthy life that lacks a clear value system, a life in which a person merely tries to survive by paying his bills and living from day-to-day instead of building financial independence he can enjoy, is a miserable preprogrammed life without a healthy self-image.

We must learn to take life a little easier. We have all experienced a situation which looked threatening one day, and then looked totally different after a good night's sleep, so much so that we could hardly believe our worries of the day before. A good relationship with our partner is just as important as excellent nutrition, regular sleep, physical and emotional fitness and a regular medical checkup. We must learn to take care of our health, nurse an illness and not go back to work until we are completely healthy. There is no advantage in trying to function with a weak body and insufficient energy. We enjoy few benefits if we lose time by repeated relapse.

## Dealing Well with Fear

We must learn to recognize fear for what it is, a warning signal to protect us. Fear can protect us in life threatening danger. We must learn to accept fear as a friend and helper, and we must learn to control our fears and not let fears control us. If you are faced with fear, first examine whether your fear is real. Question if this is real anxiety, if is it justified, and if so, why the need for protection? Is your safety in jeopardy? If you have identified the fear and you feel it is justified, focus on finding an effective solution for the problem. Do not spend more than twenty percent of your energy on identifying your fear, rather spend eighty percent on developing ways to cope and deal with the situation. The stressful situation and the threat to your mind will only disappear when you remove the dangerous situation.

People in Asia say that you must enter in the heart of your fear before you can conquer the distress. If you really face the conflict zone, you will come to the conclusion that your fear is resolved. But you must also learn to take calculated risks, because no life comes with a safety guarantee. For further development and satisfaction of your needs you must always be willing to take some calculated risks.

It is just as important to have phases of regeneration in which you give your mind and body the opportunity to restore themselves. Your energy capacity is like a battery and functions when it is regularly charged. Therefore, you must not space your phases of regeneration too far apart, you must keep your energy fully charged, just like your car.

Accept the challenges in life so that you develop your mind. Continued growth and development are the greatest stress relievers. Our self-confidence, self-esteem and self-image will increase as a result, which will help us to deal better with critical life situations.

## The Foundation for Top Performance

Strong self-esteem and self-confidence are important aspects of a good quality of life. The way we see ourselves, our self-image, and the way we view who we are and what we can achieve, determines our behavior in every area of life. And our self-awareness is the product of our experience, the result of our day-to-day behavior. Our opportunities and skills are formed by the way others see us, just as we see the success in the lives of people with whom we associate, and which inspires and helps us to believe that we can also achieve prosperity. We build in this manner a self-image that corresponds with our ability to achieve.

If we see a colleague cope calmly and efficiently with a hectic and demanding daily schedule, it opens for us to the possibility to react and behave in the same unruffled manner.

Dr. Leonard Coldwell

Our self-confidence and belief in our ability to achieve is also influenced and strengthened by the encouragement, confidence and support of others. People, who believe in us and encourage us, who recognize our abilities, values and intelligence, strengthen our self-confidence. People, who are confident that we can attain a high quality of life, will sustain our efforts with positive suggestions; this again will improve our self-image.

Other important elements in the building of a healthy self-image are physical reactions. When we hurt, are worn out and have no energy, we become convinced that we cannot do our work a hundred percent. We may believe that we cannot trust ourselves, because we cannot trust our bodies. Our emotional and physical development can, therefore, have a negative influence on the results we produce.

**To summarize:**
- To build a positive self-image, one that focuses on positive self-suggestions, you must concentrate on your success. This does not mean that you should ignore your failures and weaknesses, you must define and eliminate them. It means that you should weigh your actions and results with a problem solving orientation, so that you program a strong and positive self-image.
- Learn to see failures as challenges, as opportunities and possibilities for growth, see them simply as educational material you need to mature, a passing phase in your thought processes.
- Concentrate on examples of those people, who act and react in a way as you would like to live your life, so that you furnish your subconscious with the information that allows this type of action, reaction and the production of positive results.
- The subconscious is willing to fulfill every emotionally charged message it does not consider absurd or unrealistic. We, therefore, need the

references that we receive from examples we follow, biographies we can read and by observation and through confirmation in our communication with other people.

- Focus your attention foremost on the people, who possess the skills, talents and results you would like to have in your life.

- Surround yourself with positive people, because their immediate surroundings are a constant reminder and help us to continuously program our subconscious. When I speak of positive people, I do not mean the dreamers who float through life with a mysterious smile, rather I speak of those people who concentrate on solutions and look for answers. I think of those people, who take control of their lives and determine and shape their destinations.

- Avoid the energy robbers, I mean those people who always look at the dark side, who never take charge, and therefore cannot realize their dreams, wishes, needs and goals.

- Surround yourself only with people you enjoy, people you trust and who let you be the person you want to be.

- Never fear the future, because we know that from the 100s or even 1,000s of fears we regularly have, only a very few become reality, and those only in a much milder form.

- You will have very little influence over several future events in your life; therefore, prepare yourself for eventual crisis or difficult situations. You cannot do much else. Let the situation you fear go until the problem becomes acute, or until an explanation is warranted.

- Do not worry about illness, old age or other such uncontrollable fears because on the one hand you will program permanent images in your mind related to those fears, and on the other hand you waste so much of your energy that you will be in a permanent dis-stress situation. The quality of your life will be seriously diminished by the life-threatening emotional situation you fabricated in your mind.

- Look forward to the future because now you have been taught that you can take control of your own life. The future can only bring you that which you programmed and allowed into your life.

**Architect Not Victim**

Learn to see the future as architect, not as victim. With self-confidence, your health will grow, and when you are in good health, your strength and courage will increase and, as a result, you will get a better self-image. Your profession, the way you feel about your job, plays an integral part in the state of your health. Therefore, please do the following:

*Exercise:*

- *Define exactly and in the minutest detail what you want to do and achieve in your profession.*
- *Define your future health. How fit do you want to be, how do you want to look, how much do you want to weigh? Etc.*
- *Define exactly what professional success means to you and what you hope to achieve.*
- *Define the success you desire and how you expect to reach this height?*

**Learned Limitations**

Negative programming starts in our earliest childhood with expressions such as "We do not do such things," "That's not right," "You will never be able to do that," which are impressed into our minds. To become aware of the learned behavior that limits our life, the programming that diminishes the quality of our life and our potential to succeed, answer the following questions as accurately and as completely as you can. If you later remember something you forgot, please add it to your journal.

*Exercise:*
- *What are the limitations you were taught? What are the dreams you relinquished, because somebody told you that they were beyond your limits?*
- *What behavior and which aspirations did you never even try to realize, because you were negatively programmed that you either could not do or should not do so, because it was plain foolish or just too difficult?*
- *How did your parents, teachers, priests, nannies and others hurt your self-image and discourage you from making full use of your possibilities and talents?*
- *Which dreams slipped through your fingers?*
- *If you followed your instinct and emotions, which talents, skills, and possibilities would you say you have?*

*Please, write one more time exactly every single fact of your ideal self-image and think about who you really are. Because we come here to the most true statement: You do not know a person by the way he behaves and by the achievements you see at this point in time, but we know a man by his wishes, dreams and goals, by his needs and by the person he would like to be with all his heart.*

*You must now develop a plan of action for every goal, a step by step plan for the realization of every detail you wrote down. Please do not limit yourself, nor go overboard, and pay attention if you recognize something in your subconscious as unrealistic or absurd.*

You can reach everything in which you really believe, even if you think that it does not seem quite realistic. Therefore, do not let your rational thinking determine your needs, wishes, goals and dreams, rather let your emotions and feelings decide what you can or cannot do.

*Write down clearly, one more time in detail, which human qualities you want to possess, produce and have as a part of your life.*

## Living without Fear

As I have previously stated, in my opinion, there is nothing to fear, but fear. When we learn to cope with fear, we will conclude that we can influence every area of our life, no matter the circumstances or the obstacles. Remember, it is not "what" happens in our life, but "how" we react to what happens that determines our future. The more often we see a crisis situation as an assignment, and the quicker we work toward a solution, the stronger our self-image will become as we deal skillfully with the situation. If we do not recognize a stress situation, we must cope with the crisis while we are unprepared and will often lack the needed energy to do so.

By facing a crisis situation goal-and-solution oriented, we prepare the resources in our subconscious, so that we act skillfully in difficult life situations and will be conditioned to act without shrinking back or with self-pity. The lives of other people are not easier than ours, no matter what we like to believe. They just have learned to cope more effectively, when they face difficulties. We cannot always influence difficult situations in life, but we can decide what to do and where we want to be. We can decide how we want to use our skills and talents and which self-image we want to create of ourselves.

*Exercise:*
- *Please, define your worst fears and anxieties.*
- *Write down exactly why you are afraid.*

- *What is the dumbest thing that could happen in this situation you fear?*
- *What do you expect to happen if the worst came about?*
- *What would be the best way to avoid or prepare for this situation?*

To remove a fear you must study the situation thoroughly and act solution oriented. The surest way to remove fears effectively is a solution oriented confrontation. As soon as we learn to accept the crisis in our lives as challenges and turn them into opportunities, our lives will change.

*A person who loses hope in a crisis situation is lost. They cannot focus, nor do they see a way out. Medical research has clearly shown that people who receive a negative diagnosis of a serious or chronic illness immediately lose all defense mechanisms and their immune system plummets, if they lose hope. These people often die without a reason. Successful results in all areas of life depend entirely on a person's attitude and way of life.*

**Exercise:**

*Successful results depend on a person's own outlook and way of life. The more resources you have at your disposal, the less stress you will suffer. Therefore, I want you to list here all those situations in which you feel stressed, nervous, over burdened, overworked or tense. After you compose a detailed list, write down clearly how you could improve your reaction in the future.*

*Let this desired reaction enter your mind and run this script over and over in a positive manner, as though it were really happening. To program this desired reaction mentally, you must run this at least twenty-one times through your mind, so that you will automatically see and live this pattern of behavior. Create in this way a positive self-image and resource program, so that your mind will no longer react with stress when you face a difficult situation, because you will have enough resources to react in a positive way.*

Have a good look at people who conquer crisis situations that could have played a negative role in their lives. Find out, if possible, how those people think and react, what their thought processes are and why they act the way they do. Try to install their thought process in your own mind. Form as many reference possibilities as you can.

When you have completed and programmed a mental program that is conflict-and-problem solving oriented, give it some serious thought and write down the benefits you and the people who are important to you, are reaping from the changes in your behavior. Do not forget that you have overcome crisis before in your life.

*Write down the crisis and problems you have faced and the difficulties you have overcome.*

**Your Personal Responsibility**

Motivation and willingness are the "secrets" of success and health. You must decide and prepare to accept the responsibility by giving the time and paying the price necessary to achieve the desired success.

I am the last person to tell you that life is fair and good. That is certainly not so. Life is neutral; it is neither for nor against you. You will run into just as many positive as negative situations. Life is neither fair nor just. Your destiny is the result of your mental and physiological behavior. We can say that our future will yield the fruit of the mental and physiological behavior of yesterday and today; our life is nothing, but the reflection of all our thoughts and behavior. If you do not let a willingness to fail enter your mind, if you do not even consider this possibility, you will be guaranteed of success.

No matter what happens, you are the only person you must deal with for the rest of your life. You cannot turn in your body like you can your car or sometimes even your spouse. You are the person, who has to live for the rest of your life with your body, your personality and what you made of it, whether you like it or not. You must therefore determine who you want to be, what you want to achieve and what you will allow in your life.

Accept the responsibility and the control over every area of your life consciously, whether it is an assignment or a decision. Escape leads to stress; because the task is never accomplished you keep yourself in a stress situation, which may have disastrous results.

## Emotional and Physical Fitness

Body and spirit work together through a cybernetic cohesion, what affects one touches the other. It is not possible to work on emotional health and neglect the physical. You must work on both simultaneously, a physical fitness program and **IBMS™** sessions (for your emotional health) so that you install an excellent emotional fitness program that includes physical health, fitness and energy. Don't forget to include a proper nutritional diet, with breathing exercises for effective oxygen flow. And most importantly, pay attention to your body's warning signals the aches, pains, restrictions, etc. You must remove the source before we suffer lasting and irreversible damage.

# Section II - Chapter 6

## *Introduction to the Concept of Health*

### The Cause of every Illness

The only cause for any kind of illness is a breakdown of energy. The most damaging energy depletion in our lives comes from emotional and mental stress. The second is nutritional deficiencies, lack of exercise and oxygen. Third are physical, environmental or daily life stresses, but these are the least harmful of the three stresses.

*The first question we should ask ourselves when we get sick is, "Why did this happen?"*

If our bodies were functioning properly before we got sick, then what happened to change things? The only reason for being sick is a lack of energy; therefore, it makes sense that all we have to do is figure out what caused the lack of energy in the first place.

Stress is the main cause of lack of energy because of the stress hormones that our bodies release. These hormones trigger fight or flight responses, which put an incredible strain on our nervous system and energy level because in normal life situations, we can neither fight nor can we run! What this means is that since we cannot use the stress hormones up, they poison our system. When fight or flight hormones are released into the body, it gets a short boost of energy, but the resulting effect is that the body is drained of energy, and the immune system's ability to respond is seriously compromised.

So when we get sick, we need to figure out what emotions, such as conflict, compromise, doubt, constant worry, fear, etc. are having a deleterious effect on our health. What emotional stress is causing this drain of energy? Are we living in a relationship that we cannot take or are we living a life situation that we cannot digest? Are we afraid of the future, are we feeling helpless or hopeless? These are just some of the many questions you must ask yourself to identify the cause of your problem.

**Three Deadly Mistakes**

Many people are deluded by three misconceptions that keep them from recognizing when their health has begun to take a turn for the worse. These misconceptions cloud over the obvious signs of deteriorating health and when looked at in that light, they can be seen as some of the primary reasons for increasingly bad health in our society today.

**The first misconception: To be healthy, you only need to exercise.**

*It is a fallacy to think that simply by exercising you are and will stay healthy. Physically fit people are not necessarily healthy people. This is clearly evident from the stories we have all heard regarding some great athletes or top performers who suddenly die at the peak of their careers. Many people personally know of a fit person who was jogging or exercising and suddenly dropped dead of a heart attack.*

*There are many components to complete holistic health, of which healthy exercise is only one component. This is an important part of staying healthy, but studies have shown that a negative attitude towards work has much more of a negative impact on our health than the positive effect of working out. Excessive workouts without any thought given towards holistic health can also have a very negative impact on one's health.*

**The second misconception: Nutrition solves every problem.**

*It is a misnomer that nutrition alone is responsible for our health. While nutrition is extremely important to our overall health, it is only one of the many components necessary for a completely healthy body. Experts, such as the best selling author professor Bernhard Siegel, of Yale University, and the well-known cancer specialist Dr. Carl Simonton believe that a person's psychological attitude has between twelve to fifteen times more influence on the incident of a heart attack than nutrition does.*

**The third misconception: Avoiding stress leads to good health.**

*This is a dangerous fallacy which can lead to laziness and inactivity. Research now shows the importance of stress in human survival. Humans could not survive without stress, but there is good stress and bad stress. As such, in the same way that there needs to be a balance between exertion and regeneration, there needs to be a balance between stress and relaxation.*

*Your body is like a car, you need to take care of it. You could have the greatest car in the world, but if you do not put gas in it, the car will not run. If you do not put oil in the motor, the engine will burn out. If you run the car continuously in the red zone, it will eventually self destruct and die. Your body is the same in that it needs exercise, nutrition, and frequent stress reduction in order to stay healthy.*

*There needs to be a balance between the intake and the use of energy, between nutrition and expenditure, between effectiveness and duration.*

Remark: Most people remark after using the twenty-minute **IBMS™** sessions once a day that their energy level and overall health dramatically improves.

## Lack of Energy and the Consequences

Lack of energy and lack of oxygen lead to cell weakness. Basically the higher the stress level, the greater the lack of energy which results in a high level of dead or atrophied cells throughout the body. If your immune system is too weak to get rid of the dead, atrophied or mutated cells, they can accumulate and become toxic causing acidosis or toxemia in the system, with the possible result of cancer or tumors. Cells only mutate and die when there is a lack of nutrients, energy or oxygen; the result can lead to cancer and life threatening disease. This environment does not just cause the major development of free radicals, but it also prohibits the development of new healthy cells.

*Remember that, basically, no cell in your body lives longer than eleven months. Nearly seven billion liver cells renew every second. Every six weeks you get a new liver, every eight weeks new kidneys and eight months new lungs, every four weeks new skin, every second 4,000 red blood cells are renewed in the living body.*

**Other than some cells in the bone, teeth and brain, no cell in your body is older than eleven months.** But the new cells need the best building material and optimum environment possible to be strong and healthy cells – they need good nutrition, water and enough oxygen!

What this means is that even if you are sick today, yoı not have to remain sick forever. If you have a liver prob you can fix it with proper nutrition and healthy behavior because basically, a lack of energy is the only cause of illness. The mutation of cells is caused by lack of energy and if you will remember, emotional and mental stress is the main cause for lack of energy. Diet and behavior of course also play a major role in your health development.

Physical stress is not as serious and can be repaired with a good night's sleep, eating the right foods, drinking plenty of clean pure drinking water, getting the right kinds and amounts of exercise, etc. It is the ongoing emotional and mental stresses, and the resulting internal stress that causes disease and threatens our life.

**Stress in and of itself is not really the problem. The problem is ongoing or accumulating stress.** Compare it to rubbing your hand on the edge of a table - if you rub the table for a minute nothing will happen, if you rub your hand on the table for an hour, it may begin to hurt, and if you rub the table for five hours, your hand could be seriously hurt. If you were to rub the table for ten hours, your hand could be permanently damaged.

Now if instead you rub the table and take a break every so often to regenerate and heal, you could keep rubbing the table for the rest of your life this way without any damage. You need to handle your stress in the same way. Whenever you get or produce too much pressure and stress in your life, you need to regenerate. If you overwork, party too much, or indulge in excessive drinking, smoking or overeating, you need to basically give yourself twelve to twenty-one days to recover by eating, resting and exercising properly, just to get back to normal.

I have learned that to live in any form of extreme whether with dieting, over exercising or depriving yourself of things that you love, the end result will only lead to unhappiness and lack of energy.

If you are eating in an unhealthy way today, then for the next two days you must watch what you eat. Everybody needs to drink at least ten glasses of water a day, which helps to cleanse the body of toxins and avoid dehydration. Again, any kind of carbonation is not good as it can damage your kidneys. Carbonation is what we exhale, why would you want to take it back into your body?

If possible, you should always try to drink spring water and not tap water. If your job or your relationship is killing you, you need to change them. Find a new job, work on your relationship or find a new partner that makes you happy. If you find that you have to compromise yourself to the point that you give up who you are and what you stand for, then you need to change your work or change your relationship or you will get sick.

I believe that you can get to a point where if a relationship doesn't work, it doesn't work, and to think that a marriage counselor will fix it, is – dumb! If the people involved can't fix it then someone else definitely can't fix it either. In my experience, more people develop cancer and die because of living in bad relationships than from any other cause.

**One of the main causes of cancer in both men and women is the emotional stress caused by unhealthy relationships.** "If the key doesn't fit in the hole, it never will!" And eventually from trying to make it fit, the key or the lock will break! It is the same with a relationship. It probably is neither person's fault, but if you have to forfeit who you are and what you stand for to make a relationship work, it is not worth it and more importantly, you may die from it. To stay in a destructive relationship because of religious beliefs, or because of what the relatives or neighbors will say, or because of the children, or because of fear of loneliness is, figuratively speaking, suicide.

I have heard many times people say that you have to make compromises in order for a relationship to work, but this is wrong. If you have to change who you are or compromise what you stand for to make a relationship work in the first place, then it is wrong.

Children are better off and have a better chance of growing up with a strong foundation when there is one emotionally healthy parent than they would with two unhappy and unhealthy parents. I am not referring to occasional disagreements; I mean continuously arguing over major differences.

You should stay away from mood altering drugs as they can only harm you and worse than that, they can never fix the cause of the problem in the first place. Most mood swings generally can be alleviated with proper nutrition, more energy, water, self-esteem and healthy relationships. Most importantly, you need to find and address the cause of the problem.

If you are being treated with psychiatric care, you should consult your doctor about whether or not you really need the drugs and ask if perhaps there might be a better more natural solution available. There are in fact only a small percentage of people that actually suffer from a genetic physical neuro-chemical imbalance and really need medication.

Menopausal problems can often be helped without major drugs because they are usually caused by the body's rejection of the aging process. Unplanned pregnancies can also cause similar mental and emotional problems. If you just deal with the problem using natural therapies for six months, you will find relief. The University of Utah conducted a study where they were able to naturally relieve with a simple natural supplement, the mood swings of PMS, menopause and other related problems. (For more information please visit the websites:

www.drleonardcoldwell.com or
www.instinctbasedmedicine.com

My advice is nobody should live the way other people want, tell them to, or expect them to live. You must live for yourself because you are the only person who has to live with you twenty-four hours a day, seven days a week, 365 days a year for the rest of your life, and you are the only person who has to live with all the consequences of your actions. Even if people mean well, they don't know what is right for you.

Very often the people proffering advice on how to live or fix your life are the very people whose own lives are such a mess that you would not trade places with them for anything. You are the only person that can instinctively feel/know what is right for you.

*Get educated, but not manipulated!*

**I am absolutely convinced that nature has a cure for every kind of health challenge.** Most psychological and emotional conflicts can be easily solved with hope, goals for an exciting future, positive action, love, self love and self esteem!

People must learn to live with the realities of life, not in a dream world or in denial. Learn to take life by the horns and steer it in the direction you want it to go.

## The Foundation of Health

To take care of your body in the way that it deserves, you must first appreciate that it is a "marvel" of nature.

Here are two facts; there is no other person like you in the entire universe and the mathematical chance that there will ever be or ever was a person exactly like you is one in fifty billion. In addition, your body continuously regenerates, detoxifies, recovers and builds year after year, so that you have the greatest possibilities in life. However, if you do not provide your body with what it needs to recover, like the proper nutrition, rest and exercise, it cannot function successfully.

It is all up to you! You decide whether or not you will enjoy the fruits of your life's labor by staying healthy and growing old comfortably. If you do not consciously decide to be healthy, you will almost certainly sooner or later have to deal with medical problems. Every kind of illness is a result of conscious or unconscious decisions that we make over the course of our lives.

*There are no incurable diseases, only incurable people who are not willing to eliminate the cause of their illness.*

Usually, there is never just one cause, one mistake or one factor that is responsible for medical problems. To seriously damage your health, you must abuse your body over a long time, like smoking, heavy drinking, lack or rest and sleep, dehydration or bad nutrition. In the end, however, it is not simply one bad habit that leads to disaster, it is a combination of many things working together that bring about that end. We can only achieve and maintain complete health if we address and include all aspects of our life.

I am going to presume that you, the reader, are "a mover and a shaker" who wants learn from evaluating and implementing the information that I provide, so that you can actually use it in your life to become and stay healthy.

I believe that you are a doer, not simply an evaluator as evaluators are notorious procrastinators. Evaluators tend to judge before they know or try something new. Their insecurity confines them from experimenting with the new and unusual because they emotionally cannot deal with change, a new way of thinking, new technology and new information.

In order to blind themselves to their shortsightedness, evaluators and procrastinators often fight and obstruct with vigor anything that is a change. As such they can only be viewed as losers, but they also obstruct progress. Evaluators are the people, who, when offered a new food, refuse to try it simply because they don't like the color or the way it looks. Evaluators talk about life, but they do not live life! They usually see themselves as realists, but in reality they are nothing more than pessimists in disguise.

*Life is great and exciting if you expect the best outcome - then you will have the best result. That is realistic! Embrace every change or challenge as an adventure, a chance to prove to yourself how capable your really are!*

## What is Health?

**"Health is the optimum function of all biological systems!"**

Health is not a product of luck or coincidence, but the logical result of correct physical, emotional and mental behavior. Health is based on an optimum conservation and use of energy. With an adequate amount of energy, it is impossible to become ill, get the flu or the common cold. Have you ever seen a fully energized excited person with a positive attitude and optimism getting a cold or the flu?

We know from modern medical research that we only become ill when our body has insufficient energy. Illness is due to lack of energy caused by stress factors, bad nutrition, dehydration and lack of oxygen, and incorrect or lack of movement.

Many of my patients who had only a few months to live according to medical specialists, completely recovered. They are the proof of the body's unbelievable healing power, and they are the hope for all those who have seemingly incurable diseases. It has been my observation that one of the primary reasons that people with incurable diseases die is that they have no more goals, wishes or dreams; they no longer have a wish to live as life seems pointless.

*Every doctor knows about cases of spontaneous healings. These occur when the biological energy suddenly gets fully activated. Very often when hope, new goals, reasons or positive changes happen, people's health tends to get better.*

Of course, we can blame our environment, circumstances, other people or whatever for our sickness, but it changes nothing. You are the only one who can change yourself. When you believe in yourself and work with the **IBMS**™ and the information in this book, you will make yourself healthy. What do you have to lose?

Remark: There is nothing like false hope! No matter what - with any kind of hope, people do more, act and their quality of life improves, and they have a better chance of getting better than without hope!

## Health – Your Second Chance – a Fresh Start

You have the chance to get a start fresh by getting your health in order, living better and more successfully going forward in life. As soon as you master the basic health components like breathing, exercise, nutrition, and emotional and mental attitude, you will change your health for the better.

Fear of illness or being afraid to die are serious stress factors. From reading this book, you will understand that you can take charge of your health so that these types of fears can disappear. *That relieves you of a tremendous amount of stress.*

Illness is not caused by faith, genes or bad luck, it is caused by unhealthy behavior!

Ultimately you must change your attitude toward your health. You must see your body as an important instrument necessary for the realization of your talents, the fulfillment of your life. Health, youthfulness, and success are totally interdependent on your attitude.

First, we must discard our social conditioning and learn to take responsibility for our health, instead of giving it to a physician. A doctor or therapist can and should only be a coach, a helper or a guide to **help you to heal yourself.**

*There is no healing force outside the body! No medication or doctor can heal you, only your body can!*

We live with the widespread belief that there is no cure for many diseases. If a person is diagnosed with cancer, they automatically are terrified and often lose hope. Experts have shown that our immune system is drastically lowered the moment we hear a diagnosis of terminal cancer, or AIDS, and this is exactly when we need it the most to be strong. In fact, the immune system sort of stops working because of the preconditioned belief that there is no cure, help or hope for these illnesses.

Our conditioning triggers visions of death and destruction, which we simultaneously transfer to ourselves, causing lethargy, frustration, depression, helplessness and fear. This is crucial because at this time, we need the exact opposite, we need hope, optimism and confidence and the possibility to build up our energy in order to get healthy.

**I maintain that there are no terminal illnesses. For every recorded terminal illness there are cases of people, who survived the illness.** So this means that if just one person overcame a specific illness, it is not incurable or terminal.

There is living proof in the cancer and AIDS patients, who overcame their illness and survived. People's survival depends on who they want to emulate – the people who got better or those that died.

**Analogy**: *If you are in a legal battle and your lawyer tells you that you are going to lose then you need to change lawyers. The same is true if your doctor tells you there is no hope, you are going to die because you have an incurable disease, then change doctors. It is your life and health, and if what you are doing now does not lead you to the right results, you need to look for another way, find another doctor.*

Only when you allow for the possibility of surviving a terminal illness in your mind, will you then have a chance of surviving it. Your belief system and behavior determine the outcome. As soon as you allow in your mind the possibility of health, you provide the probability of attaining it. There is much evidence for this and there are many books on the subject that I recommend like Norman Cousins' autobiography or books by Bernie Siegel or Dr. Carl Simonton.

It is important that you make the effort to talk with people who have survived a death threatening diagnosis and that you surround yourself with supporters, people who believe in your

411

recovery and will help you to get better. Stay away from the pessimists! Besides you have everything to gain and nothing to lose by doing this.

People are generally willing to do everything possible to help people that are close to them. Consider what you would do if your spouse or your child or your best friend suffered from a life threatening illness. Would you just resign yourself to the sentence or would you do everything possible to find a solution? This effort that you would be willing to make for others is what we should also demand of ourselves.

The question is, "What works and what has helped others?" In the same way that it wouldn't make sense to ask a clinically obese person how to lose weight and stay slim, you do not want to ask somebody who has never been sick what to do! You do not ask a person who has been divorced five times, is lonely and alone, what his /her secrets for a happy marriage are.

You also would not ask a parent, who has not seen their children for several years because of an estrangement, how to bring up children properly. We need to learn from people who have already succeeded; no matter what their background or education, it is only the results that count! Look only for results, theories don't work! If a therapist, technique or person produces results, go with it and forget the hypothetical theories.

**The No Medicine Approach to Medicine**

*Dr. Isaac Jennings practiced medicine for fifteen years in the 1800s in the orthodox manner. Then he began a twenty-year study in which he gave patients with every kind of illness either sugar tablets or colored water as their therapy. He carefully documented every case and discovered that in twenty years he had greater success, sometimes twice as great as other physicians who administered the orthodox treatment.*

*Dr. Jennings documented his discoveries in the book "The No Medicine Approach to Medicine" in order to assist his colleagues with this valuable information concerning the activation of self-healing as a result of the placebo effect. However, he was sued and his work was discredited.*

In many instances, the main problem is not simply changing the belief system of the patient, but rather changing the mind set of the physician. I have personally encountered several instances when after the disappearance of a tumor, sometimes the size of a large fist, the doctor managed to persuade the patient to have an operation so that he, the doctor could see whether the tumor was really gone.

Many of the so-called miracles resulting from pilgrimages are the result of people believing so strongly in the cures and miraculous healing they want to occur. Their wish to be healed was already programmed in their mind and it became a reality for them by the time they arrived at the "Center of Miracles." It is important for me to talk about these issues to shake your beliefs so that you do not carry bias with you on your new path. It is important to form your own opinions and not be influenced by your environment.

To prevent any misunderstanding, I need to emphasize that it is imperative to seek the diagnosis and care of an accredited physician if you are sick. You need to work together on your healing - the physician as your coach and you as an informed self-healer.

***You are the only one who has to live with the consequences or mistakes that you or your doctor makes not your doctor.***

You should always be totally informed about your treatment so it is important to ask all the relevant questions. You should know and understand the inherent risks, why this particular treatment versus another and what it will do and will not do. You need to become an expert on your own health. **In the end, it is your body that has to heal itself.**

Dr. Ellis Huber, M.D., the President of the Medical Society of Berlin, Germany, writes in his books *Participation instead of Swallowing* and *Love instead of Valium* about the connection between physiological and mental shortcomings, and the genesis of chronic illness. This recognition is also gaining strength in classical medicine.

While I have already made the statement that all forms of extremism are wrong, I do make some extreme statements to demonstrate the full spectrum of possibilities. In this way, you have the opportunity to find what is right for you some where between.

In order for you to form your own opinion and develop your own personal concept for your ideal health, I want to recommend that you follow the suggestions in this book religiously for at least twenty-one days.

Many of our beliefs are formed from incorrect facts, which can have a negative influence on our health like:

- "Breakfast is the most important meal of the day."
- "People who do a lot of physical labor should eat more."
- "Always eat all the food on your plate."

Which of these old wives tales have you heard and lived by that now have a negative influence on your health and energy?

In the area of nutrition, it is important to know that food is either utilized or eliminated. If the food is just eliminated, it taxes the energy supply. It therefore makes sense to eat only nourishment that supplies energy. Eating more than our body needs and must eliminate as waste, taxes our body needlessly. We, furthermore, demand too much of our body, when we eat food that is hard to process.

Many people literally dig their own grave with their teeth, because digestion of our food takes more energy than most physical activities do. Many people do not just drain their body of energy with bad nutrition, but also regularly poison themselves. Allow yourself to have some doubt about your former belief system and compare the results for yourself after you learn new information about nutrition and the effect it has on your energy.

You are now aware that energy is the foundation of health, and a lack of energy leads to illness. Energy is ATP (adenosine triphosphate), which is the basic element of life. No matter what death certificates say, people fundamentally die of a shortage of ATP. The vital production of ATP is not possible without sufficient oxygen, which is why oxygen is the most basic necessity for our health. Use the **IBMS™** session.

*Did you know that you can live for six weeks without food, six days without water, but not six minutes without breathing? The quality of your health depends on the quality of your cells, which in turn depends on the amount and quality of oxygen and nutrition in your bloodstream. A lack of oxygen leads to deteriorating health because without enough oxygen, cells die as does your cell tissue. When your cell tissue dies, your organs follow and then your whole body dies.*

## Why Aerobic Exercise and Deep Abdominal Breathing Is So Important

*Otto Warburg, at the Max-Planck-Institute in Germany, took healthy tissue from rats and extracted eighty percent of the oxygen from the tissue, and the tissue died. He then extracted seventy percent of the oxygen and still the tissue died. When he conducted the experiment at sixty to sixty-five percent oxygen removed, part of the tissue cells survived, but they mutated, which is the beginning of cancer.*

*Dr. Harry Goldberg expanded on this experiment by injecting tumor cells into rats from which he withdrew different amounts of oxygen. The control rats that retained 100 percent of the oxygen remained healthy. Sixty percent of the rats got tumors when an average amount of oxygen was withdrawn, and all the rats (100 percent that had the higher amounts of oxygen extracted, grew tumors. 100 percent!*

An important way to detoxify our bodies and activate our lymph system is through deep abdominal breathing and aerobic exercise. If the lymph fluid does not move through the body, it is not possible to process and eliminate toxins, which leads to toxemia. The only way lymph fluid can move through our body is with movement, i.e., exercise and deep breathing. We have four times more lymph liquid in our body that blood and it needs to flow constantly!

Every second, thousands of blood cells die and are simultaneously produced. The dead cells form toxins that need to be eliminated. This is the function of a working lymph system which is why it is so important that the lymph system functions properly. Compare it to river, if it is flowing it constantly cleanses itself, but if it stands still it rots within a short period of time. The same is true of the lymph system! Detoxification takes place through the skin, kidneys, lungs and intestines.

It is important to note that we do not get energy directly from eating as our body first uses energy to digest the food. It is only after food is digested that it is available for our use. Fruit is the only exception to this rule as the body is able to immediately convert the fruit into sugar and provide energy, if it is eaten on an empty stomach otherwise it could cause fermentation, gas, bloating, etc.

In my" Modern Therapy Centers" ( name protected ) in Europe I trained my therapists to do a special full body lymph drainage that I developed in working with over 35 000 patients. ( number of patients estimated by a independent institute )that could be one of the most powerful tool for a fast recovery.

**Healthy Cells Never Die**

*Dr. Alexis Carrol believed that healthy cells could not die if they received sufficient energy, oxygen and nutrition, and toxins were regularly removed. He used cells from ten to twelve year old chickens, providing them with sufficient oxygen and removing the toxins. In this condition, he managed to keep the cells alive for thirty-four years after which time he stopped the experiment, convinced that he could have kept the cells alive forever under these conditions.*

*At the Rockefeller Institute, two Nobel Prize winners also concluded that cells in an artificial, ideal environment with sufficient nutrition and oxygen without toxins could live forever. This is only possible as long as the cells are not vulnerable by exposure to any outside influences such as an accident or other mishap.*

A restful sleep is of the utmost importance for regeneration, good health and the building up of energy resources, because the body can only produce the chemicals it needs during the time while you sleep. Alcohol disrupts the REM sleep, which is the sleeping state needed to restore your biochemical balance. Therefore, if you have been drinking alcohol, you cannot get the restorative benefits of a restful night's sleep since the alcohol induces a short and restless sleep. You may have already noticed that drinking alcohol leaves you feeling tired and depleted of energy the next day.

The body has its own means of fighting to eliminate poisons and toxins.

- The body naturally tries to eliminate poisons by vomiting and diarrhea.
- Fever is the body's way of burning out poisons.
- Sneezing, coughing and skin rashes are also ways that the body uses to get rid of poisons.

Medicine often fights these natural reactions forcing the body to retain the toxins, which can then lead to serious medical problems. Headaches can often be an indication of toxins in the body.

*Dr. Holger Crone, M.D., a leading physician for NAPS-Training in Europe often advises his patients to have an enema when they suffer from a headache. In more than ninety percent of the cases, the headache disappears after the first bowel movement. The reason is the detoxification of the colon.*

***Very often what we consider as illness or symptoms of illness is in fact the body's therapy or way of healing itself by eliminating poisons.***

**Energy, the Foundation of Health**

Without energy, you cannot function, but your energy level is not a result of bad genes, or your biological rhythm also known as "biorhythm." Your energy level is not linked to the waning of the mood - low energy is the result of compromised lifestyles, poor nutrition, dehydration, lack of oxygen, lack of exercise, restful sleep, etc.

In my work, I constantly hear people complaining about how difficult their life is, how badly they have been treated by others, how their parents were poor and could not help them financially to get a good start, etc. But these problems are meaningless because in this moment, right now only the present and the future matter! We cannot do anything about the past, instead chalk it up to bad luck or circumstance and move on with today and tomorrow.

Modern psychology and psychiatry have discovered that focusing on the past only drains people of a considerable amount of energy, time and strength, and it very often kills their optimism. In fact, it actually makes people feel worse. This is because the brain does not know the difference between a real experience and an imagined experience; it has no concept of time. In other words, the brain reacts with the similar bioelectrical and neuro-chemical impulses, producing the same release of hormones, the same body chemistry, the same neuro-transmitters and all the other neurological and physiological processes from the past, whether we are really experiencing or simply remembering a situation or event.

When someone thinks back to a traumatic event, and it is relived over and over again in their mind, they suffer the same trauma again and again, and they are using up an enormous amount of stored energy for nothing.

I believe that negative past experiences and failures should be addressed, defined, analyzed and evaluated and once they are, then they need to be let go so that they cannot influence the present and the future. Naturally, we should learn from our mistakes so that we may behave better and more effectively in the future. This is the only way that we grow and develop ourselves. But the only solution for dealing with past traumatic events is to let go! Get over it! Get on with your life! Stop whining and wallowing in self pity!

Because most people do not have the time to be sick, we should make every effort to invest our energy in a program that keeps us energized and, therefore, healthy and vital - otherwise we pay for it later. Better invest a little time now to stay healthy than spending all your time later to get rid of an illness!

There are many people who are fit, but not healthy. This is due to a lack of understanding how to properly exercise and workout so that your body is not stressed in a negative way. If at the end of your workout, you feel exhausted, worn out and/or are gasping for air, then this means that your body's source of energy is glycogen (instead of fat and oxygen) resulting in an anaerobic workout instead of an aerobic workout. Anaerobic means "existing in the absence of free oxygen."

Don't forget that a person with an abundance of energy will not get sick! You will never see illness, flu, or disease getting the best of a person filled with excitement, vitality and energy, or full of strength and love of life. A person needs to be worn out, tired, lacking in energy, toxic, dehydrated and/or acidic to get sick.

# Dr. Leonard Coldwell

*Respected physicians, therapists and researchers have clearly proven that a body filled with healthful life giving energy is resistant against viruses and bacteria. To prove his point, Professor Bernard went so far as to put cholera bacteria on a slice of bread, which he promptly ate it in front of his students. He did not get sick! Instead, he showed that there is nothing to fear from bacteria - if you have a healthy body.*

*Throughout medical history, there has never been any proof whatsoever that a bacteria or virus can damage a healthy body cell. Dr. Duisburg, a colleague of Gallo, the official discoverer of the HIV-virus, offered to inject himself intravenously with the AIDS virus to prove that a virus cannot hurt a healthy body. He stated that "The territory is everything, the microbe is negligible."*

In conclusion, scientists from all over the world agree that a body filled with energy will not get sick. In my personal practice, I have not relied on medicines or surgery to treat my patients, yet I have had remarkable recoveries with patients suffering from gout, rheumatism, asthma, cancer, muscle atrophy and cancer simply with the release of energy. When a patient starts to set new goals, and they are really willing to take their life in their own hands, hope and faith and positive energy comes to them. The result is their energy level changes and they soon feel and get better. ( I experienced many cases of spontaneous healing )

**Breathing is the Energy of Life**

This is what happens when we breathe:

**We get oxygen when we exhale! When we inhale the lungs bubbles fill with oxygen, then when we exhale, the lungs contract and the oxygen is compressed into the arteries. If we inhale too shallowly, only a small amount of the**

available oxygen enters the bloodstream; it is, therefore, very important to inhale deeply. **Inhale deep into your stomach and exhale until you have nothing more to exhale. The majority of air bubbles are in the lower part of the lungs.**

We know from breathing therapy that people who live in fear will minimize this fear when they inhale calmly four seconds through the nose and exhale eleven seconds through the mouth repeatedly ten times. It is, moreover, important to first inhale deeply into the belly and then up into the shoulder area, so that the lungs are filled with oxygen from bottom to top.

Again, when speaking on the telephone, concentrate on sitting or standing upright and inhaling deeply into the belly. This is very important and most helpful when and if you are involved in demanding situations or intense conversations, as it will give you the energy and oxygen you need to remain alert, calm, and in control. Use the **IBMS™** Breathing Session.

*Exercise:*

*Here is a wonderful breathing exercise that should be performed three times a day if possible: First inhale for 4 seconds through the nose, then hold your breath for 16 seconds and exhale for 8 seconds through the mouth. If this is difficult, do not force it, keep trying without straining. Repeat this sequence 12 times, 3 times a day; you will soon notice a substantial improvement in your energy level. If you suffer from respiratory problems, please consult your physician before starting this exercise.*

I need to mention that if you wear a skirt or pants with a waistband that is too tight, you create pressure in the area below your waist ultimately jamming your lungs so that you cannot inhale deeply. The body reacts to this by producing dis-stress hormones, which cause cramps or produces a fight or flight reaction. Because the body now fears suffocation it reacts by producing stress hormones. Then since the body does not utilize all the stress hormones they poison the body and lead to feelings of restlessness, anxiety, tension, cramps or lack of concentration.

Some therapists suggest a form of hyperventilating to artificially increase the oxygen content in the body. When I experimented with these techniques, I had very negative results with my patients.

Hints

- Climbing stairs is a good way to reduce stress.
- Sleeping with an open window allows our bodies to get restored with fresh air which is healthy. We exhale many toxins during the night that we should not re-inhale!

You are only as healthy as the health of your cells. If you build a house with inferior second or third rate materials, you should not be surprised if the insulation is poor, the windows do not open and close, or if the roof blows away in a storm. It is no different with our bodies; to be in top shape, we must take care of our body using the very best resources.

You can replenish and restore your vitality simply by walking daily for twenty minutes in the fresh air and/or experiencing your **IBMS™** sessions!

# Section II - Chapter 7

## *Prepare Yourself for Life*

If you are devoid of resources when you are in a crisis situation, you will panic. You must learn to prepare and program yourself, so that you can react as well as possible in an eventual stressful situation. Preparation does not mean that you should be afraid. Preparation means that you cover all the angles of what could go wrong, so that you can respond prepared to anything that could arise. Feeling helpless is the worst, because helplessness has an extreme negative effect on our health and on our performance; it affects our courage, so that we may not be able to act positively.

Studies show that patients who feel helpless die earlier. People who feel that they are in charge, even if their control is limited, have a better life expectation and a stronger immune system. Medical specialists have found that patients who could administer their own medicine and decide on their own lifestyle were living longer than so-called dependent patients, those who lived in hospitals and were virtually helpless.

We must all learn, as fast as possible, to instill a feeling of control in our subconscious, in our thought process and behavior. We must install a pattern of behavior that takes it for granted and accepts it as absolutely normal that we are in charge. To run away, ignore or avoid problems sets the beginning of catastrophes in motion.

Failures teach us to act and modify our behavior. We will unavoidably produce better and more effective results than before. When we learn from mistakes and act accordingly, our experience will direct us to the desired results. If you, for instance, know that a relationship is no longer working and that you are only hanging on out of convenience, because of others, or for whatever reason, then this relationship becomes destructive. After you have done everything possible to make the relationship work for both parties and accept that there is no hope, you must look immediately for a solution to end the partnership.

Guilt can cause incredible stress. Guilt feelings seldom disappear by themselves and people who have them can suffer their whole lives as a result. People condition themselves by searching their subconscious for errors and failures and are no longer able to function. Their self-esteem is diminished and they are no longer able to look for solutions; they keep searching for excuses for their failures. If you suffer from guilt, you must learn to face people with an apology or do something to pay your debt. You can also talk with them and come to an understanding, if this impossible, or look for another way to release your guilt.

*Exercise:*

*Write down the areas in which you feel guilty, whom did you hurt and why.*
*Write down solutions for redeeming your guilt as quickly as possible, or find out why it is absurd that you still feel guilty.*

**Taking the First Step**

If we are facing a large job and are focusing on the completed final result without subdividing the project into smaller parts, we often feel overwhelmed, or we suffer from anxiety, because we are afraid that we are not up to the task. But if we divide the job in front of us in small parts that we can handle, we will experience small successes that will strengthen our self-confidence. As a result, we will do our work better and accomplish more, and we will finish the job faster than we thought possible. By dividing the job into smaller parts we will, moreover, feel assured that we can handle the job. The first step is often the most difficult one. Once we start working on a job, the rest often becomes easy.

Asking for help, or looking for team solutions when we face a conflict or must solve a serious problem, is also important. Brainstorming, or sharing ideas, often helps us to move ahead. Using research material, changing our behavior and working with a team often help us feel more confident. Members of the team will also feel better, because they can contribute to our life; we will get a better understanding and move ahead, together. This not only works for a team, but it is also important and helpful when it involves our family.

**Personal Stress Reduction**

We must all learn to find, develop and maintain in our body a functioning system for regeneration and stress reduction. Breathing properly through the abdomen is extremely important and experiencing **IBMS™** sessions because they are the fastest way to unwind and regenerate. With **IBMS™** you develop relaxation techniques that are critical in reducing stress so that you do not end up with a health problem.

We must learn to eat healthy, avoiding food that needs too much energy to digest. We must create a life free of stress through clear goals and rules, and with a good value and belief system. We must develop a healthy life rhythm with regular sleep so that we feel that we are in control and can build a positive self-image.

**Your Value System**

If you want to live a life free of stress, it is important to understand what your personal values really are. Only through personal growth and regular successes can you form a goal oriented life. People suffer a great deal of stress simply from "uncertainty," by knowing exactly what you want, you experience far less stress. Your problems become simpler as you resolve all the challenges within the boundaries of your goals, which makes it is easier to make sensible, goal-oriented decisions. By learning to build, develop and expand your individual qualities and abilities, you also create a strong value system that ultimately will be transformed into reality.

As a side note, remember it is not necessary to prove yourself to anyone, but most especially not to those who are weaker or more ignorant than you. For instance when a person is sick or helpless, if you have self-esteem and self-confidence, you would not need to boast or build yourself up to them. What goes around comes around, so it is better to be kind and thoughtful when possible as this attitude will fill your life with wonderful feelings.

**The Importance of Team Play**

In general, we are social creatures who feel comfortable around other people. However, loners tend to be people who cannot be around other people because they remind them of what they are not, nice people! We depend on family, friends and acquaintances to cry and laugh with us when we are happy or sad, but it is important to understand the difference between sharing your feelings with people close to you and dependence! If you believe that your survival is dependent on someone else because of your life circumstances, you will suffer continuous stress. Dependency is a feeling not a reality!

Team play is an important element in stress reduction because no matter what, it is less stressful and easier to solve conflicts, difference of opinions, problems or whatever when you work together to find a solution. Loneliness or being alone causes lots of stress as nobody really wants to be lonely or alone. People want to have friends, a supportive close family, a friendly groups of contacts, and more; basically, people want to be a part of a team. It is our responsibility to make the first step by approaching people with kindness, friendship and real team spirit, all of which enrich and contribute to a healthier and more stress free life.

*Research studies have shown that in the U.S., widows and widowers who live alone suffer from a higher rate of cancer than those who live with someone else. Loneliness can lead to depression, and it also is one of the reasons for suicides. Another study, researched by the University of California, showed that people who live in a small close social environment (as in a small town in Southern Italy, where the study was done) have fewer heart attacks than people who live in large cities. Remarkably when the people moved out of the close knit environment, the incidence of heart attacks immediately increased to the high level of people who lived in big cities. Another study performed by a private institute showed that people, who suffer from anxiety, live under a high level of stress.*

Have you ever noticed that you feel so much better when you give than when you receive? The reason is that your self-esteem and self-image improve substantially simply from doing something positive for another person. Therefore, if you behave in a positive way towards others, your self-esteem and your self-image will automatically improve. When people trust you, it boosts your self-confidence and self-confidence lessens the stress in your life. The worst is being surrounded by people who are envious of you; they bring you down, so select your friends and acquaintances with care.

Being able to get along with all types, including difficult people, substantially reduces stress in your life. You cannot completely avoid difficult people, you cannot change them, no matter how much want to, but being aggressive with them only makes matters worse. Don't waste a lot of energy producing stress by fighting difficult people, instead simply accept them as they are.

**The Right Balance**

You are the only person who receives a message from your subconscious telling you that you are at the end, so only you can figure out what the right balance is between your work and your private life. This will keep you free from illness – listen to your instincts!

You can detoxify your mind and body faster and more effectively with energy rich food and regular exercise. Clinical psychiatrists concluded that negative emotional conditions and depression are reduced or even fully removed with plenty of exercise. In fact, the walking or exercising can get rid of certain types of depression. As previously reviewed, regular exercise increases the amount of oxygen in your body, which helps to make feelings of frustration and lethargy, often the result of a shortage of energy, go away or disappear completely. Remember that no diet is made especially for your body, your needs or your performance instead learn to eat only when you are hungry and try not to over eat. And don't eat hard to digest food especially when you are under stress because stress slows down the metabolism and you will gain weight. Also hunger heightens stress so it is wiser and better to eat small amounts of food to tide you over when you are hungry until the next meal, but you should not use the clock to determine when it is time to eat, learn instead to listen to your body.

Sensible, regenerating sleep is very important to reducing and avoiding stress. Small power-naps of a half-hour or an hour are not sufficient because the deep sleep cycles of the body only start after ninety minutes into sleep. These deep sleep cycles are necessary for restoration and they are repeated every ninety minutes. Again remember that alcohol has a negative effect on brain waves because it disturbs your sleep patterns, so that you cannot fully regenerate.

Here is a piece of advice: never use your bed for work; do not read work related material in your bed; only read for your enjoyment; don't study in bed; don't think about work problems; don't list or think about your work related activities – all of these cause stress. When in your bed, restrict your activities to those of a recreational nature or sleep. This is very important because otherwise your thoughts become part of your dreams and when you wake up you will feel, at the very least, tired. Have a notebook and pencil handy next to your bed so that if you get an idea you can immediately write it down that your mind lets it go as finished business.

If you have difficulties sleeping, try programming your mind with self-suggestions about a restful sleep like "I will sleep well, I will have wonderful thoughts and dreams all through the night and in the morning, and I will wake up fresh, feeling healthy and full of energy." Over time repeating this will program your subconscious for the desired sleep and regeneration. By the way, even if you are not tired at night lie down anyway so that your body relaxes and starts the process of regeneration naturally.

It is important to note that in life, everybody suffers through periods of anger or great sadness, and others of wallowing in self-pity, but beware to stop these times because the mind needs to back to normalcy or the negative emotions become a part of serious negative pattern that could ultimately lead to losing control.

## Calculated Risks

To achieve anything, you must take risks, but the risks should be educated risks. There is no certainty in life, but if you learn to assess your risk by knowing the facts and having a backup plan in the event that things do not work out then you substantially reduce the risks of something going wrong and not being prepared. This is a calculated risk. The fact that you have multiple backup plans will reassure you so that you will feel secure about taking the risk.

In other words, when you are confronted with a risk, calculate all the possibilities that could go wrong and then figure out a few ways to solve each of them. This will prepare you for any crisis that may occur. And by doing this you will be more apt to take the risk. There are no successes in life without risks, but developing clear strategies for coping with many likely consequences will assure you that your decision is right. It is crucial that you never incorporate luck as a factor because you create your own luck, so don't fall into the trap expecting luck to affect your outcome. Also, don't deny anything or pretend that something is what it is not! Only you can decide, according to your value and belief system, if a risk is worth taking, but try to be unbiased when judging the pro's and con's.

**The Importance of a Personal Vision**

To appreciate your abilities and enjoy life, you must give your vision the chance to flourish. Do not allow outside pressures to stifle or suppress your imagination and do not let rational thinking dominate all your decisions. To give your creativity a chance, you must be open-minded about thinking, exploring and testing new ideas. Then you can decide whether or not it makes sense to incorporate them in our lives.

Don't be stubborn about holding onto past thinking that is probably antiquated, ignorant or misinformed, live in the present changing and evolving as you grow and learn. Let your instincts, thoughts and feelings guide you toward the future that you want.

Be willing to try new things and experiment with new information which will produce creative results. If you dwell on negative past situations, you won't develop solutions, but if you let go then you can draw on your past experiences to develop effective new strategies and new behavior patterns!

You cannot change the past, no matter how much you want to and no matter how hard you struggle with what happened, you cannot influence today what happened yesterday, but you can influence what happens today and tomorrow. However, don't live always thinking in the future that "some day ..." because this can stop you from having a life or living. Excuses like "after I leave school..., after I get married.., when I have finished my studies..., when the kids are grown..., after my divorce..., after I retire..., etc." delay action so that you can end up suddenly finding yourself "old" realizing that you missed your life, it somehow passed you by always thinking that tomorrow would ... This produces such intense feelings of frustration and self-pity that some people even go so far as to take their life.

So live in the here and now, let go of the past and condition your mind for the future and achieving your own goals. This way you create solutions; the more creativity you allow in your life, the more opportunities you will have and the better you will be at dealing with crisis situations. Do not allow your past to limit your enjoyment of the future!

## Regeneration

Getting regenerated is not something that you do for the short term; it needs to be incorporated as a part of your every day routine for the rest of your life. When you started reading this book, if you had no energy or happiness in your life, then by now if you did everything in the book, you should have your energy back! Hopefully you were able to incorporate **IBMS™** sessions. I keep repeating it, but I cannot over emphasize that **IBMS™** sessions are the best way to quickly regenerate and get back control of your life.

*Once you achieve success and your emotional and mental frame of mind is healthy, you must continue to take time for regeneration because your energy will continue to fluctuate no matter what.*

You cannot outsmart your body thinking that if you are comfortable and workout a lot that this will be enough! Everybody needs time to regenerate, not just once a year, but every week or even every day, it depends on each person's needs, so you must figure out what works for you. It is simply a sure thing that if you do not take time to regenerate, you will fall apart in the long run.

## The Very Best Way to Regenerate

The **IBMS™** system offers the very best way to get regenerated in twenty minutes. This system provides the tools, possibilities and directions to turn your life into your masterpiece. With the **IBMS™** system, you have the possibility to achieve your goals faster than ever before. No matter what you choose to do, remember it is extremely important that you take time out of your schedule to regenerate otherwise over time, you could end up with a health problem.

Make the decision that you will never be satisfied with less than you can achieve. This means that you should not accept being less than 100 percent happy, successful, energized and healthy. Be conscious of all your possibilities, abilities and talents and use them to achieve your dreams. You have been given direction, now it is up to you to create a life full of enthusiasm, passion and success for yourself. Turn your life into a masterpiece.

*Remember, you are born to be healthy, happy and successful!*

# Section II - Chapter 8

## *A Conclusive and Scientific Look at Stress*

In the earlier days, stress was defined as "general adaptation syndrome," which means that stress signals and related stress hormones and reactions are caused by change. In these earlier times, animals and humans fought "change" in both their environment and life because it usually signified danger from "being out of control or out of their controlled environment.' It continues to be an instinct based stress reaction to change in our social status, life or environment.

Stress reactions are based on the need for survival - fight or flight reactions. The state of acute stress increases the body's capability to enhance short-term performance for running away from or for attacking an enemy.

Modern science proves that there is a very close connection between stress and obesity, diabetes, impotence, dementia, heart disease, cancer, memory loss and pre-aging. It is also well documented that stress causes ulcers and many different illnesses in animal experiments. So stress can make us gain weight, deplete our bones, shrink our brain, suppress our immune system, zap our energy levels and can even eradicate our sex drive.

Short term active stress leads to fight or flight responses and is not really a problem because we quickly recover from these feelings when we stop feeling threatened. The problem arises from *chronically* elevated stress experiences which produces *chronically* elevated stress hormones like adrenalin or cortisol with all their relative negative side effects.

In general, stress hormones are not bad because they help the body to survive short term danger by providing the person with the ability to use fight or flight reactions. While adrenalin can give the body the known so-called "runners high," it is responsible for enhanced short term excitement, vitality and energy, but when it is overused in chronic stress experiences, it can lead to burn out syndrome with a complete break down of body functions.

Cholesterol is very important for a steroid metabolism. Cortisol is more important in storing energy following stressful situations. Obesity and many chronic diseases can be caused by cortisol. The point I wish to make is that it is very important to keep our body chemistry leveled maintaining our cortisol level from rising too high or falling too low.

Addison disease makes people unable to secrete glucocorticoids from the adrenal glands, which leads to the person's inability to have an effective stress response. People with this disease go into a state of shock when they are faced with stressful events. Usually there is a significant drop in blood pressure, circulatory collapse and other problems.

While adrenalin is produced by the upper part of the kidneys, cortisol is produced through a series of different changes involving the pituitary gland in the hypothalamus in the brain. Cortisol has many functions including stimulation of glucose release, fats and amino acids for energy production. It also stimulates the breakdown of glycogen into glucose in the liver. Fatty acids are released by cortisol stimulation for fat breakdown. Cortisol promotes an amino acid release which is very important for muscles and our skeletal system and is necessary and important for short-term active stress responses, but over time it can turn into major physical damage and the creation of illness and chronic stress experiences. It can lead to an extreme increase in appetite and cravings because cortisol can be responsible for making you feel hungry all of the time.

This often leads to a huge accumulation of abdominal fat, a type of fat associated with cancer, diabetes or cardio vascular diseases. It has been scientifically proven without any doubt that there is a strong relationship between high stress levels and numerous chronic illnesses.

An artificial chemical form of the cortisol stress hormone called cortisone exists. This drug is used to reduce joint pain, swelling, inflammation, arthritis and other inflammatory diseases. The use of this drug is usually successful in short term approaches, but we know from medical applications that long-term use can lead to memory problems, depression, increased infections, weight gain and structural changes.

Most stress researchers agree that there is a strong correlation between chronic stress and the following conditions: increased depression and anxiety, mood swings, reduced sex drive and libido, learning impairment, memory loss, increased menopausal or PMS syndromes, which can lead to dramatic appetite changes and muscle cramps, night sweat or hot flashes, increased cravings, body fat, decreased bone density and muscle mass.

The clinically diagnosed type C lifestyle is characterized by chronic stress levels and consistently elevated stress hormones.

When the brain interprets an event as life threatening, whether real of imagined, it stimulates the endocrine glands in the body to release hormones like adrenalin or cortisol. Adrenalin is basically responsible for alertness and excitement enhancement; cortisol is responsible for modulating the body's fuel or energy sources. Cortisol is secreted by the adrenal cortex and is known as glucocorticoids, it increases the blood sugar level or glucose.

Stress basically knocks out our body's bioelectrical and neuro-chemical balance so that the body has to struggle to regain the natural healthy balance which is a part of the general adaptation syndrome.

When we suffer chronic stressors or repeating stressors due to our lifestyle or stimulation from our environment, our body can barely get back its balance and produces an over stimulation or production of stress hormones, which basically can burn out our entire system and energy level from overload. This overload can lead to a complete breakdown of bodily systems and functions if it is a chronic situation. It is called burnout syndrome. Associated problems related to elevated stress responses are; a suppressed immune system, depression, anxiety, weight gain, lack of energy, memory loss, inability to concentrate, ADD or ADHD problems. Chronic overload or burnout syndrome can lead to widespread tissue dysfunction, gastrointestinal ulceration and profound metabolic derange-ment.

Due to the stress triggered activation of body energy reserves, chronic stress experience can lead to a catabolic breakdown of tissues. Levels of cortisol and adrenalin are increased while testosterone and DHEA are decreased leading to muscle loss and fat gain. Some of the common effects from acute stress are increased breathing, high blood pressure, increased temperature as well as feelings of anxiety, restlessness, headaches, heartburn and sweating, PMS and strong menopausal problems. This is the result of neurotransmitters and hormones running rampant in our bodies.

In chronic stress situations, the levels of life building hormones decrease which can lead to pre-aging. Chronic stress symptoms can lead to increased appetite, fluctuations in blood sugar, carbohydrate cravings, weight gain, fatigue, muscle weakness, and a decreased functioning of the immune system. As a result, muscles and bone tissues are weaker and the sex drive dramatically decreases because of an extremely low level of growth hormones, sex steroids and DHEA. It also leads to increased appetite, fat accumulation and reduced caloric expenditure.

Research shows that women are more used to high levels of stress hormones and are usually better able to handle acute stress situations because of their predisposition to take care of children and the household. Another reason that women are more able to deal with the "after effects" of stressful situations is their ability to talk about their emotions and problems; by doing this, they release the steam built up inside.

Competitive athletes are another group in danger because they often create chronic physical stress by overtraining and over exercising. By over doing it, they disturb the delivery of nutrition and causing reduced mental and physical performance and constant fatigue.

The hormonal stimulation from adrenalin, norepanephrine, cortisol and many other hormones is responsible for many important aspects of physiology like cardiovascular function, immune system activity, brain chemistry, energy and metabolism.

It is important to remember that stress hormones are life enhancing and essential for survival. These hormonal stimulations can only create problems with our health or endanger our lives if the stress hormone levels are chronically elevated.

Cortisol is responsible for maintaining blood pressure and limiting excessive inflammation during acute stress experiences. Cortisol is also known to stimulate the metabolic process by increasing the level of glucose in the blood.

Unfortunately, fatty acids released by fat breakdown can have a detrimental effect on health because it reduces the cellular sensitivity to insulin which will ultimately lead to diabetes. Hypertension, obesity, diabetes, depression, irregular menstrual periods, decreased sex drive, moodiness and Alzheimer's disease are in a majority of cases associated with chronic stress.

Chronic stress can be responsible for the destruction of tissue and system breakdown including bone loss, brain shrinkage, muscle loss, immune suppression. An overactive cortizol level can lead to asthma, allergies and autoimmune diseases. Long-term exposure to high cortizol levels can lead to the inactivation of our immune system protection by causing the death of immune cells.

Modern lifestyle diseases like diabetes, hypertension, insomnia, headaches, migraines, ulcers, obesity, depression, anxiety, memory loss, lowered resistance to infection and all kinds of illness are scientifically connected to chronic stress.

It doesn't matter if the higher stress level is caused by emotional stress, from being angry about a traffic jam or being bothered or suffering insecurities in our relationships, or over exercising and causing physical stress, the results can still be detrimental.

We know that "walk-in" clinics are overburdened with ailing college students during exam week because this is a very stressful time for students with the resulting high degree of illness at this time of the year. Heightened chronic levels of stress due to job problems or relationship problems can cause allergies, migraines, asthma, cold and flu.

The brain cannot differentiate between an event that is real or imagined. So if you imagine scary pictures of future events or you constantly think about past negative experiences, your body will react with the same response as if you were actually experiencing it. In other words, the brain develops the same stress response whether it is caused by imagined or actual stressors.

Stress responses can be caused by lack of self-esteem, insecurity, doubts, fears, worries, injury, hunger, heat and cold. Any one of these can be triggered by imagined or real events which create the fight or flight response and, therefore, leads to an elevated level of stress hormones. If you constantly worry about your relationship with your spouse or children, or suffer constant insecurities about your job or financial situation, or if you are afraid of getting sick, you are creating a constant elevated level of stress simulation which can and will usually lead to burnout syndrome, lack of energy and breakdown of health and immune functions.

Self hatred and living with constant compromises in your private or business lives, generally leads to an extremely elevated stress level and can lead to an auto immune disease because indirectly the brain and the body want to get rid of the dangerous stressful situation, but because the person cannot just run away from their life, it tries to destroy itself. This is why it is so important to **not** live in constant compromises or chronic stress situations. So look for the cause of your insecurity, develop clear goals and action plans, and work on furthering the growth and development of your life to get the stressors out of your life.

**Note**: High levels of stress always lead to a lower sex drive and libido.

**The following is a list of Health Effects**
**Due to Chronic Stress:**
- Elevated cholesterol and triglyceride levels, increased appetite, suppressed fat oxidation, enhanced fat storage, muscle break down, reduced synthesis of brain neuro-transmitters, alterations in brain neuro-chemistry, suppression of immune cells in number and activity, insulin resistance, physical atrophy, shrinkage of brain cells and reduced levels of estrogen and testosterone.
- Chronic health conditions related to chronic stress include diabetes, Alzheimer's disease, osteoporosis, heart disease, anxiety, depression, frequent infections, cold, flu, attention deficit disorder, memory problems and suppressed libido.
- Chronic stress can also lead to so-called ACTS syndrome which is characterized by insulin resistance, abdominal obesity, diabetes, hypertension, and elevated cholesterol.
- Yale University research showed a clear correlation between emotional stress in women and weight gain.
- It is also scientifically proven that chronic stress leads to a decrease in muscle building hormones. It elevates blood fat levels. The University of California in San Francisco showed the correlation between chronic stress and depression, Alzheimer's disease, anxiety, and changes in brain

structure leading to cognitive defects. There is proof that high levels of stress over a period of time can shrink or even kill brain cells (atrophy).

Because stress hormones have a massive impact on insulin, it can cause endless problems with our health. Insulin regulates our blood sugar levels, but it is also responsible for storing fat in our fat cells and getting amino acids directed for protein synthesis which means muscle building. Insulin is also known as the starch hormone. The disturbance of the optimum levels of insulin in our system can therefore lead to a variety of health breakdowns.

- Chronic stress can lead to a condition that is called insulin resistance, one of the primary steps towards diabetes. Obesity can be caused by chronic stress because the stress hormones decreased the secretion of major metabolic hormones like DHEA. Stress makes you burn fewer calories, which can lead to stressing about overeating.
- While in the short term, stress can reduce appetite due to the secretion of CRH (corticotrophin releasing hormone), which feels like an anxiety or panic attack, but it can also lead to the stimulation of appetite after the stress attack.
- A disease called Cushing's syndrome is caused by extremely high levels of stress hormones, which leads to massive accumulations of abdominal fat and is accompanied by severe loss of muscle tissue in your arms and legs.
- With chronic stress, the cortisol and insulin levels rise and together send a message to fat cells to store as much fat as possible so that it can be used as energy the next stressful time.

## Stress and its Effect on your Metabolism

- A general drop in the basic metabolic rate.
- Decrease synthesis of protein
- Reduced levels of DHEA, growth hormone, steroid stimulation, stimulating hormone and IGF-1, breakdown of muscles, ligaments and tendons.

It also leads to increased blood sugar levels, reduced transport of glucose to the cells, and an increase in appetite and therefore, increased and redistribution of body fat in the abdominal region.

Scientific studies also show a close relationship between the high levels of stress hormones in the blood and high insulin levels as well as reduced growth hormone levels. The reason people usually gain weight during periods of dieting is because the diet itself is stressful on the system and sends a signal to the fat cells to store more fat for the ongoing or new stress or rather diet in this case.

- Chronic stress reduces the body's ability to release fat to use it for energy.

The University of Colorado performed several studies with athletes who over exercise that showed they suffer from immune system suppression, increased levels of body fat and mood disturbances the result of stress. The Swedish University of Goetheborg proved that a high fat accumulation and weight gain can be caused by stress.

The problem is that stress hormones and insulin disturb the blood sugar regulation, which increases appetite and stops the body from burning fat. This can lead to obesity and many other fat related illnesses.

Chronic stress also leads to feelings of fatigue, dizziness, depression, disinterest in sex, obesity, heart disease, diabetes, Alzheimer's and in some cases, can lead to cancer.

The University of Chicago concluded that inadequate sleep would promote the development of insulin resistance, basically the first step of type 2 diabetes. Inadequate sleepers were reported to secrete fifty percent more insulin and were forty percent less sensitive to the effects of insulin as compared to normal sleepers. This is one of the major causes of pre-aging. Inadequate sleep has a definite direct correlation to pre-aging and the development of several severe diseases because of the decreased energy level that leads to lower immune function. Also, stress is often the major cause of insomnia or sleep difficulties. There is also a direct correlation between insomnia and chronic fatigue syndrome.

Males usually experience a dramatic decrease in testosterone levels during stressful times, which is why chronic stress can lead to impotence or general sexual dysfunction. This is also the major reason for why men lose interest in sex. Women as well who experience a disturbance in levels of estrogen, progesterone, prolactin and testosterone can also experience a dramatic loss in sex drive. Stress can also be or related to some of the causes for infertility.

Certain types of stress can produce the so-called "feel good" chemical called endorphins. They produce a euphoric feeling called "runners high." But extended exposure to these feelings can be associated with lowered testosterone levels and reduced sperm count, resulting in a reduced interest in sex.

In my personal experience, chronic stress goes hand in hand with chronic conditions like arthritis, gastro intestinal ailments, asthma, allergies, IBS, Crone's disease and others.

*Extremely elevated stress hormones can lead to auto immune disease which means that the immune system starts to attack the bodies own tissues.*

Scientific studies have shown that stress can lead to the shrinkage of the thymus gland and the general suppression of the immune system. Stress hormones definitely inhibit the white blood cell production and activity. High levels of stress hormones suppress the secretion of chemical messengers called interferon, which leads to a large number of immune cells being unable to communicate with each other so that they are unable to effectively fight infection. Specifically, the stress hormone cortisol shuts down immune cells so they die.

When experiencing chronic stress and therefore high stress hormone levels, the integrity of the immune system starts to suffer. In some instances, it starts to unleash destructive properties on the body's own tissues resulting in all different kinds of auto immune disease like MS, lupus, fibromyalgia, arthritis and allergies.

*An auto immune disease or an over active immune system can attack the joints in the body or the nerve cells. In the case of lupus, it attacks the connective tissue.*

Scientific research and studies have shown that chronic stress leads to a fifty percent reduction of immune cells also called natural killer cells. These cells are very important for the immune function. Of significance is that when women get diagnosed with breast cancer, they automatically lose fifty percent of their killer cells because of the stress caused from hearing the diagnosis. This also explains why directly after a diagnosis of a disease, patients deteriorate. This is all caused by stress.

We concluded from animal experiments that stress hormones not only suppress the production and the activity of natural killer cells, but they also promote the synthesis of new blood vessels in tumors, called angiogenesis. This makes the tumor grows and shows that stress can lead to tumor growth. It can block the immune function and leads to an inability to battle disease.

Chronic stress can lead to lowered immune function with the resultant accumulation of bacteria and clostridia and entero bacteria or ecoli, which can lead to upset stomach, diarrhea, sore throat, cold, headaches, etc.

To note accountants get sore throats in April when they are filling last minute tax returns, and students catch colds during exam week. Research shows that psychological stress is related to a breakdown of the immune system, and therefore upper respiratory infections and problems like gastro intestinal health. It is safe to say that the more stressed out you are, the more likely you are to get sick. Stress can definitely cause blood clotting, higher blood pressure and can increase the risk of heart disease. Stress experts have shown time and time again that stress is directly related to heart attack and stroke.

Emotional stresses are also linked to heart disease. A risk of coronary heart disease is five times higher in people who are angry, anxious or worrisome. Researchers at the Mayo Clinic are convinced that psychological stress is one of the major risk factors for heart attacks. It can be caused by your life circumstances - I call it emotional or mental stress.

***Anger is one of the main causes of illness and early death.***

It is a fact that heart disease is the leading cause of death in the Western world caused by high blood sugar and physical inactivity.

No one can deny the direct correlation between stress and hypertension. A relief of stress can bring your blood pressure back to normal levels. Therefore, it is very important to regenerate and reduce your stress level and the accumulation of stress.

Many users of **IBMS™** sessions report fast relief from high blood pressure according to a study conducted by the Berlin Health Institute. The sessions can be used to increase your vitality, strength, health and the function of your immune system, and they can also help to prevent the effects of pre-aging.

Anxiety and depression are very often caused by modern lifestyle. In fact, between five and twenty percent of all Americans will suffer from depression severe enough to warrant medication or therapy.

Chronic stress also causes major mood swings and reduced energy levels as well as fatigue, concentration problems, irritability, feelings of panic. They are all the result of an imbalance in our neurotransmitters. Chronic stress can change the arrangement of neurons and of nerve cells in the brain. This means that stress is able to change the functions of the brain, which explains the often irrational behavior of people who are stressed out.

In my opinion, the medical industry has incorrectly concluded that neurochemistry is causing disorders like panic attacks, obsessive compulsive disorder or depression. Rather I am convinced that chronic mental, emotional and psychological stress lead to changes in body chemistry typical for patients with the above mentioned symptoms and illnesses. It is the stress that causes the change in biochemistry, which then leads to depression, panic or anxiety attacks.

Science shows that chronically overactive stress responses with an extreme heightened and active level of epinephrine and norepinephrine lead to symptoms like dizziness, irregular heart beat, sweating and fear of a heart attack.

One of the reasons why medication like Valium and antidepressants like Prozac and Wellbutrin are prescribed is because people are in constant stress living with financial pressure and worries.

Stress stimulation can cause a lower production of brain neuro-transmitters, which can lead to mood swings and depression or even bipolar disease.

Chronic stress can also lead to a malfunction of the automated leveling process after a stressor is gone. This means that the person is still suffering from the same symptoms even after the stress input is gone because the brain is unable to stabilize.

Drugs used to fight depression usually have horrible side effects; in fact, often the drug's side effects can actually be worse than the depression itself.

**Always remember:**

*No drug can or ever cured a disease because it only treats the symptoms!*

It has been proven that chronic stress is capable of disturbing the brain chemistry because repeated stress and prolonged exposure to stress hormones leads to the destruction of the neurons in the brain.

A major side effect of chronic stress is that people lose their ability to tap into their instincts and/or their feelings of right and wrong. They lose their ability to objectively evaluate people or situations and they get more and more insecure and helpless as time goes on.

*Chronic stress disturbs many aspects of the neurochemistry of the brain.*

Research shows that there is clearly a destruction of the brain in Alzheimer's patients that is caused by brain cell damage. Research has shown that Alzheimer's patients lack a significant amount of acetylchlorine. A lack acetylchlorine causes symptoms of memory loss and depression.

Medical studies have shown that all stressful events can cause digestion to completely stop. This can also be a major cause of ulcers.

It is a well documented fact that stress suppresses the immune system which is one of the reasons why ulcers thrive in stressful people. Stress provides the environment for a bacterium called helicobacter pylori to flourish. Eighty percent of people who have stomach ulcers have a higher level of these bacteria, but I believe that stress is the root cause for ulcers not the bacteria.

The majority of gastrointestinal conditions are caused or exacerbated in times of major stress.

Pre-aging goes hand in hand with weight gain and weaker muscles and loss of the ability to move freely. Nutritional deficiencies can cause damage in the connective tissues, cartilage, hair, skin and bones. There is proof that age related symptoms can be reversed with effective and regular stress reduction. Stress is the largest single cause for pre-aging, dehydration and nutritional deficiencies.

High stress hormone levels are frequently associated with osteoporosis, arthritis, bone and muscle loss and anorexia nervosa. A good diet and reduced stress with a lot of water and salt are proven to restore muscle tissue and bone.

- Penn State University proved that tissue damage in the elderly could be reversed with the proper diet, nutrition and exercise.
- Finnish researchers showed that by lowering stress hormones the results were that the aging process was slowed down by twenty-five percent; in contrast, the opposite is true with high levels of stress hormones.
- Stress is capable of dehydrating the skin, which speeds up the aging process because the elasticity of the skin dies so that wrinkles are more visible.
- Studies show that patients capable of quickly turning off **a** stress response can recover faster and show a dramatically slower growth of cancer cells. (You can learn how to handle your individual stress experience more effectively with **IBMS™** sessions.)
- High levels of stress hormones are related to hypertension, obesity, osteoporosis, depression and the feared syndrome X.

In general, the most effective way to minimize stress is to have a strong sense of self and a high level of energy so that with persistence one can get rid of the causes of the dis-stress in our lives.

Major stress to one person can be exciting to another person, which is why it is important to take charge of your own life by being ready and willing to take responsibility of your life. A lot of water, fresh juice, some exercise and a bit of sea salt should be a regular part of your daily life. Learn to listen to your instincts, to trust yourself and act accordingly so that you instinctively know what is right for your health and future.

The important elements for stress reduction, stress prevention and maintaining health are good friendships and relationships, frequent regeneration phases, experiencing fun, enjoyment, happiness and laughter, combined with a good attitude and love of self and others. Remember that stress does not exist until we feel threatened. We determine how we feel and react. Be prepared! The **IBMS**™ system can be your best defense and preparation!

*You are born to be happy healthy and successful! Use your full potential!*

# The Founder and Author

### Dr. Leonard Coldwell

Dr Leonard Coldwell is the personal physician for Kevin Trudeau in Europe and is the original Natural Cures Doctor. Kevin Trudeau is the New York times number 1 bestseller author of his Mega Best Seller: Natural cures they don't want you to know about and refers to Dr Coldwell and endorses Dr Coldwell's system nearly for every health challenge. Dr Leonard Coldwell is the most endorsed holistic and alternative doctor. His curing rate for so called incurable diseases in Europe is legendary. Prof Dr Peter Lange the President of the Charitee in Berlin ( equal to the NIH ) says: " My colleague Dr Leonard Coldwell is the David Copperfield of his field" . Politicians, Movie Stars, Presidents of many of the largest companies, Nobel Prize Winners in Medicine and celebrities from all walks of life rank among Dr. Coldwell's patients, clients and students.

*After sixteen years as a General Practitioner in Europe, Dr. Coldwell left general practice to concentrate on his applied research in stress and stress related diseases, with particular emphasis on cancer and other so called incurable diseases.. Along the way, he became a noted consultant and trainer for multinational corporations, charitable organizations and medical institutions. He retired (not practicing in the USA )*

Dr. Leonard Coldwell

*and moved to Charleston S.C. in 2000 where he still resides. He is the founder of the "Modern Therapy Centers" and the "Foundation for Crime and Drug Free Schools and Health for Children".*

*Dr Leonard Coldwell is a strong supporter of our troops. He was the keynote speaker at the Rally for the Troops – "Lets Freedom Ring". His powerful speech was broadcasted world wide by clear channel radio and because of popular demand constantly repeated. He is recognized by US President George W. Bush, the US Congress, the South Carolina Governor as well as Senators and Congressmen and the leaders of the Veteran organization and Churches around the country. His support for the MUSC ended with a standing ovation.*

*Congressman Joe Wilson presented Dr Coldwell at the US Congress with a special recognition and that stated: " Best wishes to my good friend Dr Leonard Coldwell, appreciate your promotion of Democracy." Warmest Regards Joe Wilson Member of Congress. And he is President of the "World Wellness Organization™".*

While in Europe, Dr. Coldwell was the author of nine best-selling books, countless articles, and hundreds of self-help audio programs. He remains a syndicated columnist with more than seven million readers and continues to author one of the most successful and widely distributed self-help newsletters in Europe. Over two million people have attended his life enhancing seminars. An independent statistical institute estimated that Dr Coldwell worked with over 35000 patients.

In addition to his appearances on numerous TV and radio stations around the world, he frequently appears on American TV news shows, radio shows and newspapers. Soon after the tragedy of September 11, 2001, he was called on by the U.S. Naval Weapons Station in Charleston, S.C. to address stress related problems as an expert on traumatic stress relief. He continues to develop programs for firefighters, military, police and other professionals to relieve "stress," and he is active in the community as a volunteer for charity and nonprofit activities; particularly his "Foundation for Crime and Drug Free Schools and Health for Children".

In 2000, Dr. Coldwell made the decision to invest his time, knowledge and experience in teaching and consulting to help make a better world for children and parents. Through his children's foundation, he is helping teachers, parents and children deal with stress and drugs in the local schools. Further, he is well into the planning stages for the world's largest most comprehensive health resort. His plan is to house every mainstream, alternative, holistic and integrated therapy system in one location so that patients will have access to state of the art healing arts and practices in a wellness setting unique to the world.

Finally, Dr. Coldwell is in the final stages of completing a multimedia self-help library that addresses all aspects of life and the human condition.

**Contact Information:**

www.drleonardcoldwell.com and
www.instinctbasedmedicine.com

Dr Coldwell will answer every question directed to him. Write to: Instinctbasedmedicine@gmail.com

For further publications and information go to: www.instinctbasedmedicine.com